Craveable KETO

C O O K B O O K

Kyndra D. Holley

Victory Belt Publishing Inc.
Las Vegas

First Published in 2018 by Victory Belt Publishing Inc.

ISBN-13: 978-1-628602-71-5

The author is not a licensed practitioner, physician, or medical professional and offers no medical diagnoses, treatments, suggestions, or counseling. The information presented herein has not been evaluated by the U.S. Food and Drug Administration, and it is not intended to diagnose, treat, cure, or prevent any disease. Full medical clearance from a licensed physician should be obtained before beginning or modifying any diet, exercise, or lifestyle program, and physicians should be informed of all nutritional changes.

The author/owner claims no responsibility to any person or entity for any liability, loss, or damage caused or alleged to be caused directly or indirectly as a result of the use, application, or interpretation of the information presented herein.

Front and Back Cover Photography by Hayley Mason and Bill Staley
Interior Design by Yordan Terziev and Boryana Yordanova

Printed in Canada

TC 0418

To my husband, Jon,

my partner in life, my best friend, and the most compassionate and giving human I know:

Thank you for always giving me the freedom and the space to chase my dreams and explore all my crazy ideas and business ventures. Without you by my side, none of it would be possible. Most of all, thank you for always believing in me and reassuring me that I can do it, even when I think I can't. You make me believe that I can move mountains.

Your patience and kindness know no limits, and I am infinitely lucky to call you mine.

Thank you for being you.

I love you.

BEFORE

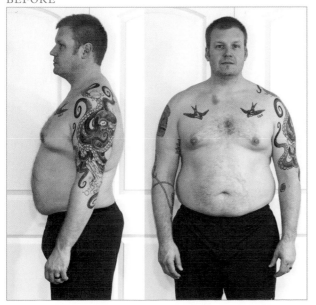

AFTER

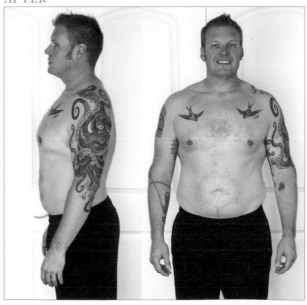

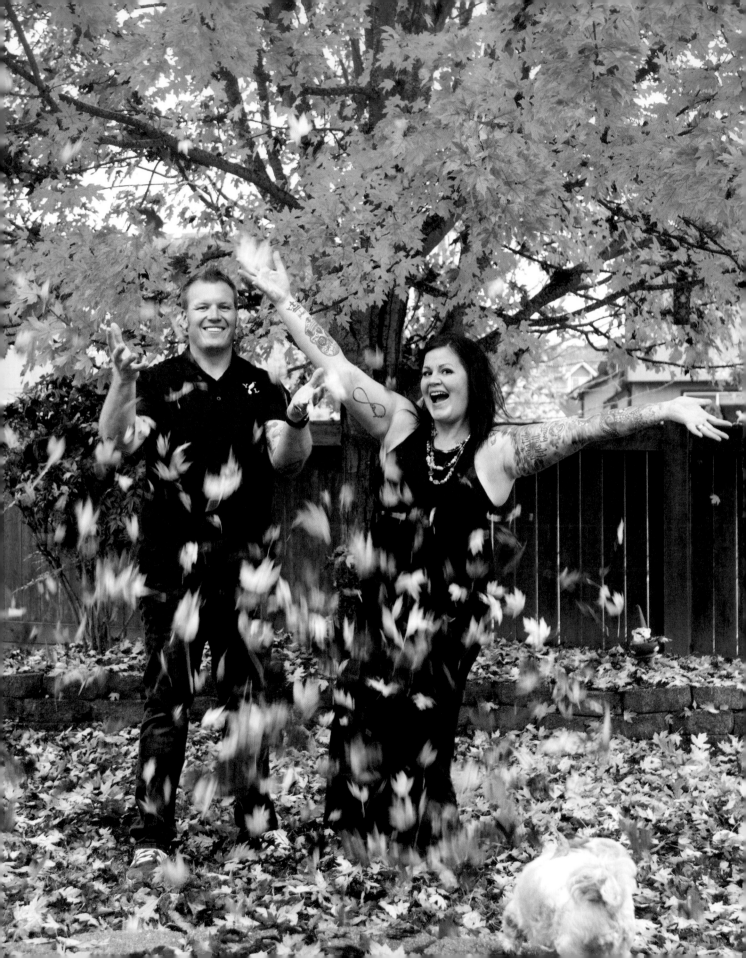

Table of Contents

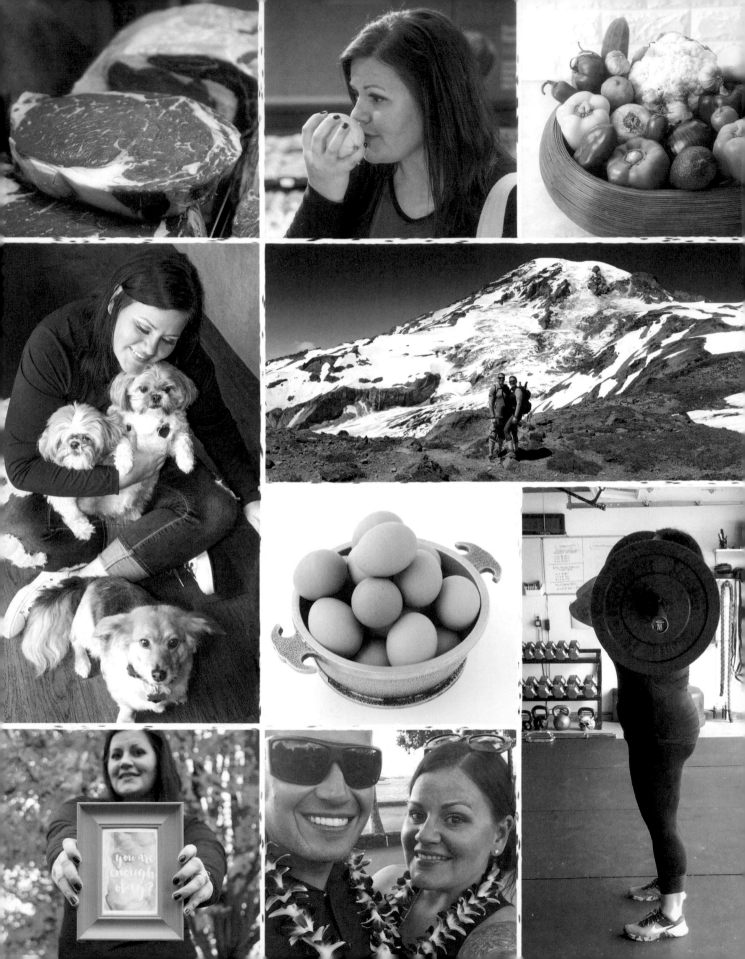

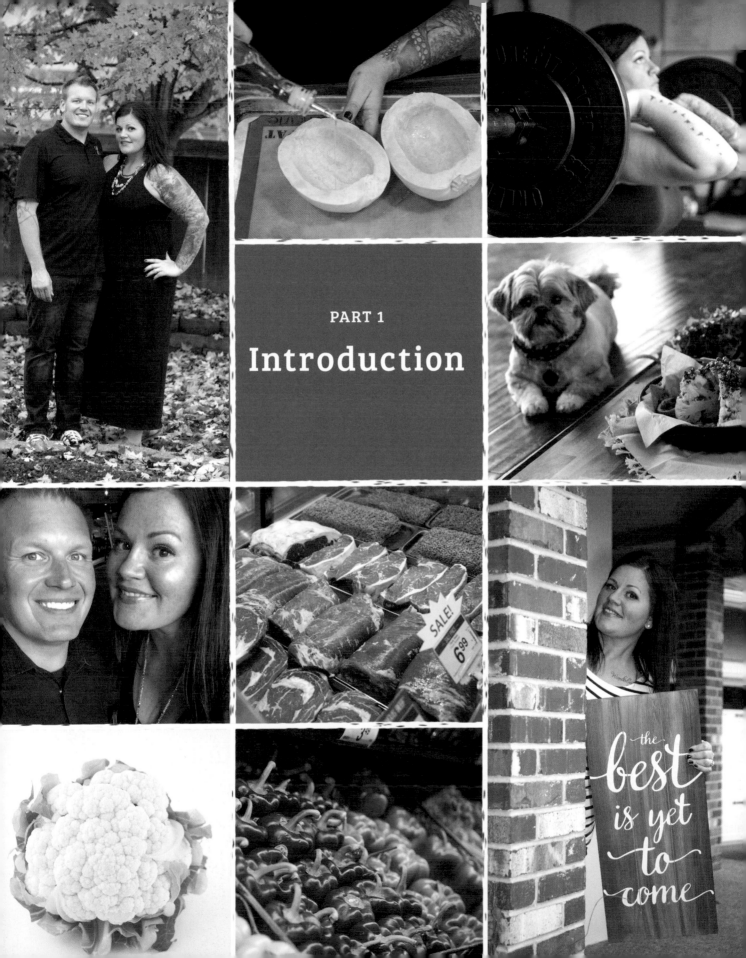

PART 1

Introduction

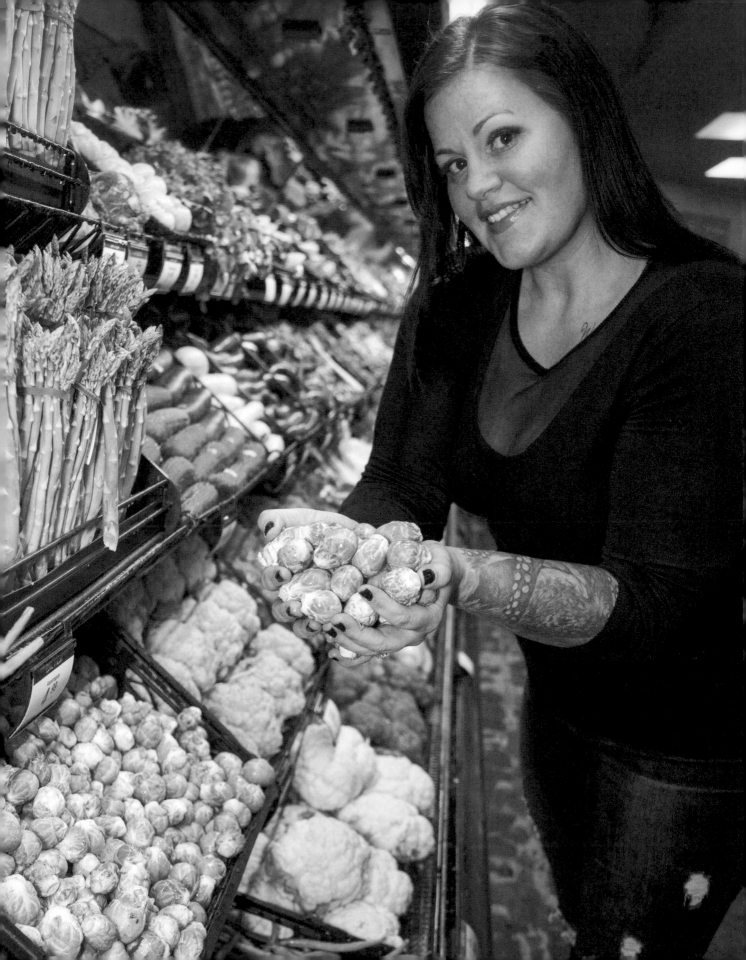

Letter to the Reader

Hey there! I'm Kyndra. I am a cookbook author, the creator of *Peace, Love and Low Carb,* and a girl with a weight problem that has spanned nearly her entire adult life. I am not a doctor or a scientist, nor am I a nutritionist. But I do have a lot to bring to the table. The low-carb table, of course.

I am not one of those bloggers or cookbook authors who has never struggled with her weight and therefore cannot possibly understand the true struggles of her audience. I am with you. Right beside you. Down in the trenches. Going through it at the same time as you. I have learned a lot along the way, and if I can share my story and help even one person feel less alone in their weight struggles, then this book will already be a smashing success in my eyes.

So if you are looking for someone who knows your plight because she has also lived it, then this is the book for you! If you are just looking for a ton of delicious and creative low-carb recipes, then this is also the book for you. If the latter is true, feel free to skip all of my rambling and jump ahead to the mouthwatering recipes.

This book may read like part journal, part cookbook, but I wanted to create a one-stop resource for those looking to find peace, self-love, and wellness through their weight-loss journey. I want this book to serve as a roadmap as you navigate the physical and the emotional sides of weight loss. They are important, overlooked pieces in the wellness puzzle.

Where a lot of traditional nutrition and "diet" plans fail is that they concentrate solely on food. While food is a great place to start, there is so much more to weight loss and wellness.

Focusing solely on food is like building a puzzle by piecing together the outer frame first (because let's face it, that's how we all start a puzzle, isn't it?) and then never going back to put all the pieces together inside the frame. Without the work on the center portion, all you have is a fragile frame that could be bumped and come apart at any time. As it pertains to this analogy, that center piece of the puzzle is *you,* and all of the components that make you, you outside of your food choices.

If you are struggling to put the pieces of your life together, my hope is that this book can be the glue that helps you finally secure them into place. As you continue on your weight-loss journey, I hope that this book not only helps keep you on track with your food, but also has you on the road to spiritual and emotional wellness, body positivity, and self-love.

I think that much like life, when it comes to how you eat, there is no one-size-fits-all approach. What works for some people may not work for others. It doesn't mean that we can't all walk parallel paths while supporting one another along the way to the same destination.

I wanted to write a book my whole life. Yes, really, I did. I just never knew that my gig would be writing cookbooks. If the front section of my book reads more like a journal, GOOD, because I want you to hear this. All of it. You, yes, YOU! The person who feels alone. The person silently struggling. The person who feels destined to struggle with weight forever. I've got you! You are not alone. You can do this. *We* can do this!

When I was in the first grade, our end-of-year project was to write a story. Maybe I'll share it with you sometime. It's the kind of story that might warrant a call home in today's world. But as I look back on it, I can't help but think of the time I grew up in: we drank out of the hose, played by the train tracks, and stayed outside until the streetlights came on. Ahhhhh, the '80s—but I digress. We first-graders wrote our stories and drew the pictures, and then our teacher laminated and spiral-bound our books for us to present to our parents. On the last page of each book was an "About the Author" page. Mine read:

> *My name is Kyndra. I am seven years old. I live with my dad, mom, sister, 2 cockatiels, a dog and a cat. I like to play outside and ride my ten-speed. I like Easter. I like to do many drawings and write stories in my spare time. When I grow up I want to be an author-illustrator.*

Wasn't I so eloquent and articulate at seven? Apparently I wrote only in lists. It all makes so much sense now. Okay, back on track, Kyndra....

That was 1986. Fast-forward more than thirty years, and who would have thought that all the twists and turns and stops and starts in my life would have led me to my dream? I guess you could say that if I never got fat, I might never have followed my dream. I was meant to endure the fat years in order to become the person I am today and truly live out my childhood dream. As much as my weight struggles brought tears and a great deal of heartache, they also gave me my voice. They gave me an outlet to write about. Through the struggles, I also found my victories. Every day I make a conscious choice to love who I was back then just as much as I love the woman I am now. Every individual chapter of my life has contributed to my story—much like every section of this book came together to form a cookbook.

As much as I love to cook, I've always loved to write. When I began writing recipes for my blog, it felt like two passions were colliding in a beautiful, harmonious crash in the kitchen. Sometimes I feel like my life is just one giant journal entry where I get to express my feelings and emotions through food. Each time I step into a freshly cleaned kitchen, it's like I am being given a blank slate. A chance to start over and create something beautiful. A place to mute the madness of the world. A place where I can just be myself. A place where I don't think about my weight or my work or the burdens of daily life. It's a place where my cup runneth over with creative juices and amazing scratch-made sauces.

In my kitchen, I work through the deepest and darkest problems. It's the equivalent of a chaise longue in a shrink's office. When I need to process something, I take it to the kitchen. The smell of fresh ingredients, the sounds of the knife rhythmically striking the cutting board, and the roar of a searing-hot pan are my medicine. They clear my mind and set my soul on fire. It was in my kitchen that I learned to love myself. It was through healthy cooking that I learned I can change my own life and the lives of others. Food gave me a voice. It gave me a platform to share my personal experiences with other people. It became so much more than food. It's a lifestyle. It's a job. It's a hobby. It's my life's mission.

Throughout *Craveable Keto Cookbook*, I will share pieces of my own weight-loss story with you: the good, the bad, and the carb-laden. I will provide you with my best tips and tricks for feeling whole and putting all of the weight-loss and wellness pieces together. I'll take you on a trip through my kitchen and show you some of my favorite low-carb creations, so buckle in and get ready for the ride.

This book may be finished, but my story is still being written. So is yours. Let's go write them together, shall we?

Peace and Love,

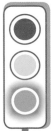

“Owning our story can be hard but not nearly as difficult as spending our lives running from it. Embracing our vulnerabilities is risky but not nearly as dangerous as giving up on love and belonging and joy—the experiences that make us the most vulnerable. Only when we are brave enough to explore the darkness will we discover the infinite power of our light. ”

—Brené Brown

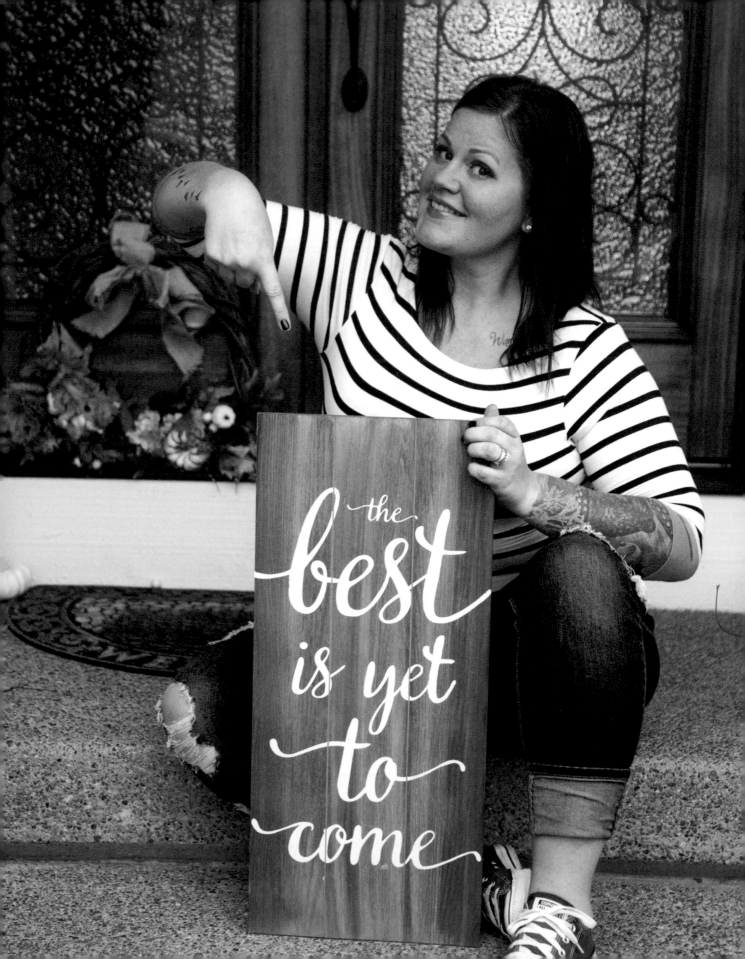

My Story

My story with weight issues probably started at birth. Okay, not really, but I was a big, healthy baby, weighing in at 8 pounds, 10 ounces. I don't think we need to go back quite that far, though.

I think, in my late thirties, I've only just begun to grasp how much my upbringing and subsequent lifestyle choices as a young adult contributed to my weight struggles and my poor relationship with food. The hardest thing about it is that you don't know what you don't know, you know? And by that I mean, while I was growing up I didn't know that Ding Dongs, potato chips, and cans of soda were bad for me. I just knew that I liked them, and they were always in the house. My parents bought them to pack in my dad's lunches for work. Since they were for his lunches, they wouldn't let me have any. And so began my obsession with them. I remember so clearly trying to sneak one single Ding Dong out of the house when I was spending the night at a friend's house. My bag was packed, and we were getting

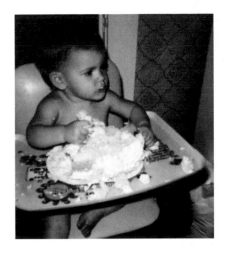

ready to leave. Children aren't the greatest at pulling off high-level crimes like Ding Dong theft, so when my mom walked by my bag and that shiny foil wrapper caught her eye, I knew I was in for it. Not only did I not get to keep the Ding Dong, but I didn't get to spend the night at my friend's house, either.

From the time I was very young, food started being both a reward and a punishment. When I should have been learning to fuel my body and eat only until I wasn't hungry anymore, I was trying to steal sweet treats and being forced to remain at the dinner table until I cleaned my plate and drank every last drop of my milk. Sometimes I would cry at the table and try to convince my parents that I was full, but I had to finish my food or just sit there. I don't really blame them for this. It's not like they were intentionally trying to torture me; it was just how things were at that time. They parented the way they had been parented, and food was just not something that was ever left on a plate. But I will say that the simple act of being forced to eat all of my food was a stepping-stone to much larger food issues that would come for me later.

I grew up in a meat-and-potatoes household. Lots of mashed potatoes, boxed stuffing mix, and whatever the cheapest cut of meat was at the grocery store that week. In fact, potatoes were the first thing I learned to cook for myself. Fried potatoes drenched in a ridiculous amount of what I then thought was butter. (I think I was already into adulthood before I realized that margarine isn't butter.) Our condiments were mayonnaise, mustard, ketchup, salt, and pepper. I remember foods as simple as olives being foods we ate only on Thanksgiving. I literally ate pieces of white bread covered in mayo as a meal—not because I was forced to, but because I was old enough to make a sandwich without hurting myself, and that is what I would make. From there I graduated to eating fried egg sandwiches every day. It's interesting that to this day, I'm still a big fan of the whole "put an egg on it" craze.

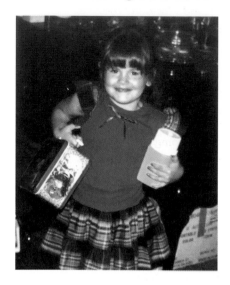

One year for Christmas, I got a *Dark Crystal* lunch box and Thermos. It was my favorite movie at the time, and I remember being so excited to pack a school lunch in my snazzy new lunch box. I've always been a visual person, and as soon as I ripped open that Christmas wrapping paper, I could see myself at the cafeteria table proudly eating a homemade lunch. Eating my white bread bologna sandwich and drinking my Thermos full of now-warm milk made me feel so cool. My lunch-packing days were numbered, though; it wasn't long before I was on the school lunch program. As my dad left the house with a packed lunch each day—one that I usually had to pack as part of my chores—I went to school to collect my free lunch. This was back in the 1980s, and there was no hiding that you were a part of the free lunch program. I went through the line and said my name, and they pulled my card out of the Rolodex, stamped it, and gave me my little aluminum lunch tray with some random food slop on it. Most of it was gross. But Friday! Oh, Friday! Friday was pizza day. I remember being so jealous of my friends who got to pack their own lunches every day. But on Fridays, they were all jealous of me, because if there is one thing that all small children have in common, it is a love of pizza.

Even at a very young age, I also loved pens, pencils, erasers, and all art supplies in general—so many of the things that I still love today. I vividly remember getting a set of those scented pencils with changeable leads. You pulled the dull lead from the bottom and pushed it through the top, and it pushed a fresh sharpened lead back out through the bottom. The pencils smelled like grapes and strawberries. I have the clearest memory of sitting outside at recess with a McDonald's Halloween bucket loaded up with all of my coolest school supplies and then selling them. I would take the money and go buy ice cream sandwiches in the cafeteria. It's such a funny memory, you know? I guess you could say that I was born with an entrepreneurial spirit. I was dealing in supply and demand in only the second or third grade! I still love pens and pencils. In fact, as I write this, I am looking at three mason jars on my desk filled with colored pencils, markers, and highlighters. Unfortunately, though, none of them smell like grapes. And I don't think I will be selling them anytime soon.

Eventually I was no longer on the free lunch program, and I headed to school each day with $2 to buy my lunch. I went to a babysitter in the morning before school. I would always ask her if I could give her my $2 and have her make me a sack lunch instead. At least once a week, she would say yes. She was the sweetest old lady and was very health-conscious. Not only did she pack me a healthy lunch, but she would put it in a cool brown paper bag, complete with a napkin and a sweet little note.

Fast-forwarding to junior high and high school, not much had changed. When I look back on it, I wasn't overweight…yet. I was just bigger than all of my friends, and that made me stand out. I was always the tallest, banished to the back row of every school photo. It didn't help that I had petite friends who immediately got noticed by boys, and I was always just kind of there, standing out like a giant. Have you ever looked at a picture of yourself taken during a time in your life when you thought you were fat, only to think, "I wish I was as thin as I was when I thought I was fat"? Yep, me too. That is pretty much the story of my life as it pertains to my weight and body issues. I never really felt comfortable in my skin, and I let the opinions of everyone around me shape my opinion of myself.

I grew up fast, or so I thought. I left home early and had my own apartment by age seventeen. I started working in restaurants, experimenting with drugs and alcohol, and generally having no regard for my health. I joined countless gyms only to pay and not go—or to go for a couple of weeks and then make some excuse to stop going. I stayed out late and slept in even later. Some days all I ate were french fries and chips, and wasn't life grand, because there was no one there to stop me. I could buy my own Ding Dongs now.

I continued working in restaurants throughout my twenties, and as my waistline grew, my self-esteem withered. I allowed a lot of people to treat me poorly. I mean, why wouldn't I? I was treating myself the same way. At age twenty-one, I started bartending. That meant a lot of late work nights and even later nights of eating and drinking with friends. Fried foods and copious amounts of beer were pretty much my two main food groups.

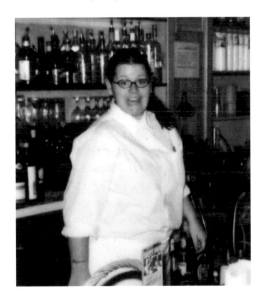

Have you ever had one of those memories that cut so deep it became burned into who you are, like your heart has been branded with a hot iron? I sure have. I remember like it was yesterday. One Friday night, while I was working behind the bar at an Italian restaurant, one of the servers decided that I was going to be the target of his bullying. Every time I moved or took a step, he would act out the motions of bracing himself for a major earthquake, as if just by walking, I was going to cause catastrophic damage. To add insult to injury, he would also make loud Godzilla-like sounds. He did it in front of everyone, and no one attempted to stop him or even hint at the fact that what he was doing was awful and cruel. At a time when I should have been learning to love myself, I was being torn down and learning to believe the words and actions of others. I started measuring my self-worth based on experiences like these. At that same restaurant, one of the chefs called me Tundra instead of Kyndra. You know, because clearly I was the size of a Toyota Tundra pickup truck. Whenever I would approach the kitchen window to get food for one of my tables, he would puff out his cheeks and flail his arms out to the side in giant half-circles, doing his best impression of the Michelin Man. He would alternate between doing that and pointing at me, just to let me know, in case there was any confusion, that he was talking about me. He did this every day. I felt anxiety and shame swell throughout my body each time I had to pick up an order for the guests in my section. This chef would also poke me in the side when I walked through the kitchen to the dish area just to point out my love handles. If he could get a good enough grip as I scurried by, he would even try to pinch me to really drive his point home.

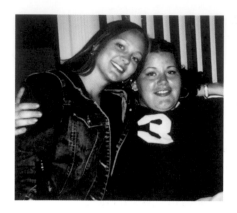

I tried to fight these experiences with humor. Cracking jokes, often at my own expense, became my defense mechanism. I learned to become the funny, engaging girl while out in public or at work, and I saved the tears for when I got home. If I was making everyone laugh, they couldn't possibly notice my weight, right? I was one of the guys. Always in the friend zone. In fact, there was a good friend of mine whom I really liked. We hung out often, and I'm fairly certain he knew exactly how I felt about him. In fact, not only did he know, but it became pretty clear that he was exploiting my feelings. One night over several cocktails, he told me that aside from my body, I was the perfect girl for him. He listed all of the things that made me perfect for him, but my every thought hung on the "aside from your body" part. He even went as far as to tell me that my hair would be a lot prettier if it wasn't so curly. It was crushing. When I think about it, it still feels like it is happening right now, in real time.

Fast-forwarding again, this time to my mid-twenties. I started working at a late-night fine-dining restaurant. I seriously thought I had arrived. The money was amazing (even more Ding Dong funds now!), and it came with a little bit of clout because it was really hard to get a job there. In fact, it was a union house, and many of the servers had quite literally worked there longer than I had been alive. This restaurant was an institution, and I thought I was pretty damn cool for landing a job there. Hidden somewhere in this book like an Easter egg is the real reason I am forever grateful to have worked there all those years ago.

Being low man on the totem pole, I worked the graveyard shift for the first few years. It was brutal. Vampire-like hours, surrounded by amazing food that I could eat whenever I wanted. As if that wasn't bad enough, the chef and I would hit up first call after work. 6 a.m. cocktails. It might sound crazy, but once you get used to it, getting off work at 6 a.m. doesn't feel any different than getting off at 5 p.m. You do the same things as everyone else; you just do them at crazy hours. I started putting on even more weight.

A coworker of mine told me all about the Atkins Diet and asked if I wanted to do it with her. I immediately bought the book. Wait, you mean to tell me that I can eat bunless bacon cheeseburgers with tons of ranch all day long and still lose weight? And I did—very quickly, in fact. I still had age and hormones on my side, and the weight melted off. I wasn't even working out. Before I knew it, I had lost about 50 pounds, and my body had bounced back beautifully. I started to love the body I was living in for the first time in my adult life. Shopping for clothes became something I actually wanted to do and not a shameful, sweaty tear-fest in the fitting room. I started going on more dates and actually being pretty selective about whom I gave my time and attention to. It seemed like life was finally turning around for me.

You see, when you struggle with weight your whole life, it is the focal point of everything you do. Everything in your life takes a backseat to your weight problem, which lives front and center in your mind. You wear it like a scarlet letter, and it starts to define you. Or so *you* think. But when you get a taste of what it's like to live without weight ruling every decision you make, you don't ever want to go back. You start to feel whole and less broken. Dare I even say "fixed"?

This first go-round with substantial weight loss gave me a false sense of what being healthy means. At the time, I equated health solely with weight. The number on the scale was the only benchmark I cared about. I still hadn't repaired my relationship with food. I still didn't know anything about nutrition. I still wasn't on any sort of consistent fitness regimen. I still hadn't fixed my relationship with myself. I still didn't love myself. Basically, I had just put a bandage over the bullet hole that was my emotions.

Can you guess what happened next? Yep, I put the weight back on. All of it and then some. I hadn't bothered to fix any of the issues that had contributed to my weight problem in the first place. But at the time, I still didn't realize that there was anything to address besides the weight. Even though I knew it worked for me, I was constantly in and out of a low-carb diet. Part of the problem lies in the last word of that sentence: *diet*. I still viewed it as a diet and not a lifestyle. Another thing I didn't realize was that you can't have only one foot in and expect it to work. You can't just dip your toe in the low-carb waters. You can't eat low-carb *some* of the time and expect to get results. In the beginning, my approach to low-carb was a lot like taking an antibiotic to cure a cold. I would do it just until I started to feel better, and then I would stop. I would start to see results and then think it was okay to start eating bread and pasta again. But that's just not how it works.

It wasn't until 2011 that I decided to get serious. I was ready to give low-carb another go and to do it right this time. Throughout all those years of working in restaurants, I had developed a real love of whole foods and the art of transforming them into beautiful dishes for people to enjoy.

Even though I never worked in the kitchen in any of those restaurants, I spent a lot of time in the kitchen because I loved watching the process unfold. Working in a handful of fine-dining establishments exposed me to ingredients and cooking techniques that I never knew existed. And as I tasted these new ingredients for the first time, it was love at first bite. My palate grew more sophisticated over time. I was able to go out for a nice meal, analyze the flavor profiles, and identify the ingredients. I began cooking at home a lot more. Each time I created something new and it was a hit, my passion was fueled even further. Food was no longer a torture device. It was no longer this thing that weighed so heavily on me—literally and figuratively.

With strength and conviction, I decided that I was going to change my life once and for all, and I resolved that it wasn't going to come at the sacrifice of the foods I loved. I set out on a mission to create healthier low-carb versions of all of my favorite high-carb comfort foods. I knew that low-carb worked, and I knew that I loved to cook. Why couldn't I combine those two things and find true weight-loss success? I started by re-creating mac and cheese, then pizza, and then lasagna, and my passion caught fire from there. I started taking pictures of my cooking adventures, and this habit gave way to the birth of my blog in July 2011.

Peace, Love and Low Carb started as a way to document my weight-loss journey and keep a record of all of the delicious foods I was eating, but it quickly took on a life of its own. As I gained followers, I was also losing pounds and inches. Cooking became my release: the very thing that freed me from the negativity I felt a lot of the time. I felt inspired and happy.

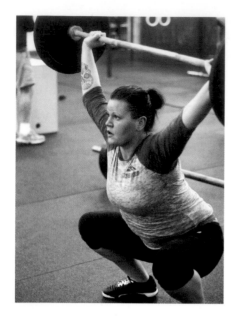

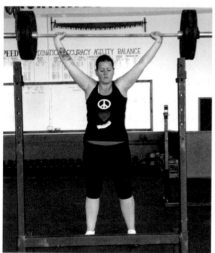

By this time I had married Jon, the love of my life. He was doing low-carb right alongside me, and before we knew it, we were both down about 50 pounds. At the end of 2012, we found CrossFit. I was all in. I drank the juice BIG TIME. CrossFit lit a fire in me that I never felt coming. I found a power within myself that I never thought I would feel, let alone feel comfortable enough to show to the world. I felt so strong and empowered. I finally found my love of fitness. I began craving it. I was the healthiest and strongest I had ever been, both mentally and physically. I was blogging full-time, maintaining my weight loss, and about to self-publish my first cookbook. By 2013 I had my CrossFit Level 1 certification (the certification required to begin coaching other athletes). My self-published cookbook was out, and it was a huge success. I was even in talks with a publisher to write my first full-length, professionally published print cookbook. Life was good. Really good. Until it wasn't.

My relationship with our CrossFit gym came to an abrupt and painful ending. The owners simply decided that they didn't like me, and they weren't afraid to let me know it. They also made it clear that they very much liked Jon and that he was welcome to stay. They later told a mutual friend that sometimes you have members of your gym whose personalities you just don't like, and it's okay to clean house. The day it all went down, I left the gym feeling heartbroken. In fact, I sat in the parking lot in a pile of tears, too distraught to drive.

You might be thinking, "But it's just a gym," and to that, I would say that you have obviously never been a part of a CrossFit gym. It's not just a gym; it's a family. It's a community. It becomes your tribe. It becomes what you eat, sleep, and breathe. Before you know it, you are either thinking about CrossFit, going to CrossFit, thinking about going to CrossFit, or hanging out with your CrossFit friends, talking about CrossFit. Pretty much every meme you have ever seen about CrossFit is spot on. It's a lifestyle and a culture as much as it is a workout. It was like I had been voted off the island, cast aside by my tribe. It tapped right back into my feelings of shame and unworthiness.

I was instantly brought back to that friend zone, Godzilla, earthquake, Tundra, Michelin Man time in my life. What was wrong with me? Was I so fatally flawed that no one could love me? Admittedly, I slipped into a bit of a funk. I stopped working out. Even though I knew how to program my own workouts and had a fully outfitted garage gym, I just stopped. Instead of training myself and pushing myself, I shut down and channeled all of my energy, anger, sadness, and sense of betrayal into my business instead. Great for my business, not so great for my body. I let the end of that "relationship" take away the love I had for fitness and, quite honestly, some of the love I had for myself. Somewhere deep inside me, those two things were so inextricably linked that I was unable to separate them. The owners of the gym might as well have told me that I was the perfect girl for their gym, aside from my personality. The experiences were different, but the emotions they stirred up inside me were of the same theme. If the people in my life couldn't accept me with a weight problem, and now I was being dismissed for my personality as well, where was I supposed to fit in?

I never should have let that experience derail me. In fact, the day it all went down, I came home in tears, sat down on my couch, and opened my MacBook. In my inbox was an email from a publisher offering me a book deal. That was the day my first print cookbook, *The Primal Low Carb Kitchen,* was conceived. One door closed and a much larger door opened. I was beyond excited to walk through it. It gave me something to channel all of my time and energy into. But my lifestyle was about to change in a big way, and my waistline was going to pay for it.

I went from lifting heavy three to five days per week to cooking and writing all day, some days for twelve to fifteen hours at a time. I barely saw daylight, let alone the gym. The only time I saw a plyo box was when I stood on one to take overhead shots of the food I had made. The only plates I was lifting were the kinds with food on them. The distraction of writing my book and growing my business made it easy to lock everything else away and not deal with it properly. Isn't that exactly how so many of us become overweight to begin with? Emotional baggage turns into physical baggage.

The weight came on slowly at first. A few pounds here, a few pounds there. Nothing a pair of yoga pants couldn't hide. (Helpful hint: If you work from home and pretty much live in yoga pants, it is a good idea to try on your jeans periodically just to make sure they still fit. It gets away from you faster than you know.) One bad meal turned into one bad day, which spawned one bad weekend, and before I knew it, I was eating more bad meals than good meals. All the while, I was still preaching the message of weight loss and wellness via a healthy low-carb lifestyle. By the time my book released, I had put on about 60 pounds. I started to feel like a fraud. I found myself wanting to hide. I wanted to be the girl behind the camera, not the one in the photos. I no longer wanted to see friends I hadn't seen in a while because I didn't want them to see how fat I had gotten. I was skipping family functions. I even forfeited all the money I had paid to attend a huge Paleo conference because I was too ashamed. I told people I wasn't going because I was too busy. There was some truth to that, but the biggest and truest reason was that I didn't want to meet some of my most admired blogging peers for the first time in person in the body I was living in. How sad is that? It's like I was wearing a fat suit that I couldn't take off. I looked in the mirror and wondered who the girl staring back at me was.

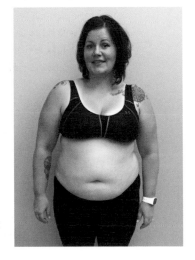

I knew that I needed to come clean—to live my best, most authentic life and to send a message to others out there who might be struggling in silent shame along with me. I wrote a post on my blog entitled "I am a healthy living blogger with a secret...I got fat again," and I put it all out there for everyone to see. The response was overwhelming and for the most part very positive. There were, of course, some keyboard cowboy trolls slinging fat-shaming insults at me over the interwebs, but I refused to let them knock me down. I had spent enough time being knocked down, and it was time to get up. I faced a lot of closed doors before I got to my open door.

> 66 You have to come to your closed doors before you get to your open doors.... What if you knew you had to go through 32 closed doors before you got to your open door? Well, then you'd come to closed door number eight and you'd think, 'Great, I got another one out of the way'.... Keep moving forward. 99
>
> —Joel Osteen

In some ways I feel like *I* was the only thing standing in my way, running ahead of myself and closing all the doors. The mental side of weight loss is hard. Being fat is hard. You know the worst part about it? People don't see you. You take up all that space and yet no one sees you. It's almost like they are afraid to look. As if being fat is contagious and contracted by a glance or a friendly smile.

When I lost all my weight for what I thought was the last time, I remember asking one of my friends if I had something on my face. I asked why everyone was staring at me. Was I being a paranoid weirdo? She said, "They are looking at you because you are so pretty." She was being sweet, lighthearted, and funny, but it was at that very moment that I realized they weren't staring; I was just visible again. My thick-stitched cloak of shame wasn't there anymore. They were no longer afraid of contracting "big giant fatty-itis" from me, and it was safe to look at me again. I was no longer invisible.

Did society make me invisible in the first place, or was it my shame? Was I the heavy girl with the slumped-forward shoulders who stared at her feet and made herself invisible in a sea of beautiful people, or was I the girl with bright eyes and her head held high, with a large personality to match her even larger frame? I think I was both of those girls. Maybe I didn't *want* to be seen. It was easy not to be seen, just as it was probably easy for people to avert their eyes.

After I lost all my excess weight, being seen made me feel more naked and exposed than being fat ever did. What was I supposed to do with that healthy, "normal"-sized body, anyway?

Well, when I get back there, I'll tell you exactly what I do with it. But for now, as I embark on this whole weight-loss journey again, my mission is simple: I want to help as many people as possible to come out of hiding. To love themselves. To feel less alone. To know that they can do this. To know that they are ENOUGH.

Life isn't just about food, and my hope is that this book helps you understand that. I hope that this book provides you with some of the tools you need to find peace and love as you heal yourself inside and out.

Please know that your worth isn't in your weight. There are a million other things that make you uniquely and beautifully *you*. What if we all celebrated those things instead?

Today, I wear my inner fat girl as a badge of honor and always carry her in my heart. She made me who I am today—from the little girl selling her school supplies for ice cream money to the young woman who caused earthquakes as she bartended and every version in between. She lives within me, reminding me of my strength, fortitude, and tenacity. I am a spirit that cannot be broken. You are, too! You just might not know it yet.

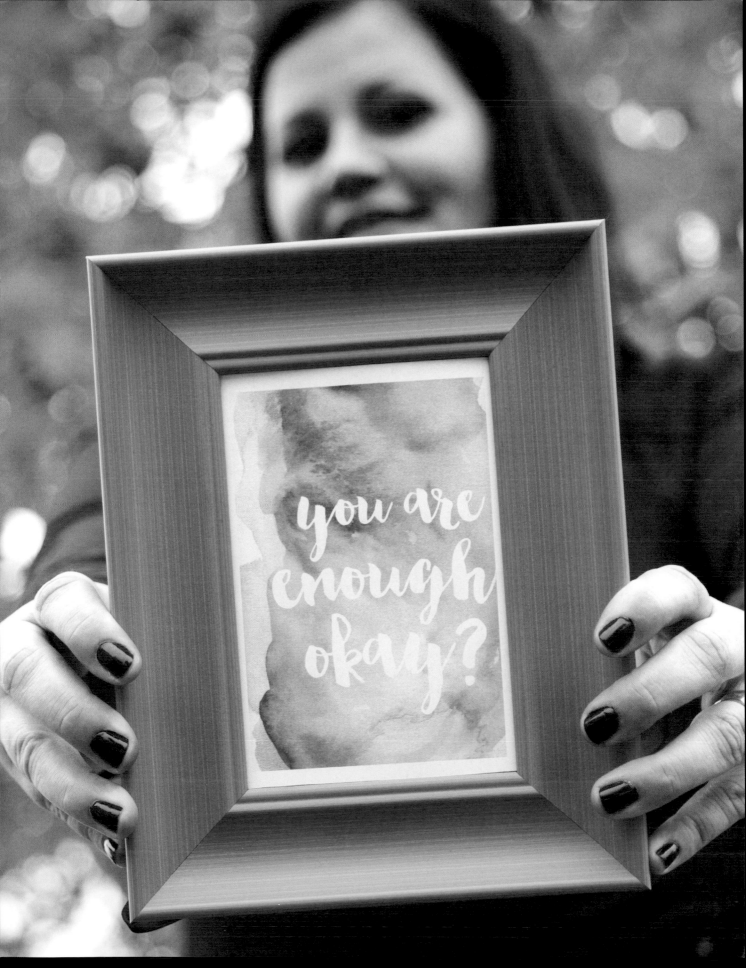

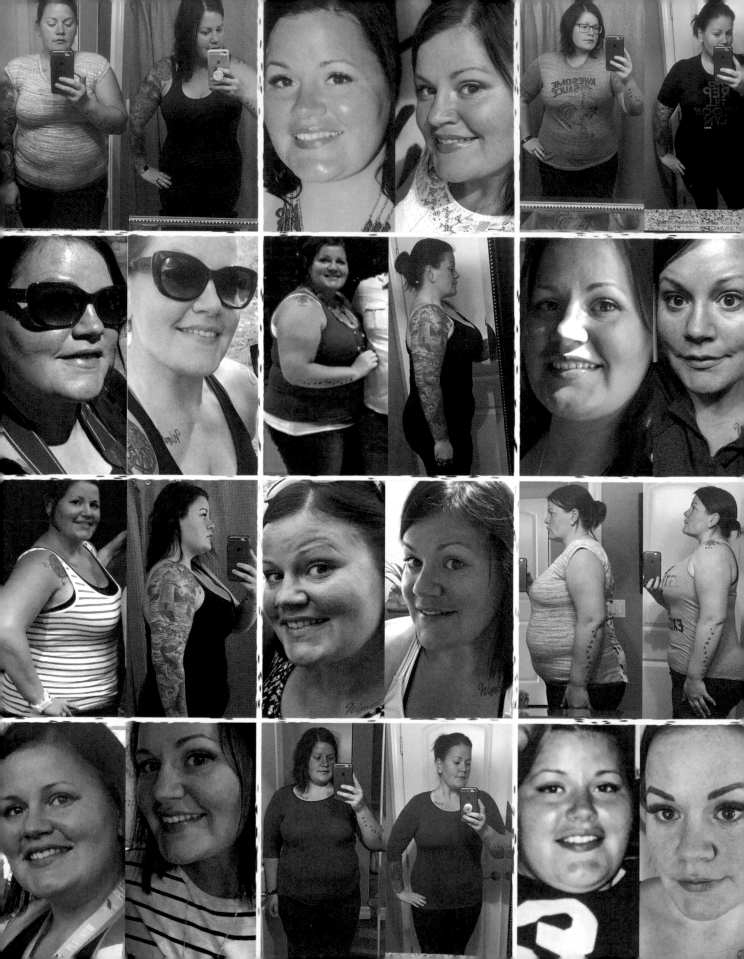

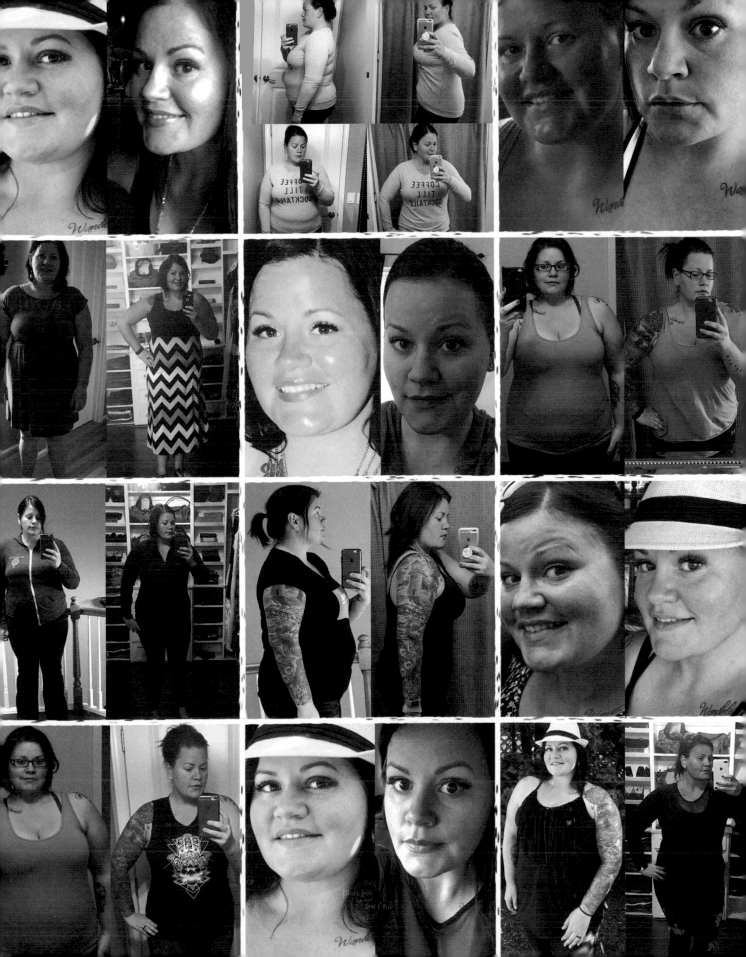

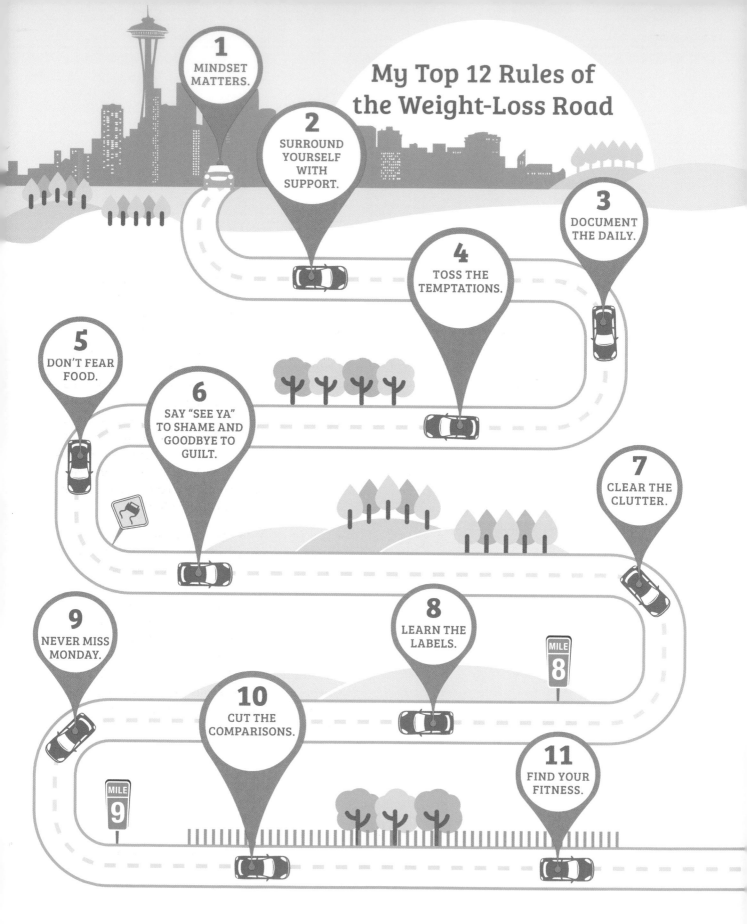

1 MINDSET MATTERS.

The body achieves what the mind believes. Let me repeat that for you: the body achieves what the mind believes. What are you telling yourself about yourself? You can't tell yourself that you will never lose weight and then expect that you will, just like you can't find happiness in saying you will never be happy. Is the story you are selling yourself a work of fiction or nonfiction? Envision the person you want to become. Imagine how it will feel to be that person and what it will look like. As you work toward becoming that person, give yourself permission to just *be*. Love yourself exactly as you are through each step of your journey. What if every day you just woke up and told yourself, "I am enough"? Nothing more, nothing less. Enough. I think we often lose sight of just how important the way we speak to ourselves is. After all, if you can't build yourself up, you can't expect others around you to do the same.

2 SURROUND YOURSELF WITH SUPPORT.

Think about your circle of influence—the people you associate with most frequently. What do the characteristics and traits of those people say about you? Nothing, you might say. Well, I love this quote by Jim Rohn, and I reflect on it often, both personally and professionally: "You are the average of the five people you spend the most time with." Let that sink in for a moment. It is such a powerful sentiment. Now, think back to that circle of influence. Who are the five people you spend the most time with? This doesn't have to mean face-to-face interaction. Who are you chatting online with the most? Who are you talking on the phone with? Who is in your car and on your heart?

Do you have your five people in mind? Are these people lifting you up and elevating you? Are they supportive, loving, and nurturing? Do they inspire and motivate you? Do they have qualities and characters that you admire and hope to emulate? If you aren't answering yes to these questions, you may need to reassess your circle of influence. Negativity breeds negativity. The same is true with positivity. So why not surround yourself with positive, supportive people? You deserve to be in the company of people who love and support you no matter what life throws your way.

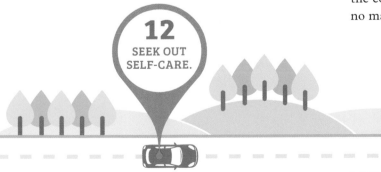

12
SEEK OUT SELF-CARE.

> 66 Grace means that all of your mistakes now serve a purpose instead of serving shame. 99
> —*Brené Brown*

③ DOCUMENT THE DAILY.

If you have struggled with your weight for quite some time, then you probably know what it's like to get rid of every picture of yourself that makes you feel bad. To always insist on being the one behind the camera and demand to see every photo taken of you so that you can make sure you don't look fat. Sound familiar? I can't stress to you enough how much you are going to wish you had kept those photos later in your journey. As I began to lose weight and document my progress, I realized how few pictures I had of the old me. To keep a clear vision of where you're going, it's important to remember where you've been.

Start taking pictures on day one. As you begin to make progress, you can compare the photos side by side to see just how far you have come. This time around, I am documenting everything, and on those days when I feel like my body hasn't changed at all, I pull up an old picture and compare it with a current photo. Small changes add up over time, and seeing the difference is astounding. It can be exactly the pick-me-up you need on a rough day.

④ TOSS THE TEMPTATIONS.

I don't mean just food-related temptations, but let's start there. Go through your cupboards, your fridge, your pantry, and your secret food stash and get rid of everything that is not a part of your healthy low-carb lifestyle. Hanging on to it is a form of slow torture. Why test your willpower when you don't have to? If you keep only good food in your house, then you will eat only good food. I know that probably sounds oversimplified, but doesn't it seem like a pretty reasonable place to start?

While you're at it, ditch that candy bar and bag of chips that you plan to reward yourself with when you reach a certain milestone. Don't reward yourself with food; you aren't a dog. Wouldn't a smaller jeans size be a much more fulfilling reward for all of your hard work? By that same token, don't hang on to clothes that are too big for you. It's like telling yourself that you know you will gain the weight back. Don't look back; you aren't going in that direction. Keep looking forward to the version of yourself that you wish to become.

⑤ DON'T FEAR FOOD.

Food should be neither a reward nor a punishment. But just like the scale, we tend to give food a lot of control over our emotions and how we feel about ourselves. As you transition to a low-carb ketogenic lifestyle, you might feel like some of the foods you are eating couldn't possibly be good for you. We spent so many decades being brainwashed by the low-fat culture that to start eating an abundance of butter, bacon, avocado, meat, cheese, coconut oil, and so on can feel like somewhat of a shock. We've come a long way from the days of rice cakes and fat-free yogurt. Let the results of your new lifestyle speak for themselves, and eat up! That is not to say that food should be a free-for-all or that you should eat with reckless abandon as long as you are watching your carbs. Quality and quantity still matter. Let food be your fuel and not your foe.

6 SAY "SEE YA" TO SHAME AND GOODBYE TO GUILT.

Can you honestly tell me one good thing that shame or guilt has brought into your life? I didn't think so. Yet it is so easy to fall into a shame spiral and feel burdened with self-imposed guilt. Forgive yourself. Think of all of the people you have forgiven in your lifetime. What allowed you to forgive them, but not yourself? In order to set yourself free from shame and guilt, you might need to let go of who you *think* you should be. Powerful stuff, right? I certainly think so. What if we all just lived without fear of shame, blame, judgment, and heartache and agreed to live unapologetically, vulnerably, and true to ourselves? I continue to work toward this goal every day. It's okay to be imperfect. No one is expecting you to be perfect except you. Give yourself permission to live as your authentic self, and amazing things will start to happen. Try practicing mindfulness, joy, and gratitude each day. It can really help keep you out of the shame game.

7 CLEAR THE CLUTTER.

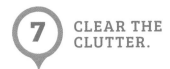

I am a firm believer that physical clutter equates to mental and emotional clutter. When my home is cluttered or my workspace is in a state of disarray, everything else starts to feel like it is systematically breaking down. I feel anxious and stressed, and everything seems a little harder than it needs to be. But when my living spaces and work areas are clean, organized, and free of clutter, everything feels a little lighter and easier to manage. It's amazing how the simplest things can have the most profound effects.

If you need to start clearing some of the clutter from your life, don't let the process overwhelm you. Start with one room at a time. If that feels overwhelming, then start with one drawer. Commit to working on it a little bit each day, even if you have only ten minutes to spare. Once you begin purging the clutter from your home, I think you'll find that you feel a little lighter and a lot happier.

8 LEARN THE LABELS.

Read everything. Everything! You are going to have that message drilled into you by the time you've finished working your way through this cookbook. How can you know exactly what you are putting into your body if you aren't paying attention? Learning how to make sense of the information displayed on a nutrition label will be a great asset to your weight-loss journey. For example, it is so disappointing to down a snack that you think is one serving only to find out after the fact that you just ate *three* servings in one sitting. Scouring labels is also a great way to identify hidden carbs and sugars. Once you start reading labels, you will be shocked to find out how much sugar is hiding in plain sight in everyday foods. For more information about how to spot hidden carbs, check out "Those Evil Little Hidden Carbs" on pages 37 to 39.

9   NEVER MISS MONDAY.

Mondays can be tricky to navigate. After a fun Saturday with friends and family and a Sunday Netflix binge-fest, you can wake up Monday morning feeling a little freedom hangover—freedom from the Monday-through-Friday grind. Monday morning is a great time to set your intentions for the week ahead. I always feel a sense of renewal. If I start the week with proper nutrition and physical activity, I am far more likely to continue this trend throughout the week. Feeling good makes you want to keep feeling good. You will smile more, feel less anxious, have better energy and mental clarity, and be ready to tackle whatever the week throws at you.

10   CUT THE COMPARISONS.

> **"THE REASON WE STRUGGLE WITH INSECURITY IS BECAUSE WE COMPARE OUR BEHIND-THE-SCENES WITH EVERYONE ELSE'S HIGHLIGHT REEL."**
>
> —*Steven Furtick*

That is one of my favorite quotes, and I remind myself of it often. We live in a digital age in which we are bombarded with the highlight reels of people's lives. Five minutes on social media can make you feel like a failure: Not worthy enough. Not pretty enough. Not thin enough. Not a good enough parent. Not a good enough friend. It's easy to forget that we are seeing carefully crafted versions of people's lives scrolling by. Comparison creeps into our deepest insecurities and infects everything like a virus. You are uniquely you. You are the only person on the planet qualified to fill your own shoes. You have unique and original gifts and talents. You are irreplaceable. More importantly, you are enough!

11   FIND YOUR FITNESS.

Yes, it is possible to lose weight through diet alone, without exercising. However, I don't recommend it. I view proper nutrition and movement as a retirement plan for the body. When I work out, I am doing it for eighty-year-old me—the spry granny who still wants to be chasing her crazy pups around or going on hikes. The weight loss that comes along with it is just icing on the low-carb cake. So where do you start?

Starting a new fitness regimen can be a daunting endeavor, but it doesn't have to be. Find what works for you. So what if everyone around you is doing CrossFit and you are doing water aerobics? You are still lapping everyone on the couch.

Can't afford a gym membership? No problem! There are so many free workouts that you can do at home without any equipment at all. Check to see if your cable provider offers an OnDemand fitness section. Don't have a cable package? Again, I say no problem. There are thousands of free full-length workouts on YouTube. Let's say that you don't have cable *or* internet. Still not a problem. Walking is free. Do some squats, push-ups, jumping jacks, planks, lunges, burpees, and so on in your living room. The options are there; you just have to decide to exercise them. Pun intended!

You can accomplish a lot by simply committing to move your body each day. Fitness doesn't have to come in the form of a daily structured workout. Small changes in your activity level can really add up over time. Here are some simple things you can do to get in a little extra intentional movement throughout the day:

- Walk instead of driving whenever possible.

- Park a little farther from store entrances to get in some extra steps.

- Take the stairs instead of the elevator.

- Crank up some tunes and dance your way through your house as you clean.

(12) SEEK OUT SELF-CARE.

This is a really big, important point that I learned way too late. Self-care doesn't have to mean spending a bunch of money on massages and pedicures. It comes in many forms. Sometimes it lives in the quiet moments that you take for yourself in the morning. Make sure to carve out time each day for you and you alone. Take a bath, meditate, read a book, do yardwork, go for a walk, or do yoga. These are all things you can do at home to practice self-care without spending any money. And these are just a few ideas. Figure out what you love and what fills your cup. Then carve out time to do some of those things. I cannot stress enough how important it is to take care of yourself. You wouldn't run your car into the ground and skip all of the necessary maintenance, would you? No, you want to protect your investment. Why should it be any different with your body? Keep those doctors' appointments. Get to the dentist. See a chiropractor if you need to. Invest in yourself. You are your biggest asset.

But perhaps most importantly, JUST KEEP GOING!
Keep fighting the fight.

> " It is not the critic who counts; not the man who points out how the strong man stumbles, or where the doer of deeds could have done them better. The credit belongs to the man who is actually in the arena, whose face is marred by dust and sweat and blood; who strives valiantly; who errs, who comes short again and again, because there is no effort without error and shortcoming; but who does actually strive to do the deeds; who knows great enthusiasms, the great devotions; who spends himself in a worthy cause; who at the best knows in the end the triumph of high achievement, and who at the worst, if he fails, at least fails while daring greatly, so that his place shall never be with those cold and timid souls who neither know victory nor defeat. "
>
> —*Theodore Roosevelt*

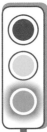

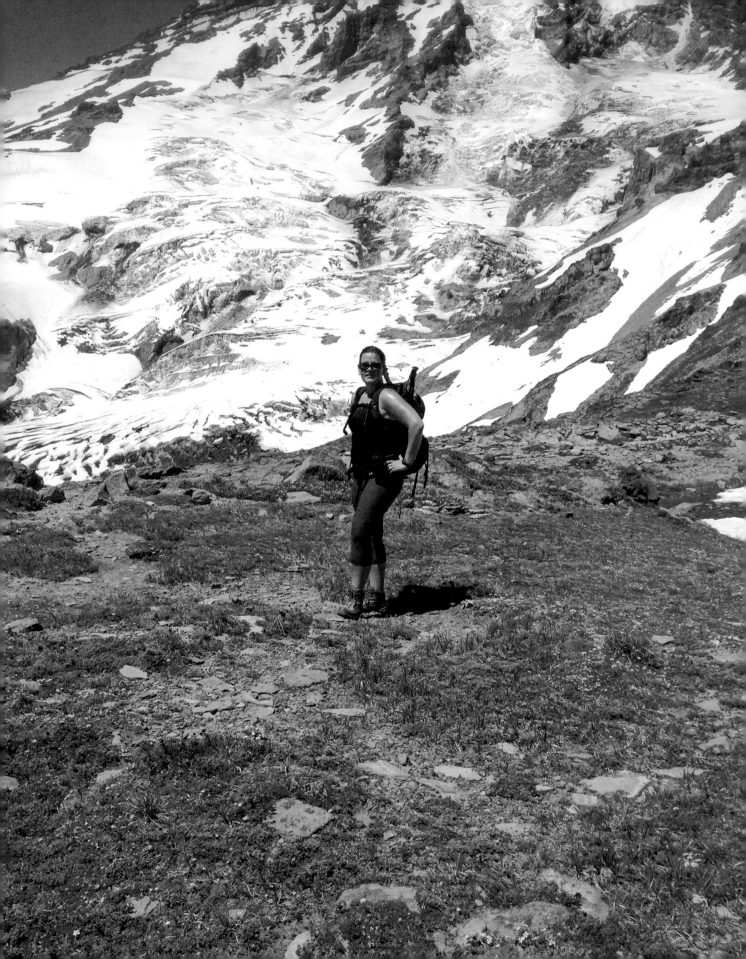

Breaking Up Is Hard to Do

I, like many of you, spent years and years in an abusive relationship with my bathroom scale. Instead of using it as a tool, as just one method of measuring my progress, I became a slave to it. I let it define me, and it came to dictate my self-worth and how I felt about myself from day to day. I let a glowing number from a digital device fill me with doubt, insecurity, and shame. I knew I had to find a way to break the cycle of abuse—abuse that I was inflicting upon myself.

Do any of these scenarios sound familiar? Could this be you?

- Do you use the bathroom right before weighing yourself?

- Do you weigh yourself completely naked, removing even your socks?

- Do you weigh yourself first thing in the morning?

- Do you exhale as deeply as you can and then hold your breath as you stand on the scale?

- Do you weigh yourself multiple times a day, knowing full well that natural fluctuations will occur, and then still beat yourself up about them?

- Do you weigh yourself after elimination in hopes of seeing a smaller number than you saw in the morning?

How do I know about all of these habits? No, I don't have a mirror into your bathroom! I know these are your habits because they were once mine, too. They are the habits of anyone who has a terrible relationship with the scale. You are not alone. But trust me when I tell you that there is life on the other side.

Stay with me here as we get a little imaginative. I'm going to tell you a breakup story from my own personal experiences. You might be wondering what a story about a breakup has to do with your relationship with the scale? Well, here is some keto food for thought: Imagine that your scale was your life partner. If your partner made you feel the way your scale does, would you stay with that person?

I had to leave this abusive relationship. I let it go on for so long, and it was slowly killing me inside. It was stealing my joy and teaching me to tear myself down instead of lifting me up. I kept trying to make it work, but nothing I did seemed to make things any better. He brought out the worst in me, and I didn't like the person I was when I was around him.

The last year or so was when our relationship started to get really rocky. Things took a real turn for the worse. I knew that if I loved myself, I needed to leave him—or at the very least, spend a lot less time with him. If I'm being honest, our relationship was never that great. He never told me I was pretty. He never made me feel comfortable in my own skin. In fact, he never did anything to boost my self-esteem or my confidence. He always took my mind to the darkest places and made me question my self-worth.

Yet I kept coming back for more. In fact, even though he always made me feel terrible, I saw him almost every day. One glimpse at him and my mood was set for the day. It was rarely a good mood, either. It was the kind of bad mood that seems almost impossible to turn around. The kind of bad day that makes you want to climb back into bed and wait until tomorrow to try again.

You could say that I was addicted to him. Like any abuser, he would throw me a bone every once in a great while. He would show me a glimpse of himself that made me think that maybe, just maybe, things were starting to turn around, and we would be okay. That we would magically have a healthy and honest relationship going forward. Then, like clockwork, he would be back to his abusive ways, and I would be back in my shame spiral.

I decided that we should take a break—try to find ourselves and see if we really wanted to be together. It was hard at first. He was so embedded in my daily routine that I almost didn't know how to not see him. Each day became a conscious choice to not be around him, to not be under his influence, and to not let him be the measuring stick for my self-worth. I didn't notice a big difference at first. I still felt pretty bad, and things didn't seem to be changing at all. Even without seeing him, I was still telling myself all of the negative things that he would constantly tell me.

As the days passed, I slowly began to feel that familiar sense of self creep back into my heart and fill my spirit. Hello, old friend, nice to see you! I almost forgot what it felt like to be around you! You see, now that he was out of the picture, my old friends Joy and Happiness came around again. We started spending a lot of time together. We laughed more than we had in ages. One night, Joy, Happiness, and I were going through my closet and trying on clothes. I picked up a pair of jeans that I hadn't tried on in quite a while. "He" never liked them and always made me feel so fat when I put them on. Joy and Happiness cheered me on as I slid them up my thighs and around my waist; they fit perfectly. They looked like they were made for my body. The three of us did a little happy dance and let out a "Yesssssss!" as we celebrated my victory.

I started to think about him less and less. Joy was around so much that she practically lived with me. When she was around, I always seemed to have better hair days, my makeup seemed a little more on point, I ate better, and I made it to the gym more often. Was I falling for Joy?

By the time winter rolled around, my habits had changed, and I really didn't miss him at all anymore. In fact, I would see him, feel nothing, and just keep walking by. Had I done it? Was I finally free of him? Had I finally realized that I didn't need him and that he was no good for me?

We got together once or twice that month. He must have missed me, because he was really nice. He showed a side of himself that I hadn't really seen before. He told me how pretty I was. He told me what a big heart I had. He listed all of the reasons there were to love me. He was wooing me big-time. I almost fell for it. We went out for an amazing dinner one night. He told me that I deserved to splurge because I had been so good for so long and the holidays were coming. It sounded logical to me. We ate and drank to our hearts' content. It was a lot of fun. But in the morning, he was back at it. He told me that I had no self-control and that I was always going to be fat. He asked me why I ever tried to leave him in the first place when I knew that I would just come running back. I knew right then and there that it was over. I couldn't let another year come to a close feeling this way about myself. So I kicked him out.

I went to see him one last time after that. I wanted closure. I wanted to tell him that he didn't break me and that his opinion didn't matter. I loved myself at all shapes and sizes. I love myself now, and I will love myself in the future, whatever it holds. I went to where he lived and climbed those familiar steps. I went into his room and walked over to him, but he didn't react. He didn't light up like he normally did when I came close. He wasn't beaming with that intensity that always brought me back. He was just sitting there, almost lifeless. As I stared at him, I couldn't understand what I'd ever seen in him. I couldn't grasp how I'd let him have such control over me. It was finally over. I breathed a sigh of relief as I walked out of his room and down the hallway, taking in a big gulp of fresh air as I stepped outside.

As the months passed, I spent even more time with Joy and Happiness. We were having so much fun. We were crushing goals together and feeling great. I knew that I would date again when the time was right, but for now, things were exactly as I wanted them to be.

See how that plays out? Sad, right? "He" is obviously the scale, not a real person. But the scale is a real, tangible item that I and so many others have allowed to control and define us. When I say that he "was just sitting there, almost lifeless," the batteries had died on my home scale. I chose not to replace them. I chose to let that dead scale sit there as a reminder that it couldn't control me and that I would decide my own fate and self-worth.

After a few months off the scale, I became less dependent on it. When I went back to weighing, I was finally able to use it as just one small benchmark of my progress—one small piece of a much larger puzzle. I began paying attention to so many other things, such as how my clothes fit, what my measurements were, how I was sleeping, and how I was feeling mentally. All of these things would come to be so much more important to me than the number on the scale.

If you are having trouble breaking up with the scale, here are some healthy habits that might help you transition away from it:

✔ Take it out back and give it an *Office Space*–style beat-down with a bat.

✔ Remove the batteries and throw them away.

✔ Have someone hide it from you until you feel you have a better perspective on it.

✔ Get rid of it altogether and donate it.

My hope for you is that you are able to find peace and freedom on the other side of the scale. Joy and Happiness are waiting for you there!

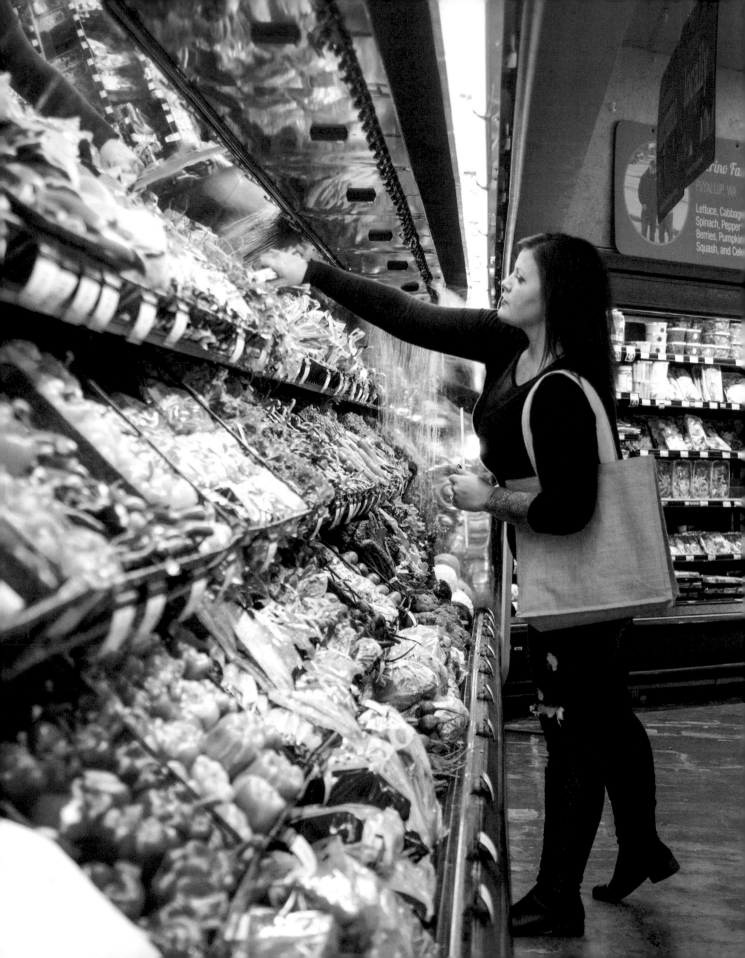

Transitioning to a Low-Carb Lifestyle

> **"TIMES OF TRANSITION ARE STRENUOUS, BUT I LOVE THEM. THEY ARE AN OPPORTUNITY TO PURGE, RETHINK PRIORITIES, AND BE INTENTIONAL ABOUT NEW HABITS. WE CAN MAKE OUR NEW NORMAL ANY WAY WE WANT."**
>
> —*Kristin Armstrong,*
> *professional road bicycle racer and Olympic gold medalist*

As you transition into your new low-carb, ketogenic lifestyle, you may feel challenged, like it just isn't for you. You are not alone in this feeling. Hang in there! You've got this. Listen to your body, give it some time to adapt, and before you know it, you will be settled in and finding ease in your new lifestyle. I've compiled some of my best tips for making the transition a little more seamless.

- Set yourself up for success by getting the people around you involved. Make it a family affair and include your whole family in your decision. Let all of your friends know about your lifestyle change. This will help them understand what you're doing and support your decisions. Ask them to help keep you accountable. Having the people who matter most to you involved in your healthy lifestyle will help you feel less alone as you navigate unfamiliar territory.

- Don't be afraid to ask questions. Join online forums. Reach out to people you view as authorities on the subjects you want to learn more about. Talk to your local grocer. When dining out, ask your servers about the menu and the ingredients used. Talk to the chef. If you don't ask, you will never know.

- Don't feel like you have to make the switch cold turkey. Some people do best with jumping right in, in an all-or-nothing fashion, while others benefit from transitioning slowly. If you fall into the latter category, work on replacing old habits with new, healthier habits one at a time.

- Scour labels. Seriously! Read the labels on everything. Even if you think you know every ingredient, read them anyway. Reading labels will help you get a better feel for the amounts of carbs in the foods you are consuming.

- Out with the old and in with the new. Get rid of all of the food that does not fit your new low-carb lifestyle. I am not saying to throw it away; perhaps you can give it to a neighbor or friend or even donate it to a food bank. Better yet, start your new lifestyle when all of the food in your house is gone and it's time to go grocery shopping. It's important to start with a clean slate so that you are not tempted to eat things you shouldn't eat.

- Get rid of temptations. There is no point in keeping foods around that you know will tempt you and make transitioning to a low-carb lifestyle harder on you.

- Always keep some prepped low-carb staples on hand—cooked chicken breasts, cooked bacon, sliced vegetables, hard-boiled eggs (see page 162), and cheeses. It's important to be able to grab something quickly in a pinch.

- Research, research, research! There are so many great books out there on low-carb and ketogenic diets. There are also some excellent blogs and websites putting out a lot of free information and recipes. Soak up all the information you can. The more you know, the better prepared you will be.

- Always have a food plan. Plan your meals ahead of time so that you aren't left reaching for anything in sight at the last moment.

- Weigh, measure, and portion your foods until you get a feel for portion sizes and the approximate numbers of carbs per serving in your everyday foods.

- Focus on whole, real foods. Keep it simple in the beginning. You don't have to turn into a master chef overnight to enjoy your meals. Try not to make it harder than it needs to be by overthinking and overcomplicating things. I like to remind myself to K.I.S.S. (keep it super simple).

- Know your Simple Low-Carb Food Swaps (see page 40) and refer to them often.

- Be prepared while on the go and pack a healthy low-carb snack or two. For help coming up with healthy snack options, refer to the Complete Guide to Low-Carb Snacking on pages 48 and 49.

- Think ahead when you know you will be dining out. Refer to the dining out guide on pages 81 to 84.

- If you slip up, don't beat yourself up. You are human. Just pick right back up where you left off and keep going. One bad meal does not have to mean a bad day. One bad day does not have to mean a bad week. One bad week does not have to mean a bad month. I think you see where I am going with this.

- When you get frustrated, think about all of the foods you *can* eat instead of focusing on what you can't eat. I know this might sound silly, but mindset matters.

- Utilize a food-tracking app. There are many different apps out there. A quick search in your app store will bring up a whole host of apps and reviews so that you can find the app that works best for your specific needs.

- Figure out what works for your body and stick to it. It might take a little trial and error, but you will get there. I promise!

- If you feel bad in the first few days, you might be experiencing what some people call the "keto flu." You might feel sluggish, have nausea, experience fatigue, or suffer from headaches. This is essentially your body detoxing from carbs. Drink lots of water, eat more fat, replenish electrolytes, take a quality magnesium supplement, and drink both broth and coconut milk. These things should help the feelings subside. Some people even report that drinking pickle juice helps them kick the keto flu. Hey, I'm all for anything pickle related, flu or no flu.

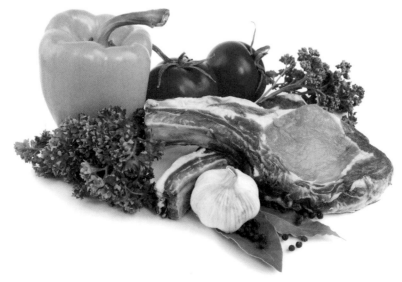

Those Evil Little Hidden Carbs

Just when you think you've got the carb-counting gig down pat, you eat something that seemed like a no-brainer only to find out later that it contained far more carbs than you thought. Sound familiar? You are not alone. It happens to the best of us. Hidden carbs are everywhere, and they can have a huge impact on your overall weight-loss success in a low-carb ketogenic lifestyle.

What are hidden carbs? They are the sneaky little starches and sugars hiding in plain sight in everyday foods. And they are hiding in a lot of places you wouldn't expect. Unfortunately, there are many labeling loopholes in the United States. If you frequent any low-carb online forums or groups, then you have likely seen several debates about whether heavy cream, cheese, and eggs have carbs. You will see people say, "Well, my brand is zero carbs." Then another person will chime in that theirs has a small amount of carbs, to which someone will always respond by educating everyone in the thread how carbohydrate labeling works in the U.S. There is a loophole of sorts that results in misleading nutrition labels. If a food has less than 0.5 gram of carbs per serving, food manufacturers are legally allowed to say that the product contains zero carbs. The "per serving" part of that loophole is what becomes problematic for people strictly tracking their carbohydrate intake.

Here's an example: Heavy whipping cream contains 0.4 gram of carbs per 2 tablespoons, but most cartons say zero. If you have a few cups of coffee with heavy cream in the morning, those hidden carbs can really add up. Not to mention if you are making a recipe that calls for 1 cup of heavy cream. That would add approximately 3.2 grams of carbs to the recipe. All that being said, that carb count is still really low. But when you are following a 20-grams-per-day lifestyle, every last gram counts. Be careful with eggs and cheese, too, as they are labeled the same way. Cheddar cheese, for example, has 0.4 gram of carbs per 1-ounce serving but is usually labeled as zero.

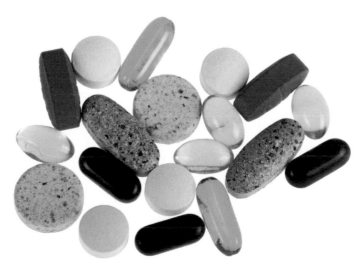

We all love surprises, right? Just not when it comes to our food. Here are some sources of hidden carbs to be on the lookout for:

POWDERED BOUILLON—Powdered bouillon is a concentrated flavor enhancer. It is often used for making rich broths, soups, and sauces. Most brands contain not only MSG, but also a variety of forms of sugar. Bouillon comes in at about 1 gram of carbs per teaspoon, and at that rate, the carbs can add up fast. Look for a cleaner-ingredient brand and use it in moderation. Better yet, use homemade stock, sea salt, and seasonings to flavor your dishes instead.

PRESHREDDED CHEESE—Many preshredded cheeses contain powdered cellulose to keep the cheese shreds from clumping. The cellulose adds minimal carbs, but it is worth noting, as it can cause weight loss to stall in some people.

PROCESSED CHEESE SLICES—Processed cheese is exactly that: highly processed. It contains a very small amount of real cheese mixed with a variety of emulsifiers, vegetable oils, food colorings, sugar, and so on. That American single you grew up eating is not real food and can contain as much as 3 grams of carbs per slice. Steer clear.

PREPARED COLESLAW—Many coleslaw dressings are packed with added sugars. Unless you made it yourself and know exactly what's in it, skip it. A half cup of prepared coleslaw has approximately 14 grams of carbs.

CONDIMENTS—Many condiments are packed with added sugars. This is fairly easy to control by simply reading labels before you purchase or consume any condiments you haven't used before. As far as controlling added carbs in restaurant condiments, refer to the dining out guide on pages 81 to 84.

COUGH SYRUP—It's hard to stop and think about carbs when you can't stop coughing, but did you know that one dose of Nyquil contains approximately 19 grams of carbs? There are natural brands of sugar-free cough drops on the market that are much lower in carbs.

OTHER MEDICINES AND VITAMINS—If any of your medications or vitamins are candy coated, flavored, or chewable, there's a good chance you are taking in extra carbs. Many medicines and supplements contain sugar or artificial sweeteners. Even your daily multivitamin might contain as much as 3 grams of carbs.

IMITATION CRABMEAT—"Krab with a K," as I like to call it. Don't be fooled by this impostor. Many people assume that because real crabmeat contains zero carbs, imitation crabmeat is the same, but this is simply not the case. Only 3 ounces of imitation crabmeat contains approximately 13 grams of carbs.

PROCESSED MEATS—Processed meats are meats that have been smoked, salted, cured, dried, or canned. This includes sausages, hot dogs, salami, bacon, and ham. A lot of times, the processing methods include adding sugar to the meat.

MILK—Many people fail to think of milk as a carb and are unpleasantly surprised when they hear just how many carbs are in milk: approximately 12 grams in one 8-ounce glass of 1% or 2% milk. Whole milk is approximately 11 grams, and half-and-half is approximately 10 grams. Thankfully, once we get to the higher-fat milk products like half-and-half and heavy cream, we are using only 1 to 2 tablespoons at a time. Heavy cream is a great choice for low-carbers because it comes in at less than 1 gram of carbs per 2 tablespoons (or about 6.5 grams in 8 ounces).

MILK SUBSTITUTES—Many milk alternatives, such as almond milk, coconut milk, and cashew milk, have hidden carbs. Well, they are actually hiding right there on the label, but it is easy to grab the wrong brand. It is really important to read labels. Make sure to purchase an unsweetened variety with no added flavorings or sugars.

RESTAURANT OMELETS—This one is always surprising to me. Fun fact: a lot of restaurants add pancake batter to their omelets to make them fluffier. Well, they may be nice and fluffy, but they are no longer low-carb or gluten-free.

SAUCES AND GRAVIES—A lot of sauces contain flour, sugar, or both. Always read labels before buying, and when dining out, be sure to ask your server or the chef about the restaurant's sauces.

SEASONINGS BLENDS AND PACKETS—Always read the labels on store-bought seasoning mixes. You would be surprised at how many different brands contain added sugars, which are just added carbs.

SHELLFISH—Many people assume that, like meat, all seafood is free of carbs. While many types are, including halibut, salmon, crab, and lobster, some shellfish is not. There are approximately 4.5 grams of carbs in 3 ounces of scallops. Twenty medium-sized clams contain 8 to 10 grams of carbs. There are approximately 6 grams of carbs in 3 ounces of mussels. Six medium oysters contain 2.5 to 4.5 grams of carbs.

GLUTEN-FREE FOODS—While many low-carb, real foods are naturally gluten-free, the term *gluten-free* does not automatically mean that an item is also low-carb. The terms are not synonymous. For example, take white rice. It is gluten-free but packs a whopping 45 grams of carbs per prepared cup. For keto substitutes for these higher-carb foods, check out the Simple Low-Carb Food Swaps on pages 40 and 41.

LOW-FAT AND FAT-FREE VERSIONS OF FOODS—Remember, the lower the fat content, the higher the carb count. In making low-fat versions of foods like yogurt, cheese, and salad dressing, most manufacturers simply replace the fat with sugar to make the product taste good. One more reason not to fear fat. Nix the low-fat products and stick to delicious and healthy whole-food fats like avocados, olives, and coconut oil.

SUGAR-FREE FOODS—Don't make the mistake of thinking that sugar-free is synonymous with low-carb. They are not one and the same. Many of the sugar-free foods on the market are actually quite high in carbs.

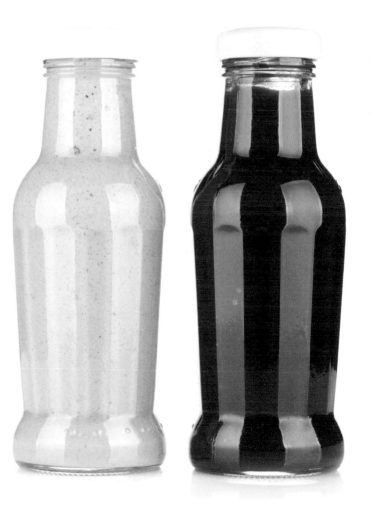

Simple Low-Carb Food Swaps

Finding success in switching to a low-carb, ketogenic lifestyle relies heavily upon your willingness to get creative, keep an open mind, and have realistic expectations about the substitutions being used. Cauliflower rice doesn't taste exactly like rice. Only real rice tastes like rice. But I rather enjoy cauliflower rice, and at times I even prefer it. When prepared correctly, it is a very close match in taste and texture. I'll take the weight-loss and health benefits from eating cauliflower rice over the tired, full, bloated feeling I would get after a giant serving of mashed potatoes any day. It's about making consistently good food choices and learning to love the food you are eating for exactly what it is.

Six or seven years ago, you couldn't pay me to eat cooked cauliflower, and now I love it so much that I actually crave it. In fact, there are very few foods that I miss from my old lifestyle. I have been able to seamlessly transition into healthier food choices without feeling deprived by thinking outside the box when it comes to my food choices. I think you will see a lot of that throughout the recipes in this book. I've done all the creative thinking for you. You can just sit back, relax, and cook delicious, healthy foods. I'm not one of those people who is going to try to hand you a piece of celery and convince you that it is chocolate. I am a realist and you should be, too. It will make your low-carb lifestyle a lot easier. Notice that I never use the word *diet*? Lasting success comes in thinking of this as a lifelong change and not as a quick fix or a patch. I hope that these simple swaps and recipe suggestions help ease your transition to a low-carb lifestyle.

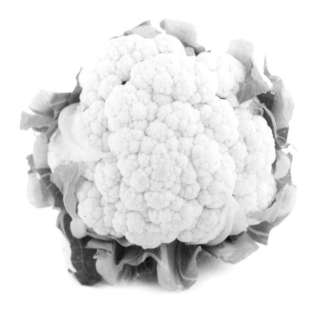

BREADS AND BUNS—lettuce wraps, portobello mushrooms, gluten-free wraps and tortillas, Asiago Rosemary Bacon Biscuits (page 172), biscuits from Reuben Biscuit Sandwiches (page 226), cloud bread (there are lots of recipes online)

CRACKERS AND CHIPS—pork rinds, sliced vegetables, pepperoni and salami chips (see page 146), Garlic Parmesan Cheese Crisps (page 198), Garlic Dill Baked Cucumber Chips (page 158), cabbage chips, dried seaweed snacks, kale chips, crispy bacon, flax crackers

FRENCH FRIES—Baked Avocado Fries (page 170), crispy Parmesan zucchini fries

HIGH-CARB BREADING—Savory Breading Mix (page 354), Nut-Free Keto Breading Mix (page 355)

LASAGNA—"Just Like the Real Thing" Lasagna (page 240), lasagna-stuffed peppers, eggplant lasagna, zucchini noodle lasagna (There are recipes for all of these dishes on my site, peaceloveandlowcarb.com.)

MILK—heavy cream, almond milk, coconut milk, cashew milk

PASTA—cauliflower, vegetable noodles, shirataki noodles, shredded cabbage, spaghetti squash, kelp noodles, Creamy Pesto Chicken Zucchini Pasta (page 250), Chicken Zoodle Alfredo (page 252)

PIZZA CRUST—chicken crust, cauliflower crust, Pizza Crust (page 356), Nut-Free Pizza Crust (page 358)

POTATOES—For mashed potatoes, substitute Creamy Herbed Slow Cooker Cauliflower Mash (page 284) or celery root mash. For roasted potatoes, substitute radishes like in the Butter Roasted Radishes recipe (page 292). For breakfast potatoes, substitute radishes like in the Radishes O'Brien recipe (page 116). For crispy hash browns, try a mixture of grated radishes and cauliflower. For home fries, try the Garlic and Herb Oven-Roasted Home Fries on page 122.

RICE—cauliflower rice, grated zucchini, shirataki rice, Basic or Fiesta Cauliflower Rice (page 282), Cranberry Pecan Cauliflower Rice Stuffing (page 286)

SUGAR—granular erythritol, powdered erythritol, brown sugar erythritol, stevia, stevia glycerite, xylitol, monk fruit

THICKENERS—xanthan gum, guar gum, pureed vegetables, heavy cream

WHEAT FLOUR—almond flour, coconut flour, sunflower seed flour, flaxseed meal, protein powder, psyllium husk powder (*Note:* Most of these are not 1:1 substitutes for wheat flour. There are some thorough guides online that can help you figure out how to convert some of your favorite recipes to use low-carb flour substitutes.)

YOGURT—plain coconut milk yogurt, sour cream, full-fat ricotta cheese, cream cheese mixed with coconut milk, Almond Joy Chia Seed Pudding (page 326)

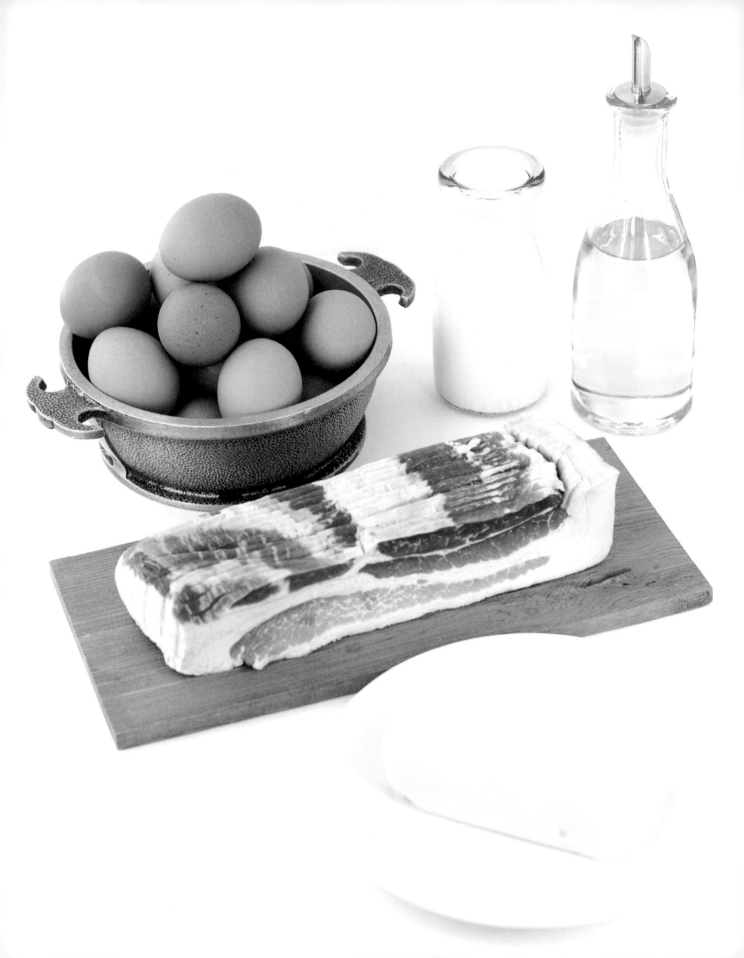

Stocking Your Keto Kitchen

If I were to collect all of the low-carb refrigerated and frozen items that I eat, this is what the list might look like. This is not a complete list of low-carb, ketogenic foods; rather, it is a list of the foods that I eat regularly and the ingredients used in the recipes in this book.

You can refer to the meal plans on pages 71 to 75 to determine which of these foods you might want to have on hand at one time.

FRIDGE AND FREEZER STAPLES

DAIRY PRODUCTS

Grass-fed butter

Heavy cream

Full-fat sour cream

Asiago cheese

Blue cheese crumbles

Full-fat cream cheese

Feta cheese

Goat cheese

Mascarpone cheese

Mozzarella cheese

Parmesan cheese (both grated and shredded)

Provolone cheese

Full-fat ricotta cheese

Sharp cheddar cheese

String cheese

Swiss cheese

REFRIGERATED CONVENIENCE FOODS

Capers

Dill pickle relish

Dill pickles

Green olives

Kalamata olives

Pepperoncini

Roasted red peppers

Sauerkraut

MILK SUBSTITUTES

Unsweetened almond milk

Unsweetened cashew milk

Unsweetened coconut milk

Unsweetened macadamia nut milk

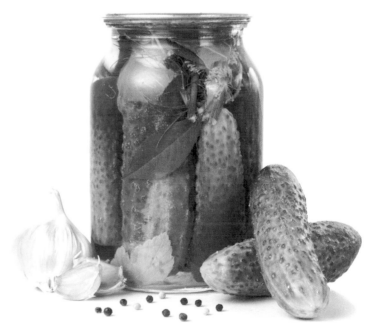

PROTEINS

Pastured eggs

Chicken breasts

Chicken thighs

Whole chicken

Ground chicken

Ground turkey

Ground beef

Steak (multiple cuts)

Ground pork

Pork belly

Pork chops

Pork tenderloin

Deli meats

Grass-fed hot dogs

Bacon

Breakfast sausage

Ham

Pancetta

Prosciutto

Pepperoni

Salami

Wild-caught clams

Wild-caught cod

Wild-caught halibut

Wild-caught salmon

Wild-caught scallops

Wild-caught shrimp

FRUITS AND VEGETABLES

Asparagus

Avocados

Bell peppers

Brussels sprouts

Cabbage

Cauliflower

Celery

Chives

Cranberries

Cucumbers

Eggplant

Fresh herbs

Garlic

Green beans

Green onions

Jalapeños

Kale

Lemons

Lettuce (several varieties)

Limes

Mushrooms

Onions (red and white)

Radishes

Rainbow chard

Shallots

Spaghetti squash

Spinach

Sun-dried tomatoes

Tomatoes

Zucchini

CONDIMENTS AND SAUCES

Dijon mustard

Garlic and Herb Marinara Sauce (page 344)

Garlic Dill Tartar Sauce (page 339)

Ranch Dressing (page 332)

Reduced-sugar ketchup

Spicy brown mustard

2-Minute Mayo (page 336)

Walnut Avocado Pesto (page 340)

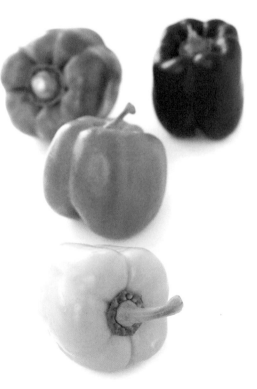

PANTRY STAPLES

If you came over to my house right now and opened the doors to my pantry, these are the items you likely would see at a glance. I like to shop sales and stock up on nonperishable items that I use frequently. My pantry is typically bursting at the seams.

VINEGARS AND FLAVORINGS

Apple cider vinegar

Balsamic vinegar

Red wine vinegar

Unseasoned rice wine vinegar

Coconut aminos

Cooking sherry

Hot sauce

Toasted sesame oil

Worcestershire sauce

HEALTHY COOKING FATS

Avocado oil

Coconut oil

Duck fat

Olive oil

Ghee

Grass-fed butter

Grass-fed tallow

NUTS, NUT BUTTERS, AND SEEDS

Raw almonds

Raw cashews

Raw pecans

Raw walnuts

Pine nuts

Reduced-sugar peanut butter

Unsweetened almond butter

Chia seeds

Pumpkin seeds (pepitas)

Sunflower seeds

BAKING PRODUCTS AND COFFEE BOOSTERS

Collagen

Grass-fed gelatin

MCT oil powder

Protein powder

Almond flour

Coconut flour

Brown sugar erythritol

Granular erythritol

Powdered erythritol

Baking powder

Baking soda

Pure almond extract

Pure lemon extract

Pure orange extract

Pure vanilla extract

Sugar-free maple extract

Sugar-free dark chocolate chips

Unsweetened cocoa powder

Xanthan gum

CANNED AND JARRED GOODS AND CONVENIENCE FOODS

Artichoke hearts

Black olives

Boxed beef stock

Boxed chicken stock

Crushed tomatoes

Diced tomatoes

Diced tomatoes and green chilies

Stewed tomatoes

Tomato paste

Diced green chilies

Pork rinds

Sustainably caught canned salmon

Sustainably caught canned tuna

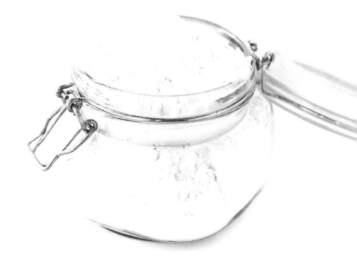

Let's Get Spicy

Spice every dish with a little peace and love and you will please every palate. They say variety is the spice of life, but I say spice is the variety of life!

My spice collection is one of my favorite parts of my kitchen. With a protein, a cooking fat, and a collection of spices, I can make some serious magic happen. Spices are what take food from bland and boring to extraordinary. Spices add flavor and aroma, enhance the taste of food, and even change or enhance the color. Don't believe me? Check out the beautiful color of the Egg Drop Soup on page 184, which comes from turmeric powder.

Seasonings and spices can seem a little intimidating if you are not used to cooking with them, but I will break down some of the basics for you and show what I keep on hand in my kitchen. These are all spices that you will see throughout the recipes in this book as well.

CHOOSING YOUR SPICES

Not all spices are created equal. Many of the less-expensive brands you see in stores may already be near the end of their shelf life. The less-common spices could sit on the shelves for months before anyone buys them. There is also a good chance that these products were sitting in a warehouse for many months before they even hit the store shelves. Spices aren't something you are going to will to your children; they have expiration dates and need to be replaced regularly. Most spices have a shelf life of between one and two years if stored properly (see below).

Here are some of my best tips for choosing the best-quality spices without breaking the bank:

- Buy your everyday spices from the bulk section. I'm not saying to buy a pound at a time; I'm just saying that ounce for ounce, you can save a lot of money going the bulk route. And you can usually find great per-ounce prices on organic spices and seasonings.

- Shop local. You can find great prices on locally sourced organic spices and seasonings at farmers markets.

- Order online. A lot of reputable companies sell spices in bulk on their websites. The savings are passed on to you because buying online cuts out the middle man (the store).

- Buy whole spices and grind them yourself using a spice grinder or mortar and pestle. Doing so will save you money and get you the freshest spices possible. It also ensures that there aren't any additives in your spices.

STORING YOUR SPICES

Store your spices lying flat in a drawer so you can always see each spice at a glance. This helps you know what you have on hand and prevents you from buying the same spices over and over again. Who needs four bottles of lemon pepper seasoning? That was me when I still kept my spices in a cupboard. Now all three drawers in my center island are filled with my spices and homemade seasoning blends, and I can easily see what I have and what I need to buy or make more of.

Store spices in airtight jars to preserve their freshness, ensure fuller flavor, and extend their life. Do not store them above the stove or in direct sunlight. Heat, moisture, and sunlight can all shorten the shelf life and potency of spices.

Now that we are feeling spicy, let's have a look in my spice drawers, shall we?

Basil (dried)	Cloves (ground)	Himalayan pink salt	Rosemary leaves (dried)
Bay leaves	Coriander (ground)	Italian seasoning	Rubbed dried sage
Black pepper (ground)	Cream of tartar	Lemon pepper seasoning	Sea salt
Black peppercorns	Cumin (ground)	Mustard powder	Sesame seeds
Caraway seed	Curry powder	Mustard seeds	Smoked paprika
Cayenne pepper	Dill weed (dried)	Nutmeg (ground)	Tarragon leaves (dried)
Celery salt	Dried minced onions	Onion powder	Thyme leaves (dried)
Chili powder	Fennel seeds	Oregano leaves (dried)	Turmeric powder
Chinese five-spice	Garlic powder	Parsley leaves (dried)	Vanilla beans
Cinnamon (ground and sticks)	Ginger powder	Red pepper flakes	

Let us not forget all the amazing spice blend recipes in this cookbook!

- Barbecue Dry Rub (page 353)

- Cajun Seasoning (page 351)

- Everything Bagel Seasoning (page 352)

- Mexican Seasoning Blend (page 350)

- Seasoning Salt (page 349)

tip:

Don't forget that spices aren't a free food, as many people seem to think. They do have carbs. After all, the foods they come from contain carbs.

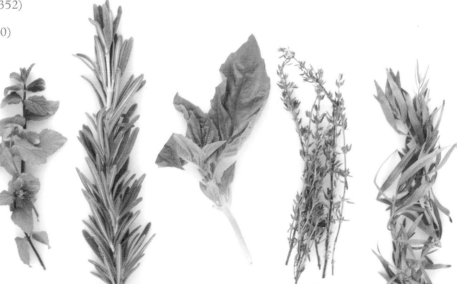

Complete Guide to Low-Carb Snacking

For me, having high-quality, low-carb–friendly snacks on hand is a major component of staying on track. I am far less likely to grab something I shouldn't eat if I have healthy snacks readily available. When I travel, I always pack my own snacks. I fill my backpack with healthy, nonperishable foods to take on the plane or on a road trip. Not only does it keep me prepared in a pinch, but it saves me money, too. Have you seen the prices of in-flight meals and roadside gas station snacks lately?

PORTABLE SNACKS—NO PREP REQUIRED

Avocados

Boxed bone broth

Canned tuna or salmon

Cheese sticks

Dehydrated broccoli chips

Dill pickles

Dried seaweed snacks

Flax crackers

Jerky

Kale chips

Meat sticks

Mixed nuts and seeds

Mixed olives

Nut butters

Pork rinds

Salami or pepperoni

Sardines

Unsweetened coconut chips

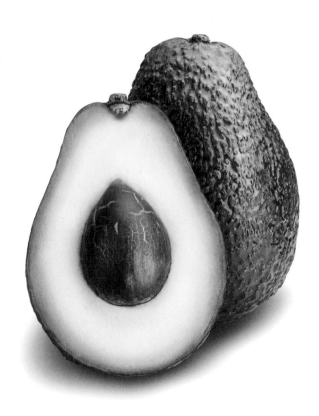

WINE

Wine is typically your safest bet when dining out. It ensures that you know exactly what you are getting and that you aren't accidentally getting a high-carb mixer or the wrong type of liquor.

Note: Be sure to take note of the size wine pour you are ordering and figure out the carb count based on the 5-ounce pours listed below.

RED WINE	Carb Count in 5 Fluid Ounces
Pinot Noir	3.5 g
Merlot	3.7 g
Cabernet Sauvignon	3.8 g
Syrah	3.8 g
Zinfandel	3.8 g

WHITE WINE	Carb Count in 5 Fluid Ounces
Sparkling white	1.5 g
Brut Champagne	2.5 g
Sauvignon Blanc	2.8 g
Pinot Grigio	3 g
Chardonnay	3.1 g

SWEET WHITE WINE	Carb Count in 5 Fluid Ounces
White Zinfandel	5 g
Riesling	5.7 g
Moscato	8 g
Sangria	10+ g
Late-harvest Riesling	12 to 18 g
Port wines and sherries	13+ g
Wine coolers	20 to 50 g

BEER

There are hundreds, if not thousands, of different beers on the market. Here is a list of some of the lowest-carb beers out there. These beers are easy to find at your local grocery store. Please note that none of them are gluten-free. If you are living a strict gluten-free lifestyle, I would steer clear. Check out brands like Omission that are crafted to remove gluten. If you have a higher carb allowance or are at a maintenance weight, hard cider can be a delicious option as well.

BEER	Carb Count in a 12-Fluid-Ounce Bottle
Bud Select 55	1.9 g
Miller 64	2.4 g
Michelob Ultra	2.6 g
Bud Select	3.1 g
Miller Lite	3.2 g
Busch Light	3.2 g
Michelob Ultra Amber	3.7 g
Amstel Light	5 g
Coors Light	5 g
Corona Light	5 g
Bud Light	6.6 g
Heineken Light	6.8 g

You will notice that not everything listed here can be considered low-carb, but I wanted to give you a thorough guide to help you make informed decisions.

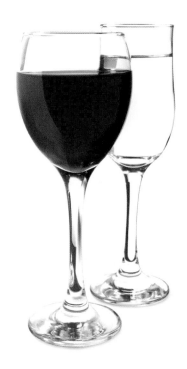

PREPARED SNACK IDEAS

Almond Joy Chia Seed Pudding (page 326)

Asiago Rosemary Bacon Biscuits (page 172)

Bloody Mary Deviled Eggs (page 166)

Boosted Coffee (page 140)

Creamy Avocado Pesto Deviled Eggs (page 162)

Deviled Ham and Egg Salad Lettuce Wraps (page 204)

Dill Chicken Salad (page 194)

Garlic Dill Baked Cucumber Chips (page 158)

Garlic Dill Pickled Brussels Sprouts (page 156)

Garlic Parmesan Cheese Crisps (page 198)

Salted Caramel Nut Brittle (page 302)

Sour Lemon Gummy Snacks (page 152)

Tuna Salad Pickle Boats (page 148)

Bacon

Bone broth

Chopped fresh vegetables

Cucumber slices

Dark chocolate

Fat bombs

Guacamole

Hard-boiled eggs (see page 162)

Low-carb hummus (you'll find several recipes on peaceloveandlowcarb.com)

Meat and cheese roll-ups

Minute muffins

Protein shakes

SNACKING TIPS

- Bring your own healthy snacks to the movies. Theaters aren't nearly as strict with outside snacks and beverages as they used to be. Whenever I go to the movies, I bring a big bottle of water and something healthy to nosh on if I'm feeling hungry. Better yet, forgo the snack altogether. As a society, we are programmed to feel like we can't watch a movie without eating. It is only at the theater that I think about snacking when watching a movie. When I sit down to watch a movie or TV show at home, I don't automatically feel the need to eat something.

- Keep a healthy nonperishable snack in the glove box or center console of your car to avoid ending up in a hangry snackcident.

- Keep a stash of healthy low-carb snacks in your desk drawer at work. You never know when you might forget your lunch or have to work late. It just might save you from hitting up a fast-food restaurant on the way home.

- Stash a couple of snacks in your gym bag. This will help you eliminate hunger or a lack of energy as a reason not to work out.

- Before snacking, ask yourself if what you are feeling is true hunger or if something else is at work—stress, boredom, high emotions, and so on. If you aren't sure, try drinking some water and waiting it out.

- Portion out your prepared snacks so that you don't overdo it. It is easy to lose sight of portion control with snacks. Also, pay attention to the serving sizes on packaged foods. Sometimes even the smallest package contains multiple servings. Don't accidentally consume extra carbs by forgetting to scour the labels.

  While snacking, we tend to ignore our standard eating behaviors, like sitting at a table or portioning out our food onto a plate. Instead, we're standing in the kitchen, driving in the car, sitting at a desk, or chatting up a friend while chowing down mindlessly on whatever is in front of us. Practice conscious eating behaviors when snacking and you are far less likely to overdo it. Portion out your snack, put it on a plate, and put the rest away. You are likely to feel more satisfied if you are making conscious food decisions and not just mindlessly eating.

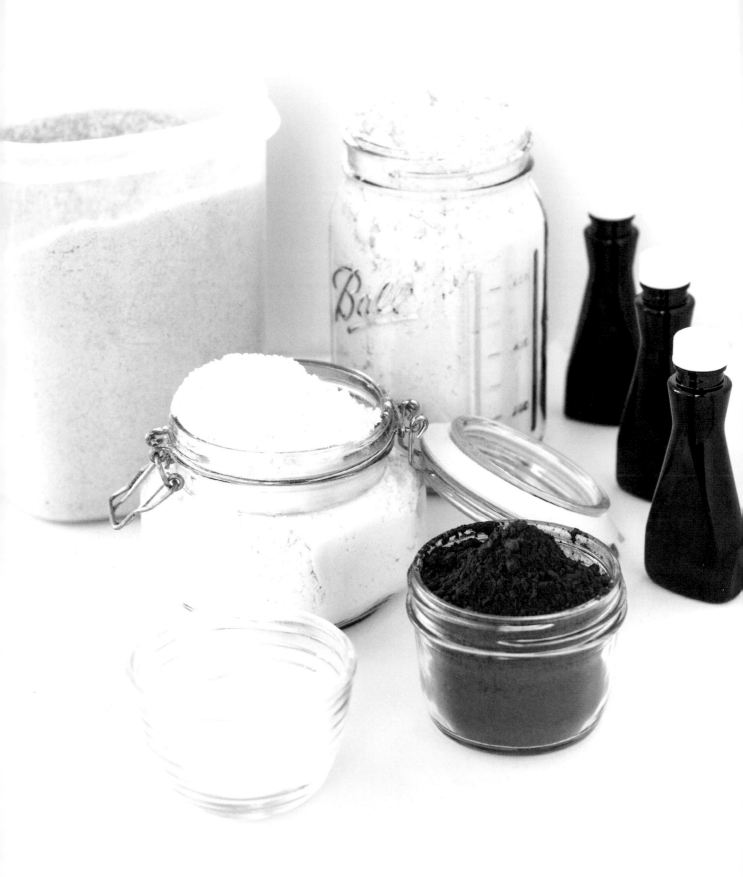

Ingredients Used in This Book

In this section, I am going to highlight some of the specific products and brands that I used to create the recipes in this book. I am not typically a brand-specific person, but I always look for the best-quality ingredients with the best price points. Do not feel like you have to buy a whole bunch of specialty ingredients to maintain a low-carb, ketogenic lifestyle. Anyone who tells you that you need to do so probably has a hidden agenda, so steer clear.

In this book, you won't find any ingredients that you can't readily find at a typical grocery store. I want to make this lifestyle as easy as possible for you. That being said, I do buy a lot of products online from sites like Amazon and Thrive Market because the prices are often much lower than they are at the grocery store.

I firmly believe in working with what you have and doing the best you can in any situation. For example, if you can't afford grass-fed butter, just get the best-quality butter you can afford, and stay away from margarine! If you are looking at almond flours and the store brand has the same nutritional info as the brand-name version, by all means buy the store brand. It just might save you the money you need to get that grass-fed butter.

ALMOND FLOUR—For the recipes in this book, I used finely ground blanched almond flour. A couple of my favorite brands are Anthony's and Bob's Red Mill.

APPLE CIDER VINEGAR—When selecting a brand of apple cider vinegar, look for a raw, unfiltered version. My favorite brand is Bragg.

AVOCADO OIL—Avocado oil is my favorite oil for cooking. I use it for almost everything. It is right up there with butter and ghee for me. Refined avocado oil has a smoke point of over 500°F, making it excellent for high-temperature cooking and frying. It also has a very light and neutral flavor, making it perfect for my 2-Minute Mayo (page 336) and a variety of salad dressings. My favorite brand is Chosen Foods.

BACON—Many brands of bacon are loaded with multiple forms of sugar. Look for sugar-free, clean-ingredient brands. Some of my favorites are Fletcher's, Hempler's, and Pederson's Natural Farms.

BROTH AND STOCK—It's easy to make your own stock and bone broth. Not only will making your own save you a lot of money, but homemade versions pack a nutritional punch. That being said, it is perfectly fine to go the stock-in-a-box route. I typically do. But look for a brand that is organic and has no added sugars. The only ingredients in a box of chicken stock should be chicken, water, spices, and vinegar.

CANNED TUNA AND SALMON—You might not know this, but many popular brands of canned tuna and salmon contain soy. It's another one of those surprising ingredients that doesn't quite seem like it belongs. Those same brands often use really low-grade farm-raised fish or fail to practice sustainable fishing methods. I love the brand Wild Planet. Not only is all of their seafood wild-caught, but it is sustainably pole- and line-caught as well.

COCONUT AMINOS—I use coconut aminos in place of soy sauce for just about everything. My favorite brand is Coconut Secret. If you're going to use soy sauce, make sure to look for a gluten-free variety, like tamari.

COCONUT FLOUR—I use finely ground coconut flour. My favorite brand is Nutiva. I buy it on Amazon to save a few dollars.

COCONUT MILK—When selecting coconut milk, canned is typically the way to go. I am not brand specific on this one, but make sure to look for brands without added sugars; the only ingredients should be coconut, water, and a natural stabilizer, such as guar gum.

ERYTHRITOL (Granular, Powdered, and Brown Sugar)—Many of the sweet treat recipes in this book call for granular, powdered, or brown sugar erythritol. The two brands that I use and love are Swerve and LC Foods Company. I highly recommend both. Ordering online from LC Foods Company will likely save you some money. That is the only place I go for brown sugar erythritol.

GHEE—Ghee is a form of clarified butter in which the milk solids are separated out. You are left with a golden liquid that has a nutty, caramel-like aroma and taste. It has a longer shelf life and a higher smoke point than butter, making it a great option for cooking at higher temperatures. It is usually tolerated by people who have lactose and dairy sensitivities, as the milk solids have been removed. That being said, those with severe dairy allergies should probably still steer clear. I use ghee in place of butter in a lot of my recipes. My two favorite brands are Tin Star Foods and Fourth & Heart.

GRASS-FED BUTTER—I always buy grass-fed butter. I prefer my butter to come from cows that are not fed GMO corn and soy products or pumped with growth hormones and antibiotics. For me, it is a matter of voting with my dollars. It is a splurge I will always make. My favorite brand is Kerrygold. For the recipes in this book, I used salted butter unless otherwise noted.

LEMON JUICE—I use fresh-squeezed lemon juice whenever I have lemons on hand, but where it is called for in the recipes in this book, you can always substitute bottled lemon juice. Just make sure that it does not include any added sugars and is 100 percent lemon juice.

MEATS—Whenever possible, I buy grass-fed meats from small family farms (preferably local): grass-fed beef, organic pastured chicken, and pasture-raised heritage pork. It is important to me to know the history of my meat and to support companies that put the ethical treatment of animals at the forefront of their mission, vision, and values. I have a monthly subscription to ButcherBox and absolutely love it.

PASTURED EGGS—Why pastured eggs, you might ask? Well, for me there are several reasons. Buying local farm-raised, pastured eggs enables me to support local farmers and saves me money. Farm-fresh eggs are cheaper than factory-farmed eggs from the grocery store. They have rich, deep orange yolks and are much higher in omega-3 fatty acids and vitamin E. The difference in taste is remarkable. Once you eat a farm-fresh egg, there is no going back. Most importantly, I refuse to support factory farming practices. Happy chickens lay happy eggs.

PORK RINDS—I feel like I need to start out by telling you that I have never been a fan of pork rinds. The smell, the texture, the taste, and even the *idea* of them were a huge turnoff to me. But I have been able to successfully mask them in my breading mixes (pages 354 and 355) so that I can't taste them at all. It wasn't until very recently that I actually began to like them. I quickly learned that not all pork rinds are created equal and that there is a lot of variation between brands. I will use a lot of different brands for breading foods, but there are only two brands that I will actually eat as a snack: Epic and 4505 Meats.

SEA SALT—Sea salt supplies vital minerals that help support a healthy body. I used fine sea salt in all the recipes throughout this book, except where another type is noted.

SPICES AND SEASONINGS—I go into much more detail about spices in my "Let's Get Spicy" guide on pages 46 and 47, but my favorite brand of store-bought spices and seasoning blends is Simply Organic. I buy them online to save a few dollars.

SUGAR-FREE DARK CHOCOLATE CHIPS—Some of the sweet treat recipes in this book call for sugar-free dark chocolate chips. My favorite brand is Lily's. They are sweetened with stevia.

UNSWEETENED COCOA POWDER—Unsweetened cocoa powder has an intense dark flavor. Make sure to steer clear of cocoa mix and sweetened cocoa powder, which contain added sugars.

VANILLA EXTRACT—Not all vanilla extracts are the same. Many of the brands you see in stores are actually imitation vanilla extract, meaning that they could have artificial colorings, artificial flavors, sugars, and even corn syrup added to them. Saving a dollar or two just isn't worth it. I always opt for pure vanilla extract. My favorite brand is Simply Organic. You can save a couple bucks by purchasing it online from a site like Amazon or Thrive Market.

25 Tips for Reducing Food Waste

One of the things that I dislike the most in this world is food waste. I work very hard in my own kitchen to ensure that we use all of our food and none of it goes to waste. How many times have you had a plan for that ground beef in the fridge only for life to get in the way, and before you know it, it has turned brown and smells a little off, and you have to throw it away? Trust me, we've all been there. With a few small lifestyle changes, though, you can be well on your way to becoming a waste-free household.

Often, the keys to making food go further and eliminating waste lie in proper food storage. If you constantly find yourself with small portions of unused food or food that goes to waste before you can use it up, these tips might help you get the most bang for your buck when it comes to fresh foods.

GENERAL TIPS AND TRICKS

1. Know the difference between sell-by, best-by, and use-by dates. Also, make sure to keep up-to-date with changes to food labeling regulations.

   Sell-by date lets retailers know the date by which the food should be sold or removed from store shelves. This does not mean that the product is expired or unsafe to consume. (*Note:* Many stores have a discounted area with items that are close to or past this date. It is a great way to save money. Approximately one-third of the shelf-life of a product occurs after the sell-by date.)

   Best-by date is a suggestion to consumers as to when a product should be consumed to ensure maximum quality and freshness.

   Use-by date is also for consumers. This is the suggested date by which a product should be eaten. It does not mean that eating it after this date will make you sick, but its quality will start to decline, and food safety could decrease.

2. Freeze anything that is nearing its use-by date before it goes to waste so that you can use it later.

3. Make sure that your refrigerator and freezer are set at the ideal temperatures to prevent spoilage.

4. Save vegetable scraps in a resealable plastic bag in the freezer and continue adding to the bag until you have enough scraps to make homemade stock. You can then use that stock in recipes instead of store-bought stock.

5. Utilize small amounts of leftovers to repurpose into new meals, like frittatas or casseroles.

6. Store fish and poultry in airtight containers to ensure maximum freshness.

7. Keep the fridge clean and organized. Doing so makes it easier to keep track of what you have on hand and reduces waste and spoilage. No more buying things you already have only to see them go bad.

8. Invest in a vacuum sealer to ensure proper storage. This gadget will help you portion out leftovers or products bought in bulk.

9. Plan your meals so you know exactly in which order to use your ingredients and prevent spoilage.

10. Take leftover scraps of meat and vegetables, add broth and seasonings, and turn them into a delicious soup.

MEATS

11. Use leftover bones to make homemade bone broth.

12. Buy meat in bulk, portion it out, and freeze the individual portions. This will help prevent freezer burn and keep you from over-portioning your meals.

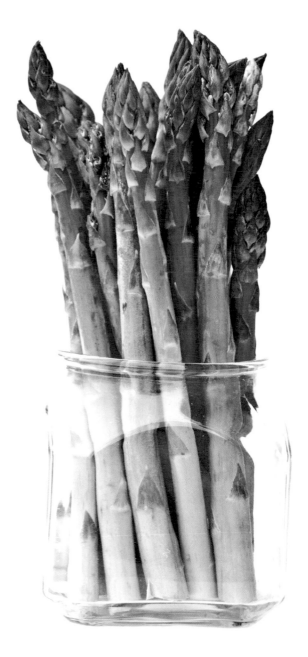

PRODUCE

13. Store fruits and vegetables separately. Most fridges have a designated drawer for each, with separate temperature and humidity controls.

14. Know which produce should be stored on the counter and which should be stored in the fridge. Proper storage will ensure that you get the longest possible life out of your produce.

15. Store mushrooms in a paper bag to extend freshness.

16. Use extra-ripe produce for making homemade sauces.

17. When buying fresh-cut herbs or delicate greens, store them with a paper towel in the packaging to reduce moisture and the chance of mold.

18. When produce is not in season, frozen is more economical and will last longer.

19. Don't wash your produce before putting it in the refrigerator. Wash it right before using it.

20. Freeze leftover sauces and stocks in individual containers for later use.

21. Buy an ethylene gas absorber and store it with your produce to prolong life.

22. Brush the cut sides of avocado halves with lemon juice or olive oil to extend their life.

23. Chop up extra herbs and freeze them in an ice cube tray with olive oil or melted unsalted butter for later use.

24. Store chopped green onions in a jar in the freezer.

25. Store asparagus upright in about 1 inch of water. You will be amazed at how long it stays fresh in the fridge when stored this way!

Keto on a Budget

One of the things I hear most often from people who are transitioning to a low-carb, ketogenic lifestyle is that eating this way is "so expensive." While real food isn't always as cheap as packaged ramen and mac and cheese, there are a lot of little things you can do to make your money go further. Besides, would you rather fill your body with highly processed, wheat-filled Frankenfoods or fuel it with healthy, nutritious, real foods? I'm pretty sure the answer to that question would be unanimous.

With a little creativity and a willingness to put forth some effort, you should be able to keep your grocery bill close to, if not lower than, what you currently spend each month. You will be pleasantly surprised to see that real food isn't, in fact, "so expensive." Packaged foods are often *more* expensive because you pay more for the convenience.

Ridding your fridge and pantry of high-carb processed foods and replacing them with low-carb whole-food options can seem like a big upfront expense. But if you use the tips listed here along with the information in the section "Transitioning to a Low-Carb Lifestyle" on pages 35 and 36, you should find making the switch a lot easier and more affordable than you initially expected. As you build up the staples in your refrigerator and pantry, you'll spend less and less over time.

Just to drive home my point, let's do a little comparison, shall we? Keep in mind that prices obviously vary by region, but I tried to make this list as accurate as I could. I priced ingredients at several different stores to come up with the lowest costs, and I even pulled the prices based on store brands, not brand-name products.

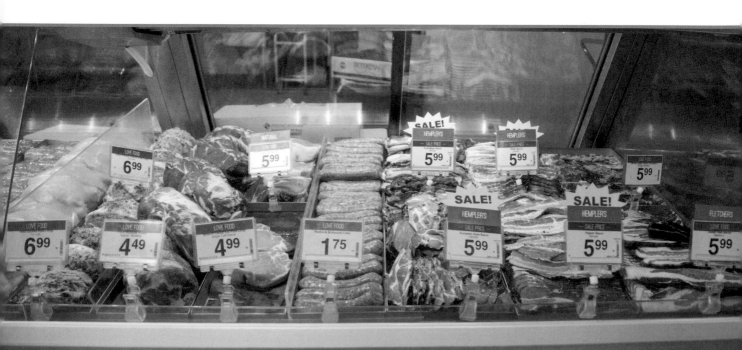

HIGH-CARB, HIGHLY PROCESSED MEAL:

Hamburger Helper with Corn and Salad

$2.50 box of Hamburger Helper

$2.99 carton of milk (for the boxed meal)

$1.09 margarine (for the boxed meal)

$3.99 1 pound of ground beef

$0.89 can of creamed corn

$3.29 bagged salad mix

$1.99 store-brand ranch dressing

Total for 4 servings: $16.74
($4.19 per serving)

LOW-CARB, REAL-FOOD MEAL:

Chicken Zoodle Alfredo (page 252) with Garlic Parmesan Cream Sauce (page 342) and Parmesan Roasted Broccoli (page 281)

$1.96 four large zucchini

$2.99 1 pound of boneless chicken thighs

$2.00 shredded Parmesan cheese

$4.99 1 pound of real butter

$3.09 carton of heavy cream

$0.79 head of garlic

$0.49 bunch of fresh parsley

$1.99 1 pound of fresh broccoli

Total for 4 servings: $18.30
($4.58 per serving)

Now let's break a few things down. The low-carb, real-food meal comes in at a slightly higher cost per serving, but it is low-carb, gluten-free *real* food. It utilizes three easy recipes from this book and leaves you with leftover cheese, butter, cream, garlic, and parsley for future meals. I left out the salad because this meal is already packed with vegetables. You could bring the price down even further by skipping the butter, which is the most expensive item on the real-food list. The recipe calls for only a couple tablespoons of butter, yet we were able to splurge for a whole pound. If you already had olive oil or another healthy cooking fat in your pantry, you could use that instead of butter, and then this whole real-food dinner would come in at only $3.32 per serving. Now, can you still tell me that eating healthy is "so expensive"? I think not.

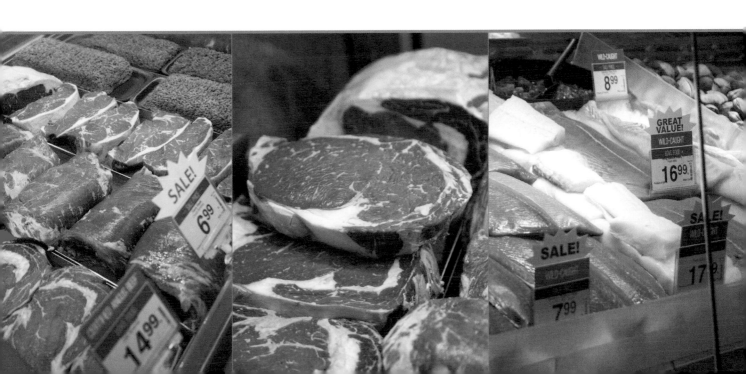

HERE ARE SOME OF MY BEST TIPS AND TRICKS FOR SAVING MONEY ON YOUR GROCERY BILL:

- Plan ahead for the week and make a grocery list before heading to the store. It might sound simple, but you wouldn't believe how many people I talk to who just go to the store without a plan and wing it.

- Stick to your list. If an item isn't on your grocery list and isn't part of your meal plan, you don't need it. Ignore that little voice inside telling you that you do.

- Use a meal plan for the week and stick to it. (See pages 71 to 75 for some examples.) This will cut back on waste and extra expenses.

- Never buy groceries with a credit card if you can avoid it. If you don't pay off your bill at the end of each month, the interest will have you paying for those groceries long after they're gone.

- Don't be afraid to shop multiple stores. Doing so may be a little more time-consuming, but it can save you *a lot* of money. Also, check out local stores that offer delivery. Many times the delivery is free and the prices are the same as they are in the store. Taking advantage of this service is a great way to help you stick to your grocery list.

- Stick to the perimeter of the store, which is typically where the healthiest foods are. There are obviously some quality foods in the interior aisles, too, but don't fall prey to advertising gimmicks. The brands placed at eye level are always the most expensive. Check the top and bottom shelves for the best deals.

- Check weekly ad circulars and shop according to store sales.

- Use coupons whenever possible and always ask for price matching. Many larger companies offer printable coupons on their websites.

- Now that we are all familiar with what the use-by, sell-by, and best-by dates mean (see page 54), don't be afraid to buy discounted meats and freeze them for later. I can't tell you how much money this tactic has saved me over the years.

- Take advantage of sales on nonperishable items that you use regularly and stock up.

- Skip the packaged foods. They are usually filled with ingredients you don't need to be eating, and you pay a convenience fee for its being prepackaged. Fresh food is a much healthier option, anyway.

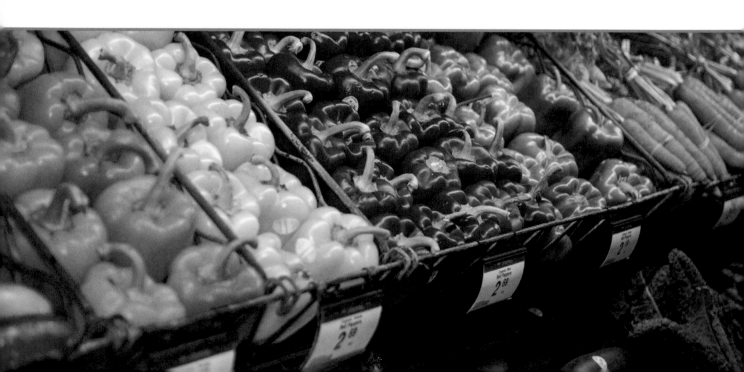

- Skip the bagged salads and cut your own lettuces. Store them with a paper towel to make them last longer.

- Shop the bulk food section for items like everyday spices, nut flours, and raw nuts and seeds.

- Buy meat in bulk, portion it out, and freeze it for later.

- Shop online at sites like Amazon and Thrive Market for items like spices, condiments, and baking supplies. You can usually snag some great deals with free shipping, and many of these items are far less expensive than they would be at your local grocery store.

- Skip the brand names and go for their generic equivalents. Many times the generics have the exact same ingredients, but they always cost less.

- Whenever possible, buy produce at farmers markets. Not only are you supporting your local community, but you can also save a lot of money. Depending on your local market, you can usually snag some great deals on meat and eggs as well.

- Buy local pastured eggs whenever possible. They are much healthier for you and are typically a lot less expensive than eggs from the grocery store. Purchasing eggs from nearby farmers also supports your local economy.

- Buy fresh produce when it is in season. In the off-season, frozen produce is more economical.

- Source your meat from local butchers or farmers. You can save a lot of money, and you typically get far better cuts of meat. This is also a good practice for the environment. The shorter the distance your food has to travel, the less impact it has on the environment.

- Buy whole chickens and cut them down yourself. You can save a lot of money if you are willing to cut your own meat. Never done it before? Have no fear; there are a lot of awesome tutorials online.

- Skip the preshredded cheeses and grate your own. You pay a premium for having the work done for you—not to mention that preshredded cheese usually contains some sort of additive to keep it from clumping.

- Grow your own vegetables and herbs. Starting your own little garden comes with a minimal upfront expense but pays off big-time. And there is something so rewarding about growing your own food and being involved in the entire process from seed to plate.

- Join a local CSA or food co-op to save on produce costs and get better-quality produce.

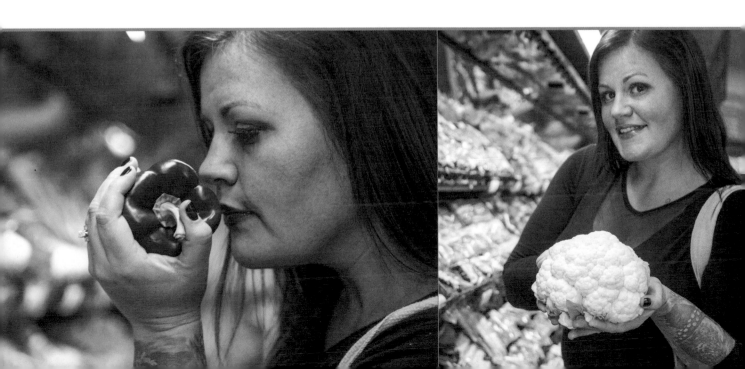

- Do the best you can with what you have. You don't have to jump right in and buy all organic and grass-fed. Over time, as you continue to save money, you will find more funds to use for splurges like organic produce, grass-fed meats and butter, and eggs from pastured hens.

- Make your own seasoning blends from the spices you have on hand. Doing so will save you money, and you can make sure that your homemade blends contain no added fillers.

- Repurpose leftovers whenever possible. Have some leftover meat and veggies from last night's dinner? Combine them with some whisked eggs and your favorite cheese and make a frittata for breakfast.

- Check dollar stores and discount grocery stores. You never know what you might find! Our local discount grocery store has a fairly large organic section, and I'm able to find some of my favorite brands for dirt cheap.

- Substitute cheaper cuts of meat where possible. Learn about all the different cuts of beef, pork, and chicken and then shop accordingly. For example, chicken thighs can be substituted for chicken breasts in nearly every dish. Not only does it save you money, but it is a great way to add a little extra fat. Win-win!

- Cut back on needless snacking. Ask yourself if you are truly hungry. If you are, skip the packaged snacks and make your own instead. There are several great recipes for snacks in this book; see Chapter 2.

- Skip the bottled water. Instead, buy a water filter; it will pay for itself over time with the savings from not buying bottled water.

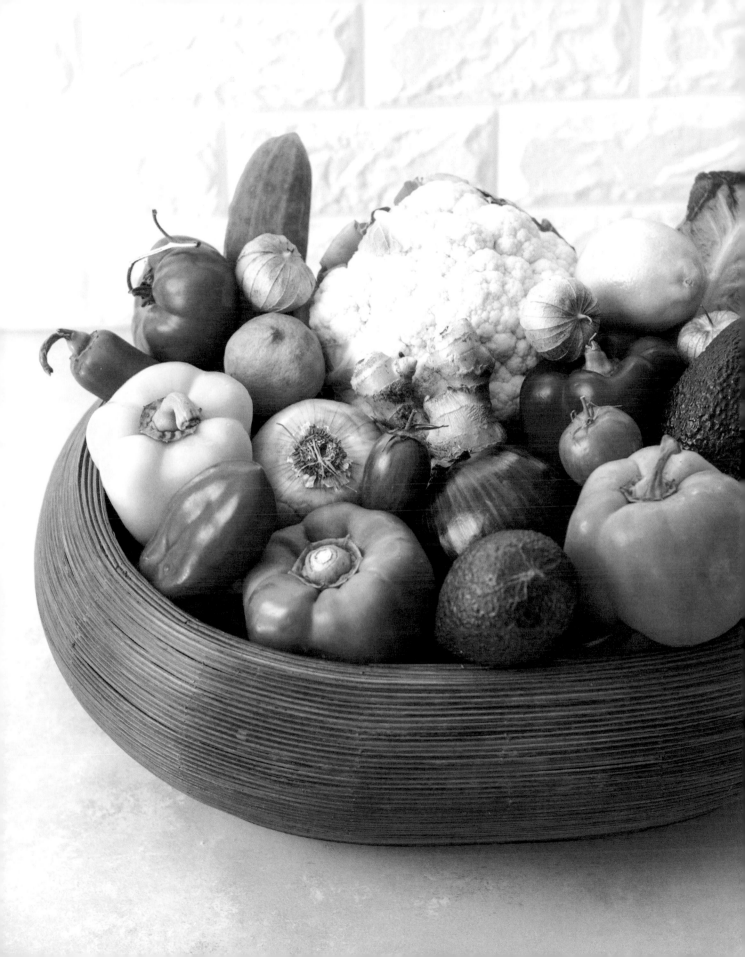

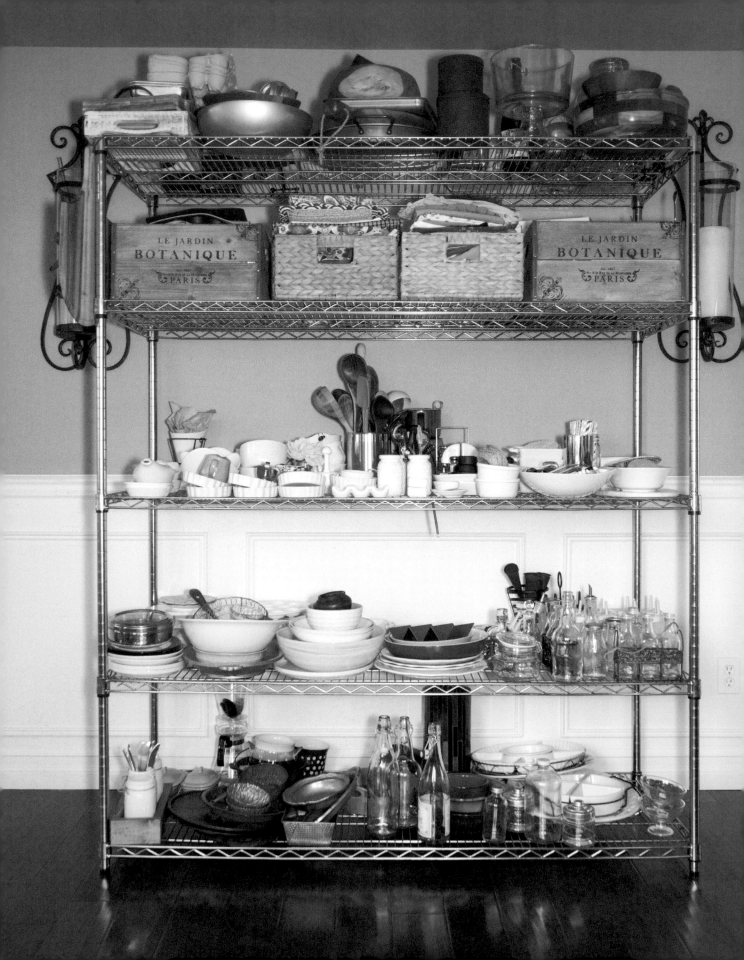

My Favorite Kitchen Tools and Gadgets

MEASURING TOOLS

MEASURING CUPS (BOTH LIQUID AND DRY) AND SPOONS—My measuring cups and spoons come out every time I cook. When following a recipe, it is important to measure your ingredients accurately. You can always add, but you can't subtract ingredients from a recipe. I have Pyrex 2-cup and 4-cup (1-quart) liquid measuring cups and two sets of measuring spoons, along with an accurate set of dry measuring cups.

DIGITAL FOOD SCALE—Not only will a food scale help you measure and prep ingredients, but it can also help you stay within your daily macronutrient targets by letting you know exactly how much you are eating.

COOKWARE AND BAKEWARE

STAINLESS-STEEL SKILLETS AND SAUCEPANS—A quality set of cookware will make your time in the kitchen a lot easier and more enjoyable. I prefer stainless steel, as many of the nonstick pans on the market can leach toxins and heavy metals into your food. I recommend purchasing a set that includes various sizes of skillets as well as saucepans. Often you can save money by piecing the set together and purchasing only the pans you need.

ENAMELED CAST-IRON PANS AND DUTCH OVEN—After I bought a few enameled cast-iron pans, I instantly wanted to update all of my pots, pans, and skillets. Enameled cast iron is naturally nonstick, cooks very evenly, and cleans up easily. These pans are a little pricey, but worth every penny.

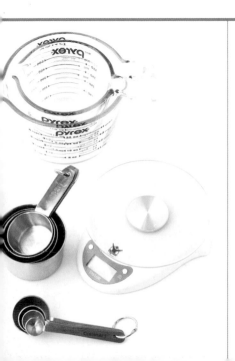

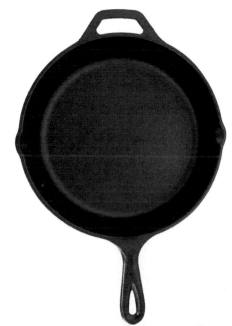

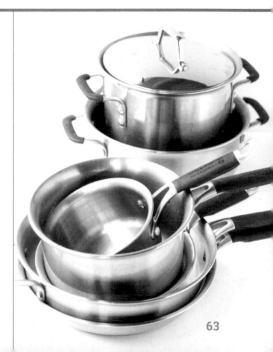

CAST-IRON SKILLET—I should probably change the name of my cast-iron skillet to frittata pan. While these skillets have endless uses, they are perfect for making deliciously fluffy, crisp-edged frittatas. They are ovenproof, making them great for cooking dishes that start on the stovetop and then are transferred to the oven. From getting the perfect crust on a hamburger patty to cooking up a deliciously juicy steak, there really isn't anything a good cast-iron pan can't do.

EGG PAN—This pan isn't a necessity, but it is how I make perfect eggs. I highly recommend investing in a good-quality egg pan. It will up your breakfast game. However, be wary of cheap, toxic nonstick pans.

SLOW COOKER—My favorite thing about slow cookers is that they are great for year-round use. They're perfect for those cold winter days when you want something warm and comforting and equally perfect for those hot summer days when you don't want to heat up the oven. Not to mention that they do all of the work for you.

BAKING SHEETS—A good set of baking sheets will easily outlive you. The sheets I have are from my very first apartment when I was a teenager. I use two types: rimmed baking sheets with about 1-inch sides, also known as "sheet pans," and cookie sheets, which are flat and have no sides. The sides of rimmed baking sheets prevent spillage, and they are great for cooking just about anything, from roasted vegetables to sheet pan meals to toasted nuts. I use cookie sheets for cookies and other foods that are not likely to produce juices and spill. If you have only rimmed baking sheets, don't let that stop you from making the cookie recipes in this book (see pages 314 and 322). Go ahead and use your rimmed baking sheets to make them.

SILICONE BAKEWARE—Silicone loaf pans and muffin pans have been a game-changer for me. You don't have to worry about food sticking to them, and they make food prep less messy and time-consuming. Cleanup is easy, and you don't have to use paper liners. These pans are soft-sided, though, so be sure to put them on top of a rimmed baking sheet to catch any spills.

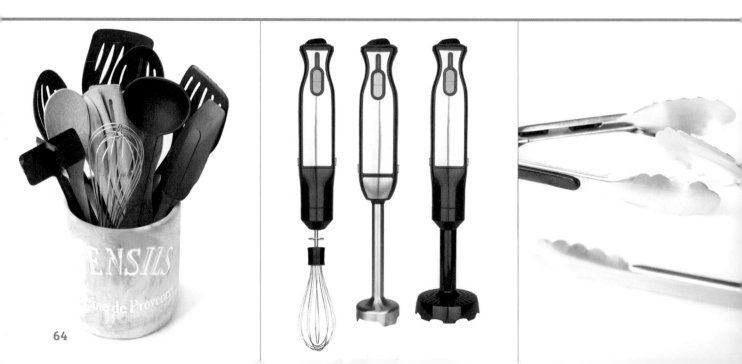

OTHER HANDY TOOLS

CUTTING BOARDS—In my kitchen, there never seem to be enough cutting boards. I am somewhat of a cutting board hoarder. Sometimes I even put cutting boards on top of cutting boards! Using separate cutting boards for different food groups is a great way to prevent cross-contamination and reduce the risk of food-borne illnesses.

FOOD PROCESSOR—Food processors are amazing for blending and chopping ingredients. Some of the larger ones even have multiple blades and can grate cheese, slice vegetables, whisk eggs, crush ice, and perform many other tasks. I have a large Magimix by Robot-Coupe, and I wouldn't trade it for the world.

GRATERS—I like to stock my kitchen with a few different types of graters. A four-sided box grater gives you the option to grate, shred, and slice. I keep a Microplane grater on hand for zesting fruits and grating fresh ginger, garlic, and onions. Then I like to have a smaller, single-blade handheld grater for use right over the pan while I cook.

HIGH-POWERED BLENDER—A good high-powered blender can be a lifesaver. I use mine for making pancake and waffle batter, pureeing soups and sauces, and even making my morning Boosted Coffee (page 140). Any gadget or appliance that serves multiple purposes is a winner in my book.

IMMERSION BLENDER—I am surprised by how many people I talk to who don't own an immersion blender (also called a stick blender or hand blender). In my opinion, this type of blender is worth its weight in gold. I use mine to make the perfect mayo every time (see page 336) and for pureeing soups and sauces. My kitchen wouldn't be complete without this tool.

KITCHEN SHEARS—My kitchen shears see a lot of action, from chopping fresh herbs to cutting crispy bacon into bits. If my tong hands ever fail (see "Tongs" on the next page), I'll replace them with kitchen shears.

KNIVES—When it comes to knives, you really do get what you pay for. A quality set of knives will last you a long time if you care for them properly. Although it might seem contrary to logic, more kitchen accidents occur from using dull knives than from using sharpened chef's knives.

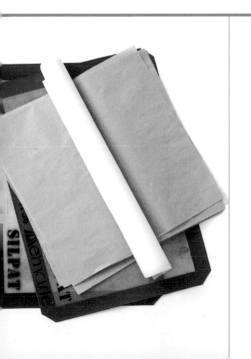
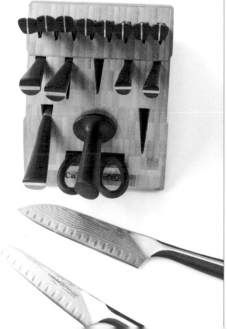
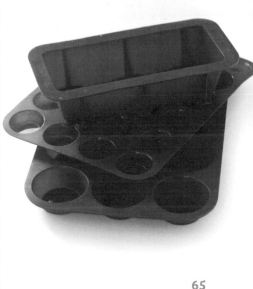

NESTED STAINLESS-STEEL MIXING BOWLS—
Stainless-steel mixing bowls are easy to clean and will last forever. I recommend getting a set that comes with lids so that you can prep foods and store them in the refrigerator without having to transfer them to another container.

RUBBER SPATULAS—Rubber spatulas are among the best multipurpose kitchen tools ever created. They come in a variety of sizes, and I like to keep a couple of each size on hand. These spatulas are perfect for getting those delicious browned bits off the bottom of the pan while deglazing and equally perfect for scraping out every last bit of homemade mayo from the jar.

SILICONE BAKING MAT AND PARCHMENT PAPER—I cook very few foods directly on a baking sheet. You will probably notice that as you go through the recipes in this book. Lining baking sheets with a silicone baking mat or parchment paper makes cleanup a breeze. Best of all, using a silicone mat is environmentally friendly and cost-effective. I've had the same one for years.

SPIRAL SLICER—The advent of the spiral slicer changed the low-carb landscape forever, putting noodles back on the menu in many different forms. My favorite tool for spiral-slicing vegetables is the Paderno World Cuisine 4-blade spiral slicer.

WIRE COOLING RACKS—These racks serve a dual purpose in my kitchen. The first one is obvious: cooling. But the second is perhaps my favorite. I like to place a rack on top of a rimmed baking sheet to raise the food I'm cooking up off of the baking sheet to help get crispy foods crispier. This setup is great for making sure that the undersides of breaded foods don't end up a soggy mess.

TONGS—After fifteen years in the restaurant industry, I often joke that if I were ever to lose a hand, I would want a pair of tongs instead of a prosthetic. From pulling bacon off of a sheet pan to flipping food on the grill, my tongs are always close by when I am in the kitchen. If you try to steal my bacon, I just might use them to pinch you.

WHISKS—A good set of whisks is an absolute must. Whisks are perfect for both wet and dry ingredients.

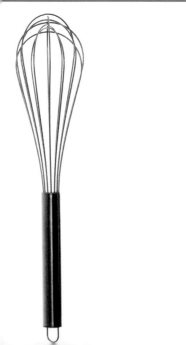
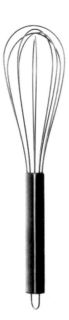
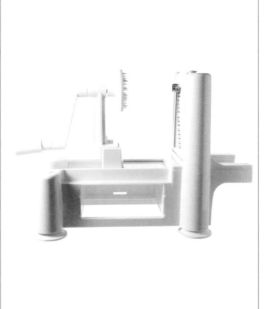
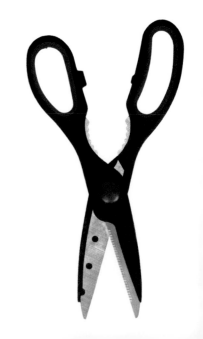

Tips for Measuring

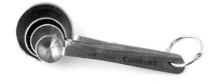

GENERAL MEASURING TIPS

- If you do not have two sets of measuring cups or spoons, one for wet and one for dry ingredients, measure the dry ingredients and then the liquid ingredients. It will save you time in between, as you won't have to dry the measuring cups in order to keep the dry ingredients from coating the cups.

- Never measure ingredients directly over the bowl. If you spill or overfill your measuring tool, you could ruin the entire recipe and be forced to start over.

- Do not mistake ounces for fluid ounces. Ounces are a unit of weight, and fluid ounces are a unit of volume.

- Precise measurements are crucial for baking recipes. Cooking is a little more forgiving.

- To keep track of which ingredients you have already added to your recipe, start by placing all of the ingredients on one side of the bowl. As you add them, move them to the other side of the bowl. This will help you remember where you are in the recipe if you get distracted.

TIPS FOR MEASURING LIQUIDS

- Make sure that the measuring cup is on a flat and stable surface.

- Most measuring cups do not measure small increments; therefore, measuring spoons should be used when a recipe calls for teaspoons or tablespoons of liquid.

- When using a larger measuring cup and filling it to a measurement line on the side, get down so that you are at eye level with the cup to make sure that it is filled just to the line.

- Fill liquid measuring cups and spoons to the rim for the most accurate measurement.

TIPS FOR MEASURING DRY INGREDIENTS

- When measuring dry ingredients, spoon the ingredient into the cup and then level it off with a knife or other flat-sided object.

- When using a measuring spoon, scoop the ingredient and then level it off.

- When a recipe calls for dry ingredients by weight, use a good-quality food scale (see page 63) to measure those ingredients.

- When using a scale, remember to tare the scale (zero it out) before measuring.

- Level the ingredient instead of packing it down in the measuring cup. Packing the ingredient changes the measurement. Do so only if a recipe calls for packing.

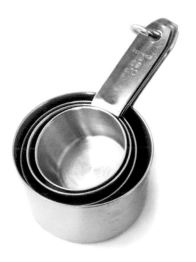

Meal Plans and Meal Prep

Meal planning has been a big part of my success. I am a firm believer that if you fail to plan, you plan to fail. Planning and prepping your meals in advance can mean the difference between having a healthy dinner and stopping for fast food on a busy weeknight.

There are five meal plans in the following pages to help you set you up for success. I've included a little something for every style of keto: Nut-Free, One-Pot, Dairy-Free, 30-Minute, and Egg-Free. Each of these plans is meant to feed four to six people and utilize leftovers throughout the week to help give you back some of that precious free time.

I know that meal prep can seem like a daunting task. People often ask, "How do I do it?" I always chuckle a little at this question because the answer is so simple. You just cook food. Plain and simple...cook food. It doesn't have to be harder than that. Cook food, portion it into single meals, and put them in your fridge and freezer. I realize that I may be simplifying things too much, but it really is that easy. If you don't have an entire day to spend cooking and portioning out meals, you can still do a little bit of food prep each day.

Here's what I do: I just cook more food. By that, I mean that if I would normally cook four servings of a meal, I double the recipe and make eight. Then I vacuum-seal the rest and put it in the freezer. I am already in the kitchen, putting in the work. Simply doubling the recipe requires no extra effort. Cook once, eat twice! Just a little tip that I hope will help you, especially if you find meal prep to be overwhelming. Just tackle it a little bit at a time. Before you know it, you will have a freezer full of ready-made meals.

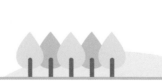

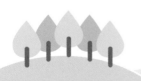

> **IF YOU DON'T HAVE A PLAN AND LEAVE YOUR FOOD CHOICES TO CHANCE, CHANCES ARE GOOD THAT THOSE CHOICES WILL STINK.**
> —*Unknown*

TIPS FOR MEAL PREP

One of the things that has helped me succeed in my own weight-loss journey is setting aside some time to prep food each week. I typically do it on Sunday mornings, except during football season, of course. I plan my meals for the week, spend the morning cooking, and then portion everything out and pack it into the fridge and freezer to eat throughout the week. Not having to worry about what I am going to eat makes those hectic weekdays so much easier and helps me stay on track with my health and fitness goals. It's just one less thing to deal with—not to mention that I have more quality time with my family in the evenings because I am not in the kitchen cooking every night.

If meal planning and leftovers aren't really your thing, you can still do a lot of prep work in advance. Setting aside time for simple tasks like cutting up vegetables, prepping salad ingredients, shredding cheese, making sauces and dressings, and hard-boiling eggs (see page 162) can cut down on the time you spend in the kitchen during the week.

Here are some of my tried-and-true meal prep tips:

- Set aside non-negotiable time each week for meal prep. Make a silent promise to yourself and your health that you keep week in and week out. Schedule this time as you would a job.

- Since we have already established how to do keto on a budget (see pages 56 to 60), let's apply some of that knowledge to food prep. If you score a great deal on fresh produce, for example, you can roast large batches of vegetables on a rimmed baking sheet, portion them into individual servings, and freeze them for reheating later. If you don't have the time to roast them all at once, you can portion them into individual freezer bags and add your cooking oil and seasonings right to the bags so that all you have to do is spread them on a rimmed baking sheet and roast them when you are ready to eat them.

- Overlapping ingredients across multiple recipes will save you time *and* money in the kitchen. If bell peppers are on sale this week, for example, cut them all down at the same time and prep recipes for the week that include bell peppers.

- Keep a stash of frozen organic vegetables on hand. They are perfect for quick and easy meals, and you don't have to worry about using them up as quickly as fresh vegetables. If you have some sort of ground meat and some vegetables in the freezer, you can whip up something pretty tasty at a moment's notice.

- Whenever possible, double the recipe. I apply this principle to just about everything I cook. If I am in between meal prep or just feel like cooking something different than what I have already prepped, I double the recipe and freeze the rest so that I am always building my stash of food in the freezer. This approach works great with freezer-friendly recipes like Fried Cabbage with Kielbasa (page 242) and Pork Egg Roll in a Bowl (page 228). Cook once and eat multiple times.

- Rice cauliflower and spiral-slice zucchini in large batches and freeze them. Then you will always have cauliflower rice and zoodles on hand for quick and easy meals, as the bulk of the time-consuming work is already done. See pages 76 to 79 for instructions.

- Invest in a good set of glass storage containers, a vacuum sealer, and various sizes of freezer bags.

- Don't forget about your slow cooker. If you don't have one, it is a worthwhile investment. Slow cookers are perfect for year-round cooking—great for those cold winter days when you want something warm and comforting, and equally perfect for hot summer days when you don't want to heat up the oven. You can cook large batches of food in them, and they do all of the work for you. What's not to love?

- Use a muffin pan to make individual-sized breakfasts like French Toast Egg Puffs (page 128). You can also bake a dish like the Cheesy Chorizo Breakfast Bake (page 102) in a muffin pan for single-serving portions for those busy work mornings. Muffin pans are also great for prepping individual-sized entrées, like meatloaf.

- Stock a mini salad bar. If you were to come to my house right now and open my vegetable drawer, you would see stacks of glass storage containers filled with salad toppings. I prep ingredients for quick salads throughout the week and line each container with a paper towel to absorb the excess moisture. Some of the ingredients I like to prep are bell peppers, cucumbers, mushrooms, olives, cheeses, meats, hard-boiled eggs (see the tips on page 162), and a variety of lettuces.

- Be sure to label and date everything that goes into your freezer. That way, you always know what you have on hand and how long it's been in there.

- When making your own low-carb snacks, portion them out into single-serving snack packs. This makes it easy to grab and go, and it will help keep you from overindulging.

- Buying rotisserie chickens from the grocery store can be a quick and easy way to do a little food prep for the week. You can portion out the chicken and pair it with a side dish, or you can use it in recipes that call for cooked chicken, like Dill Chicken Salad (page 194). You can usually get a great deal on rotisserie chickens, especially later in the evening when stores tend to put them on clearance.

- Batch-cook large quantities of meat on an outdoor grill. Then pair them with various side dishes and you are set for the week.

- Cook foods together whenever possible. Aside from the slow cooker, one of my favorite ways to cut down on time and messes is to throw together sheet pan meals. I throw my protein and vegetables on a rimmed baking sheet and cook them all together. Dinner doesn't get much easier than that! See page 248 for my Crispy Chicken Thigh and Vegetable Sheet Pan Dinner recipe.

- I usually whip up a couple of different marinades and then get some large chunks of chicken marinating in one and some large chunks of beef marinating in the other. I also prep some vegetables. Then I can combine the meat and veggies in no time to make kebabs for dinner—perfect for outdoor grilling or on a grill pan on the stovetop.

- Prep anything that you eat a lot of throughout the week. For me, it's eggs. I always have a stash of hard-boiled eggs in my fridge so that I can whip up some Creamy Avocado Pesto Deviled Eggs (page 162) or Deviled Ham and Egg Salad Lettuce Wraps (page 204).

NUT-FREE MEAL PLAN

	BREAKFAST	LUNCH	DINNER	SIDE, SOUP, OR SALAD	DESSERT OR SNACK
DAY 1	Baked Egg Jars — 108 — *4 servings*	Chef Salad Skewers — 202 — *4 servings*	Best-Ever Fork and Knife Pub Burger — 260 — *6 servings*	Roasted Cauliflower Mock Potato Salad — 192 — *6 servings*	Mason Jar Chocolate Ice Cream — 308 — *4 servings*
DAY 2	Pizza Eggs — 118 — *1 serving*	Dill Chicken Salad — 194 — *8 servings*	Steak Fajita Bowls — 210 — *6 servings*	Fiesta Cauliflower Rice — 282 — *6 servings*	Lemon Coconut Cheesecake Bites — 312 — *20 servings*
DAY 3	Baked Eggs with Chorizo and Ricotta — 106 — *6 servings*	Deviled Ham and Egg Salad Lettuce Wraps — 204 — *4 servings*	Beef Tips in Mushroom Brown Gravy — 262 — *6 servings*	Green Beans with Shallots and Pancetta — 276 — *6 servings*	Garlic Dill Baked Cucumber Chips — 158 — *6 servings*
DAY 4	13 Jon's Special — 110 — *6 servings*	Cheesy Ham and Cauliflower Soup — 186 — *20 servings*	Fried Cabbage with Kielbasa — 242 — *6 servings*	Dill Pickle Coleslaw — 280 — *6 servings*	Chocolate Chip Cookie Dough Bites — 320 — *8 servings*
DAY 5	Lemon Ricotta Pancakes — 124 — *8 servings*	Shrimp and Cheesy Cauliflower Rice Stuffed Peppers — 220 — *4 servings*	Spaghetti Squash Pork Lo Mein — 214 — *8 servings*	Charred Asian Asparagus and Peppers — 290 — *4 servings*	Dark Chocolate Mousse — 304 — *4 servings*
DAY 6	Reuben Frittata — 114 — *8 servings*	Cheesy Ham and Cauliflower Soup — 186 — *Leftover*	Crispy Chicken Thigh and Vegetable Sheet Pan Dinner — 248 — *4 servings*	Dill Pickle Coleslaw — 280 — *Leftover*	Garlic Dill Baked Cucumber Chips — 158 — *Leftover*
DAY 7	Lemon Ricotta Pancakes — 124 — *Leftover*	Shaved Brussels Sprouts Caesar Salad — 191 — *4 servings*	Sausage, Shrimp, and Chicken Jambalaya — 224 — *8 servings*	Creamy Cucumber Salad — 195 — *8 servings*	Lemon Coconut Cheesecake Bites — 312 — *Leftover*

ONE-POT MEAL PLAN

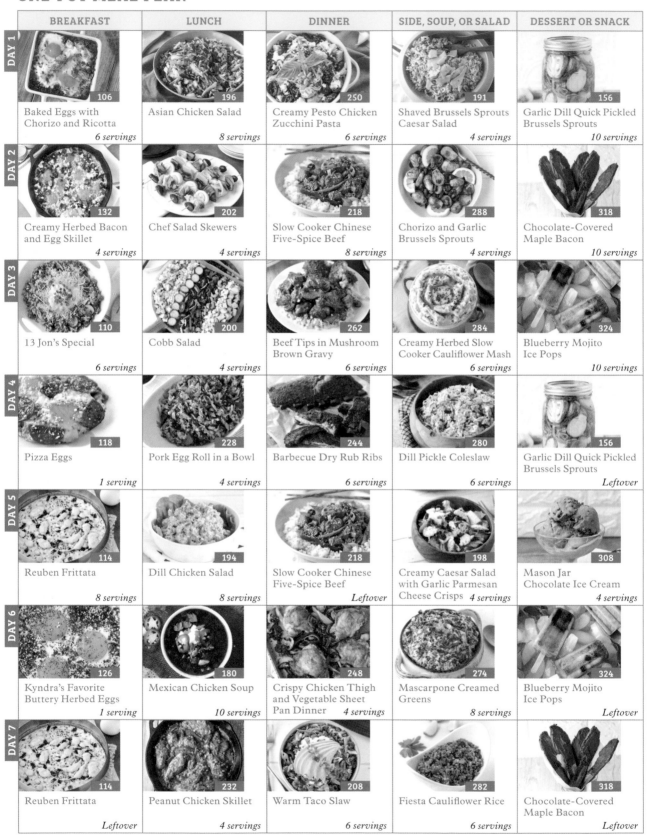

	BREAKFAST	LUNCH	DINNER	SIDE, SOUP, OR SALAD	DESSERT OR SNACK
DAY 1	Baked Eggs with Chorizo and Ricotta — 106 — *6 servings*	Asian Chicken Salad — 196 — *8 servings*	Creamy Pesto Chicken Zucchini Pasta — 250 — *6 servings*	Shaved Brussels Sprouts Caesar Salad — 191 — *4 servings*	Garlic Dill Quick Pickled Brussels Sprouts — 156 — *10 servings*
DAY 2	Creamy Herbed Bacon and Egg Skillet — 132 — *4 servings*	Chef Salad Skewers — 202 — *4 servings*	Slow Cooker Chinese Five-Spice Beef — 218 — *8 servings*	Chorizo and Garlic Brussels Sprouts — 288 — *4 servings*	Chocolate-Covered Maple Bacon — 318 — *10 servings*
DAY 3	13 Jon's Special — 110 — *6 servings*	Cobb Salad — 200 — *4 servings*	Beef Tips in Mushroom Brown Gravy — 262 — *6 servings*	Creamy Herbed Slow Cooker Cauliflower Mash — 284 — *6 servings*	Blueberry Mojito Ice Pops — 324 — *10 servings*
DAY 4	Pizza Eggs — 118 — *1 serving*	Pork Egg Roll in a Bowl — 228 — *4 servings*	Barbecue Dry Rub Ribs — 244 — *6 servings*	Dill Pickle Coleslaw — 280 — *6 servings*	Garlic Dill Quick Pickled Brussels Sprouts — 156 — *Leftover*
DAY 5	Reuben Frittata — 114 — *8 servings*	Dill Chicken Salad — 194 — *8 servings*	Slow Cooker Chinese Five-Spice Beef — 218 — *Leftover*	Creamy Caesar Salad with Garlic Parmesan Cheese Crisps — 198 — *4 servings*	Mason Jar Chocolate Ice Cream — 308 — *4 servings*
DAY 6	Kyndra's Favorite Buttery Herbed Eggs — 126 — *1 serving*	Mexican Chicken Soup — 180 — *10 servings*	Crispy Chicken Thigh and Vegetable Sheet Pan Dinner — 248 — *4 servings*	Mascarpone Creamed Greens — 274 — *8 servings*	Blueberry Mojito Ice Pops — 324 — *Leftover*
DAY 7	Reuben Frittata — 114 — *Leftover*	Peanut Chicken Skillet — 232 — *4 servings*	Warm Taco Slaw — 208 — *6 servings*	Fiesta Cauliflower Rice — 282 — *6 servings*	Chocolate-Covered Maple Bacon — 318 — *Leftover*

DAIRY-FREE MEAL PLAN

BREAKFAST	LUNCH	DINNER	SIDE, SOUP, OR SALAD	DESSERT OR SNACK	
138 Chocolate Peanut Butter Waffles *6 servings*	194 Dill Chicken Salad *8 servings*	268 Asian Beef Skewers *6 servings*	278 Ginger Lime Slaw *6 servings*	326 Almond Joy Chia Seed Pudding *4 servings*	DAY 1
126 Kyndra's Favorite Buttery Herbed Eggs *1 serving*	180 Mexican Chicken Soup *10 servings*	248 Crispy Chicken Thigh and Vegetable Sheet Pan Dinner *4 servings*	192 Roasted Cauliflower Mock Potato Salad *6 servings*	158 Garlic Dill Baked Cucumber Chips *6 servings*	DAY 2
117 Pastrami Breakfast Hash *4 servings*	204 Deviled Ham and Egg Salad Lettuce Wraps *4 servings*	246 Dill Pickle Juice Brined Fish and Chips *4 servings*	280 Dill Pickle Coleslaw *6 servings*	318 Chocolate-Covered Maple Bacon *10 servings*	DAY 3
122 Oven-Roasted Garlic and Herb Home Fries *6 servings*	228 Pork Egg Roll in a Bowl *4 servings*	244 Barbecue Dry Rub Ribs *6 servings*	272 Oven-Roasted Cabbage Wedges with Dijon Bacon Vinaigrette *8 servings*	324 Blueberry Mojito Ice Pops *10 servings*	DAY 4
116 Radishes O'Brien *6 servings*	196 Asian Chicken Salad *8 servings*	242 Fried Cabbage with Kielbasa *8 servings*	276 Green Beans with Shallots and Pancetta *6 servings*	322 Chewy Peanut Butter Cookies *18 servings*	DAY 5
112 Sausage and Egg Breakfast Sandwich *1 serving*	202 Chef Salad Skewers *4 servings*	218 Slow Cooker Chinese Five-Spice Beef *8 servings*	184 Egg Drop Soup *6 servings*	152 Sour Lemon Gummy Snacks *11 servings*	DAY 6
118 Pizza Eggs *1 serving*	148 Tuna Salad Pickle Boats *5 servings*	210 Steak Fajita Bowls *6 servings*	282 Fiesta Cauliflower Rice *6 servings*	302 Salted Caramel Nut Brittle *10 servings*	DAY 7

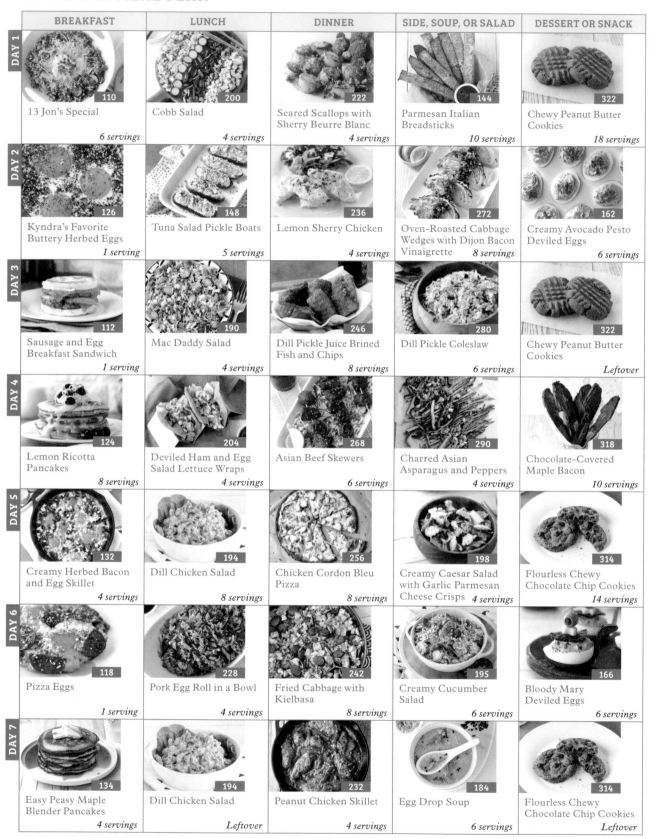

	BREAKFAST	LUNCH	DINNER	SIDE, SOUP, OR SALAD	DESSERT OR SNACK
DAY 1	13 Jon's Special — *110* 6 servings	Cobb Salad — *200* 4 servings	Seared Scallops with Sherry Beurre Blanc — *222* 4 servings	Parmesan Italian Breadsticks — *144* 10 servings	Chewy Peanut Butter Cookies — *322* 18 servings
DAY 2	Kyndra's Favorite Buttery Herbed Eggs — *126* 1 serving	Tuna Salad Pickle Boats — *148* 5 servings	Lemon Sherry Chicken — *236* 4 servings	Oven-Roasted Cabbage Wedges with Dijon Bacon Vinaigrette — *272* 8 servings	Creamy Avocado Pesto Deviled Eggs — *162* 6 servings
DAY 3	Sausage and Egg Breakfast Sandwich — *112* 1 serving	Mac Daddy Salad — *190* 4 servings	Dill Pickle Juice Brined Fish and Chips — *246* 8 servings	Dill Pickle Coleslaw — *280* 6 servings	Chewy Peanut Butter Cookies — *322* Leftover
DAY 4	Lemon Ricotta Pancakes — *124* 8 servings	Deviled Ham and Egg Salad Lettuce Wraps — *204* 4 servings	Asian Beef Skewers — *268* 6 servings	Charred Asian Asparagus and Peppers — *290* 4 servings	Chocolate-Covered Maple Bacon — *318* 10 servings
DAY 5	Creamy Herbed Bacon and Egg Skillet — *132* 4 servings	Dill Chicken Salad — *194* 8 servings	Chicken Cordon Bleu Pizza — *256* 8 servings	Creamy Caesar Salad with Garlic Parmesan Cheese Crisps — *198* 4 servings	Flourless Chewy Chocolate Chip Cookies — *314* 14 servings
DAY 6	Pizza Eggs — *118* 1 serving	Pork Egg Roll in a Bowl — *228* 4 servings	Fried Cabbage with Kielbasa — *242* 8 servings	Creamy Cucumber Salad — *195* 6 servings	Bloody Mary Deviled Eggs — *166* 6 servings
DAY 7	Easy Peasy Maple Blender Pancakes — *134* 4 servings	Dill Chicken Salad — *194* Leftover	Peanut Chicken Skillet — *232* 4 servings	Egg Drop Soup — *184* 6 servings	Flourless Chewy Chocolate Chip Cookies — *314* Leftover

EGG-FREE MEAL PLAN

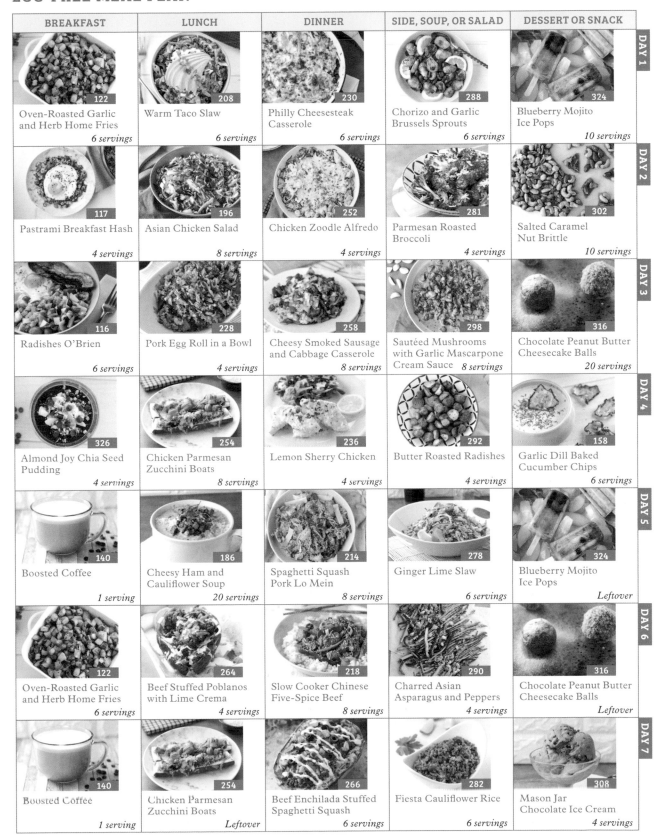

BREAKFAST	LUNCH	DINNER	SIDE, SOUP, OR SALAD	DESSERT OR SNACK	
122 Oven-Roasted Garlic and Herb Home Fries *6 servings*	**208** Warm Taco Slaw *6 servings*	**230** Philly Cheesesteak Casserole *6 servings*	**288** Chorizo and Garlic Brussels Sprouts *6 servings*	**324** Blueberry Mojito Ice Pops *10 servings*	DAY 1
117 Pastrami Breakfast Hash *4 servings*	**196** Asian Chicken Salad *8 servings*	**252** Chicken Zoodle Alfredo *4 servings*	**281** Parmesan Roasted Broccoli *4 servings*	**302** Salted Caramel Nut Brittle *10 servings*	DAY 2
116 Radishes O'Brien *6 servings*	**228** Pork Egg Roll in a Bowl *4 servings*	**258** Cheesy Smoked Sausage and Cabbage Casserole *8 servings*	**298** Sautéed Mushrooms with Garlic Mascarpone Cream Sauce *8 servings*	**316** Chocolate Peanut Butter Cheesecake Balls *20 servings*	DAY 3
326 Almond Joy Chia Seed Pudding *4 servings*	**254** Chicken Parmesan Zucchini Boats *8 servings*	**236** Lemon Sherry Chicken *4 servings*	**292** Butter Roasted Radishes *4 servings*	**158** Garlic Dill Baked Cucumber Chips *6 servings*	DAY 4
140 Boosted Coffee *1 serving*	**186** Cheesy Ham and Cauliflower Soup *20 servings*	**214** Spaghetti Squash Pork Lo Mein *8 servings*	**278** Ginger Lime Slaw *6 servings*	**324** Blueberry Mojito Ice Pops *Leftover*	DAY 5
122 Oven-Roasted Garlic and Herb Home Fries *6 servings*	**264** Beef Stuffed Poblanos with Lime Crema *4 servings*	**218** Slow Cooker Chinese Five-Spice Beef *8 servings*	**290** Charred Asian Asparagus and Peppers *4 servings*	**316** Chocolate Peanut Butter Cheesecake Balls *Leftover*	DAY 6
140 Boosted Coffee *1 serving*	**254** Chicken Parmesan Zucchini Boats *Leftover*	**266** Beef Enchilada Stuffed Spaghetti Squash *6 servings*	**282** Fiesta Cauliflower Rice *6 servings*	**308** Mason Jar Chocolate Ice Cream *4 servings*	DAY 7

Techniques for Making Low-Carb Rice and Noodles

As I mentioned earlier in the section "Tips for Meal Prep" (pages 69 and 70), I like to keep large batches of riced cauliflower and zucchini noodles on hand for quick and easy meals. They are used in the meal plans in recipes such as Slow Cooker Chinese Five-Spice Beef (page 218) and Chicken Zoodle Alfredo (page 252), and they can serve as a base for so many other dishes.

HOW TO MAKE RICED CAULIFLOWER

There are a couple of different ways to make your own cauliflower rice. Both are simple and require minimal effort and kitchen tools that you likely already have.

Start by removing the leaves from the head of cauliflower.

To rice cauliflower using a food processor, core the cauliflower and cut it into florets; discard the core. Place the florets in the food processor and pulse until the cauliflower is in rice-sized pieces.

To rice cauliflower using a box grater, leave the head of cauliflower whole and grate the florets on the largest holes of the box grater. Discard the core.

A large head of cauliflower should yield approximately 4 cups of riced cauliflower. If you are not going to use it right away, store it in the refrigerator for up to 3 days. Alternatively, you can freeze riced cauliflower for later use.

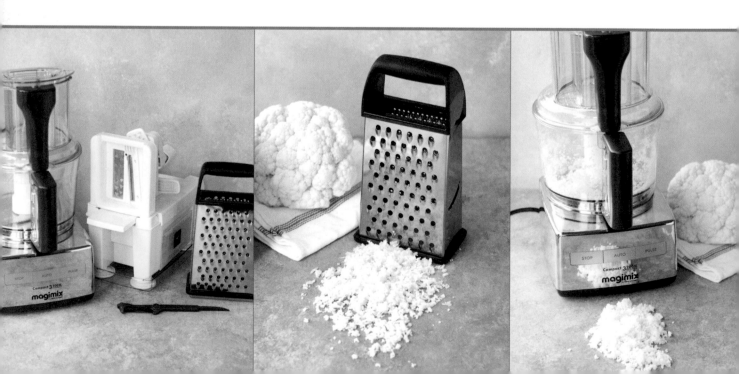

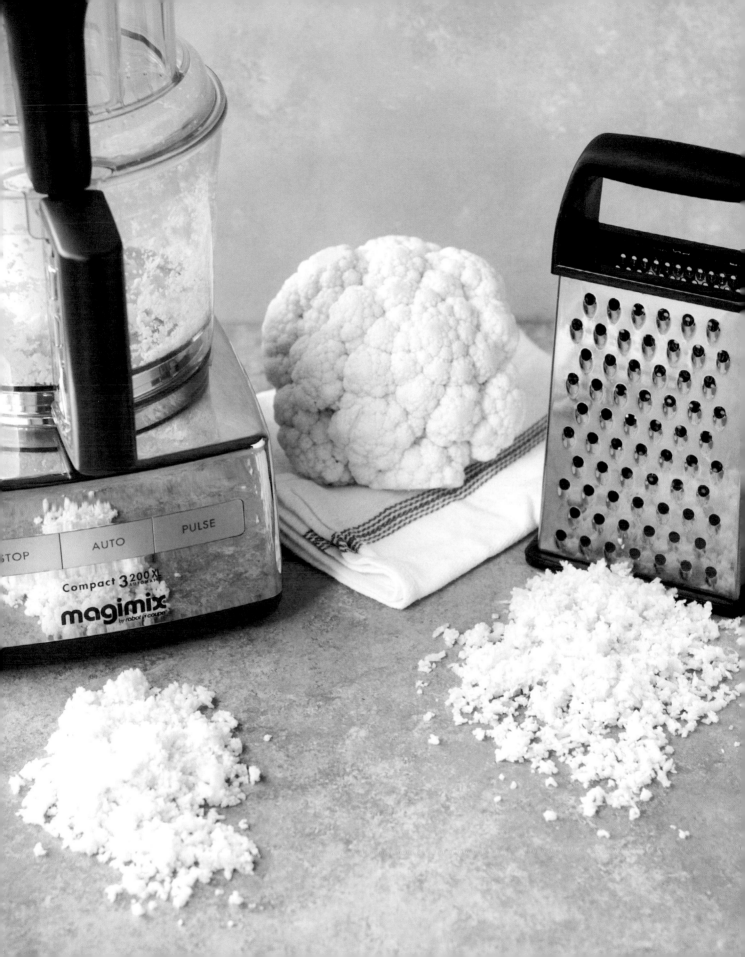

HOW TO MAKE ZUCCHINI/VEGETABLE NOODLES

There are a few different ways to achieve perfect zucchini noodles. As I mentioned in "My Favorite Kitchen Tools and Gadgets" (see page 66), my favorite way to spiral-slice zucchini and other vegetables is with the Paderno World Cuisine 4-blade spiral slicer. It is easy to use and makes noodles in four different shapes and sizes. But you don't have to have a spiral slicer to make zucchini noodles at home. A box grater or julienne vegetable peeler will also work.

One 8- to 10-inch-long zucchini typically yields 1 to 2 servings of noodles, depending on whether you are making an entrée or a side dish. If you are not using the noodles right away, store them in the refrigerator for up to 3 days. Alternatively, you can freeze the noodles for later use.

Start by slicing off the ends of the zucchini or other vegetable. For each of the methods described below, depending on your preference, you can peel the zucchini or leave the skin on. I prefer to leave the skin on, as it helps the noodles hold up to the heat while cooking.

To make zucchini noodles with a spiral slicer, spiral-slice the zucchini according to the directions provided with your spiral slicer.

To make zucchini noodles using a julienne vegetable peeler—a cost-effective and safe way to make zucchini noodles at home—scrape the peeler lengthwise down the zucchini, producing long noodlelike slices.

To make zucchini noodles using a box grater, grate the zucchini on the largest holes of the box grater.

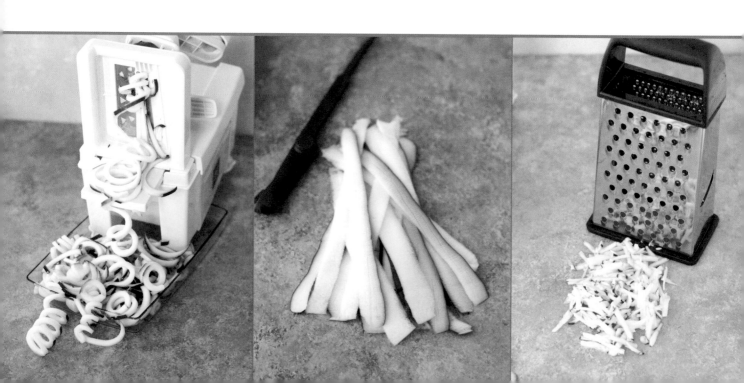

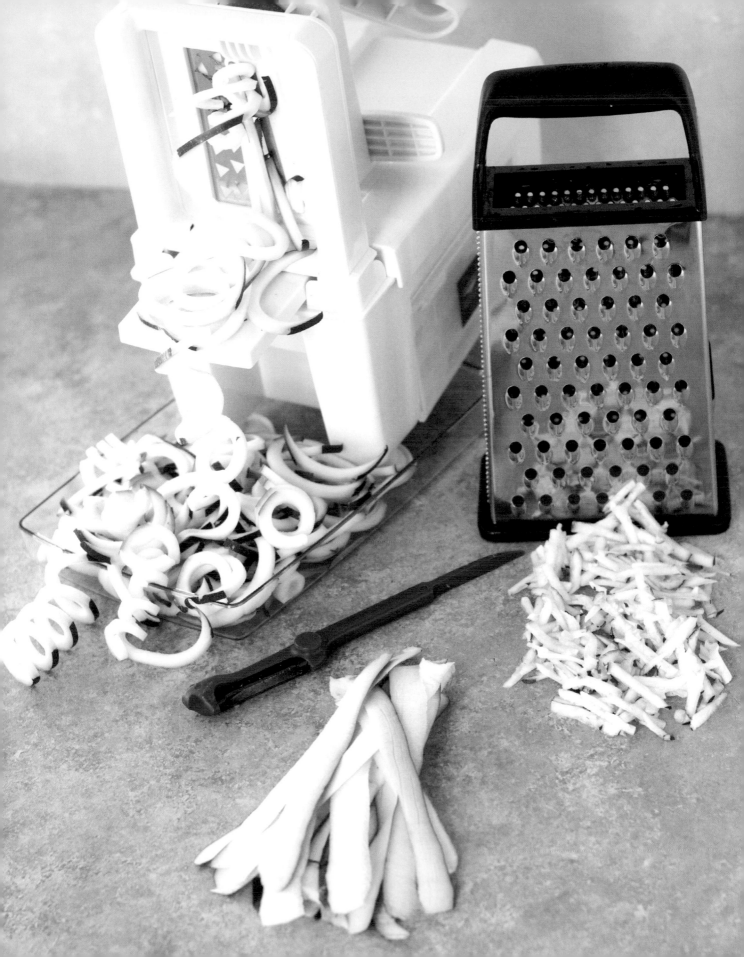

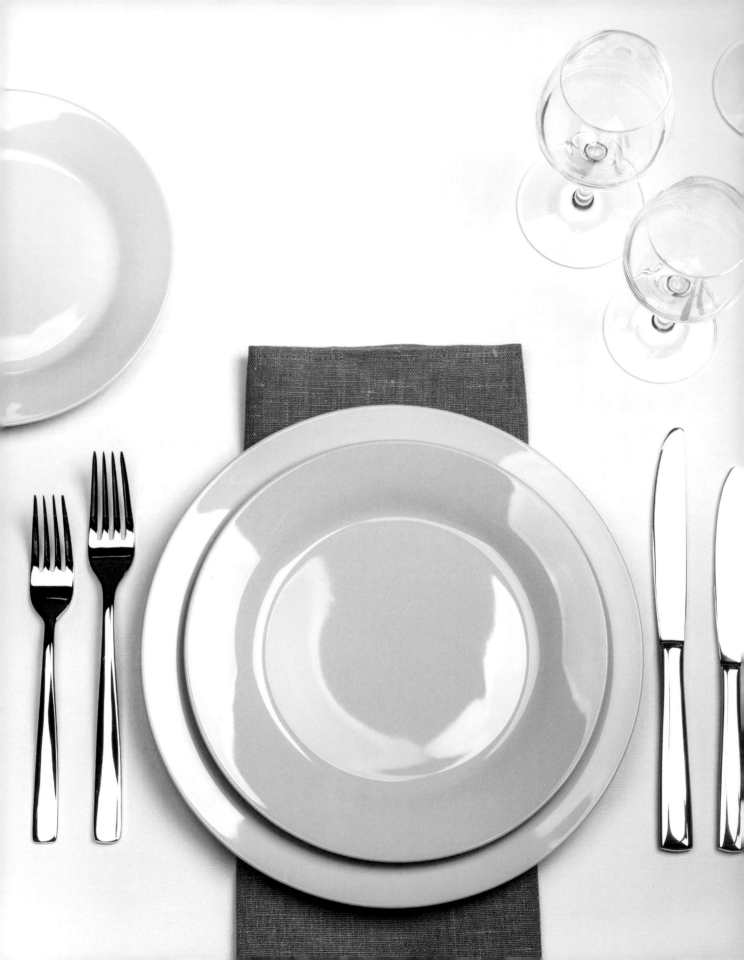

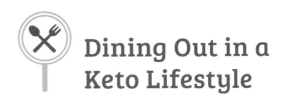

Dining Out in a Keto Lifestyle

With a few simple rules, you will be able to confidently navigate any restaurant menu and make selections that fit your low-carb lifestyle.

Many people come to feel that in order to maintain their lifestyle choices, dining out is off the table. Well, I can tell you firsthand that it isn't. I worked in restaurants for more than fifteen years. The options are there; you just have to ask for them. More often than not, the answer lies off the menu.

PLANNING IS PARAMOUNT

Look up the restaurant menu online and decide what you are going to order before you get there. Then you don't even have to open the menu and tempt yourself with dishes you know you shouldn't have.

Call the restaurant ahead of time with any questions you might have.

Look for nutritional information online. Many larger chain restaurants post that information on their websites.

It's definitely not as fun, but if you are certain that there just won't be anything you can eat, eat before you go so that you won't be tempted to order something you might regret later.

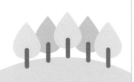

One of the delights of life is eating with friends; second to that is talking about eating. And, for an unsurpassed double whammy, there is talking about eating while you are eating with friends.

—*Laurie Colwin*

SKIP THE STARCH

- ✓ **PASS ON THE POTATOES.**
- ✓ **REFUSE THE RICE.**
- ✓ **BAG THE BREAD.**
- ✓ **FORGO THE FRIES.**
- ✓ **PURGE THE PASTA.**
- ✓ **GOODBYE TO GRAINS.**
- ✓ **SUB THE SIDES.**

Before they even have a chance to bring it, politely decline the bread. It is a lot harder to say no to the bread basket when it's already in front of you.

If you are strictly gluten-free, ask for a gluten-free menu. Many restaurants offer them even if they don't advertise them.

Most restaurant entrées are served with a starchy side. Avoid temptation by asking for a different side when ordering. Don't be afraid to ask for what you want. It may not be on the menu, but that doesn't mean the restaurant doesn't have it or won't make it.

Here are some things you can ask for instead of a starchy side:

✓ a side salad

✓ extra vegetables

✓ a cup of soup (be sure to ask for a complete list of ingredients)

Instead of sandwich bread or a hamburger bun, ask for your sandwich or burger to be wrapped in lettuce. Alternatively, ask if you can get your sandwich toppings as a salad. If the kitchen isn't willing to accommodate your request, simply ask for no bread or bun.

Anything fried is going to be a no-go. Unfortunately, most restaurants haven't yet caught on to the creative ways we low-carbers bread our food. Don't be afraid to ask for grilled, baked, or sautéed items in place of fried foods. If a salad comes with breaded and fried chicken, ask to substitute a grilled chicken breast. If an entrée comes with fried shrimp, ask if you can have sautéed or grilled shrimp instead.

If you see a pasta dish you like and it has a low-carb–friendly sauce (I will talk more about sauces here in a minute), ask if you can get everything in the dish, minus the noodles, over a side of vegetables instead.

Finally, who says you have to order a main course? You can make your own sampler platter from the appetizer menu. Get a couple of different small bites and make a meal out of them. There are quite a few low-carb appetizers available on most restaurant menus: bacon-wrapped prawns, stuffed mushrooms, spinach and artichoke dip, wings, and antipasto, just to name a few. As always, be sure to ask about any ingredients you might not recognize. The appetizers I just listed are not guaranteed to be low-carb and gluten-free at every restaurant.

Speaking of appetizers, be careful when ordering chicken wings. Don't assume that they are naturally low-carb and gluten-free. Many restaurants coat their wings in flour or cornstarch to help them get nice and crispy when fried. Don't be afraid to ask questions. You are spending your hard-earned money and treating yourself to a meal out, and you should get exactly what you want. I say this having spent many years on the other side of the dining situation. Even during the busiest shifts, we were always accommodating of food substitution requests. Just don't get crazy and ask for a steak in place of a parsley garnish! (Yes, that actually happened to me once.) Leaving a generous tip for an accommodating server always helps, too.

CHANNEL YOUR CREATIVITY

Don't be afraid to go off-menu. If you don't see something that fits your needs, ask if you can create it. Keep in mind that there are reasonable requests, and then there are requests that are a little too over the top for a busy restaurant.

Here are some ideas to help you create your own dishes:

✓ Pick a protein that you see on the menu and pair it with a side of vegetables or a salad.

✓ Get a salad and add chicken, steak, salmon, or some other protein.

✓ Add healthy fats to your meal, like avocado, olive oil, nuts, and seeds.

✓ As previously mentioned, order from the appetizer menu and pick two or three items to make your own meal.

SAY "SEE YA" TO SUGAR

Skip the soda. Decline the dessert.

I realize that for some people, drinking soda can be a really hard habit to break. Learning to decline it when dining out is not only good for your waistline, but good for your wallet as well.

Let your server know in advance that you aren't interested in dessert, either. If you see a dessert tray floating around, make it known that you don't need to see it.

Many restaurants offer a cheese plate for dessert. If you are truly still hungry, order the cheese plate and a small amount of mixed fresh berries, if available.

CAREFUL WITH CONDIMENTS AND DITCH THE DRESSINGS

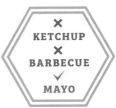

Kick the ketchup. Banish the barbecue. Mix up mayo.

Unfortunately, condiments such as ketchup and barbecue sauce are loaded with sugar, making them poor options at any restaurant.

Mustard and mayonnaise are typically safe choices anywhere you dine. I like to get creative and mix up my own sauces using mayonnaise. Try adding a little hot sauce or Worcestershire sauce to a side of mayo to kick it up a notch.

A good general rule for salad dressings is to ask for dressings on the side if you aren't sure whether they are low-carb. Ranch, blue cheese, and Caesar dressings are typically safe in small amounts, while dressings like Thousand Island, honey mustard, and French are typically a no-go because of their sugar content. Vinaigrettes are usually a great option as long as they do not have a sweet component to them. That sweet component is almost always some form of added sugar.

While not everyone is comfortable doing so, I am definitely a girl who will pull my own dressing out of my purse at a restaurant. My health is more important to me than what a complete stranger might think of me.

SIDELINE THE SAUCES

✓ **ADIOS TO ALFREDO.**

✓ **BRING ON THE BÉARNAISE.**

✓ **PAUSE FOR PAN SAUCE.**

✓ **GIVE UP GRAVIES.**

✓ **TAME THE TOMATO.**

While Alfredo sauce may seem like a no-brainer, in most restaurants the Alfredo sauces are flour-based, making them neither low-carb nor gluten-free.

Rich, buttery sauces like hollandaise and béarnaise are always a safe bet if they are made from scratch. When made from scratch, their main ingredients are butter, egg yolks, and lemon juice. When made from a powdered mix, however, they end up being higher in carbs and not gluten-free. Before ordering, be sure to ask the server if these sauces are made fresh in house.

Pan sauces require a little more digging. Sometimes they are just the rendered juices from the meat with a little stock, butter, and seasonings thrown in. If this is the case, then by all means indulge. However, if the sauce is a thicker sauce, there is a chance that flour was added during cooking to thicken it. Again, it is a matter of asking the right questions.

I have yet to see a gravy in a restaurant that is low-carb or gluten-free. Restaurant gravies are always thickened with some sort of flour. However, it never hurts to ask. I certainly haven't eaten at every restaurant in the world (although I would really love to).

Tomato sauces are usually a fine option, but in smaller portions, as tomatoes have a higher carb count than some of the other low-carb fruits and vegetables (see page 44). Just make sure that the tomato sauce doesn't have any added sugars or sweeteners and is made with only fresh vegetables, meats, and spices.

TAKE YOUR TIME AND ENJOY THE EXPERIENCE

Don't rush through your meal. If you give your stomach time to catch up with your mouth, you will feel sated sooner and not eat past the point of being full. Eating slowly also gives you more time to visit with your dining companions.

Dining out with friends and family should be fun. While it is important to make good choices that suit your lifestyle, you don't want it to come at the expense of having a good time with the people who matter most. You should eat to live, not live to eat. When you become a slave to your food choices, healthy eating stops being fun and stops being sustainable long term.

Dining In in a Keto Lifestyle

By nature, people love to dine together. There is something so intimate about sharing a meal. It is one of the most primal things you can do with another human. It is a time to gather, connect, discuss, and nourish. Some of my favorite memories took place around a table with good food and good friends. But sometimes when you embark on a new way of eating, this magical moment of connection can start to turn into a source of fear, anxiety, and isolation. "What if there is nothing there I can eat?" "What if they don't understand the way I eat?" "What if they mock my food choices?"

Here are some quick tips to help ease the anxiety of hosting or attending a dinner party:

✓ Make it a potluck. If everyone brings a dish to pass, there is sure to be something you can eat—even if it is only the dish you brought.

✓ Give the party a theme. Then you can make it a theme that naturally lends itself to low-carb dishes. Think grilling, surf-and-turf, meat and vegetables, kebabs, and so on.

✓ Don't be afraid to tell people how you eat. Give them a chance to surprise you. I'm sure that they will be far more accommodating and understanding than you give them credit for.

✓ Ask questions. Then ask more questions. It's okay to want to know exactly what is in the food you are eating. No one will be offended if you ask, I promise.

✓ Host the get-together yourself so that you are in control of the food selections.

✓ Label the food at the party with the name of the dish and its ingredients, and suggest that others do the same. That way, you have a good idea of the carb count of each dish and whether it is a dish you can eat.

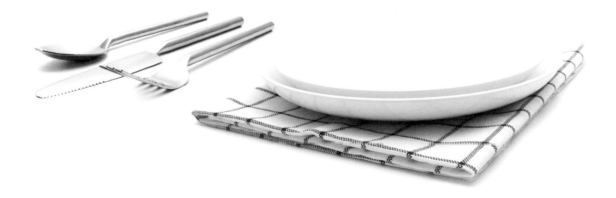

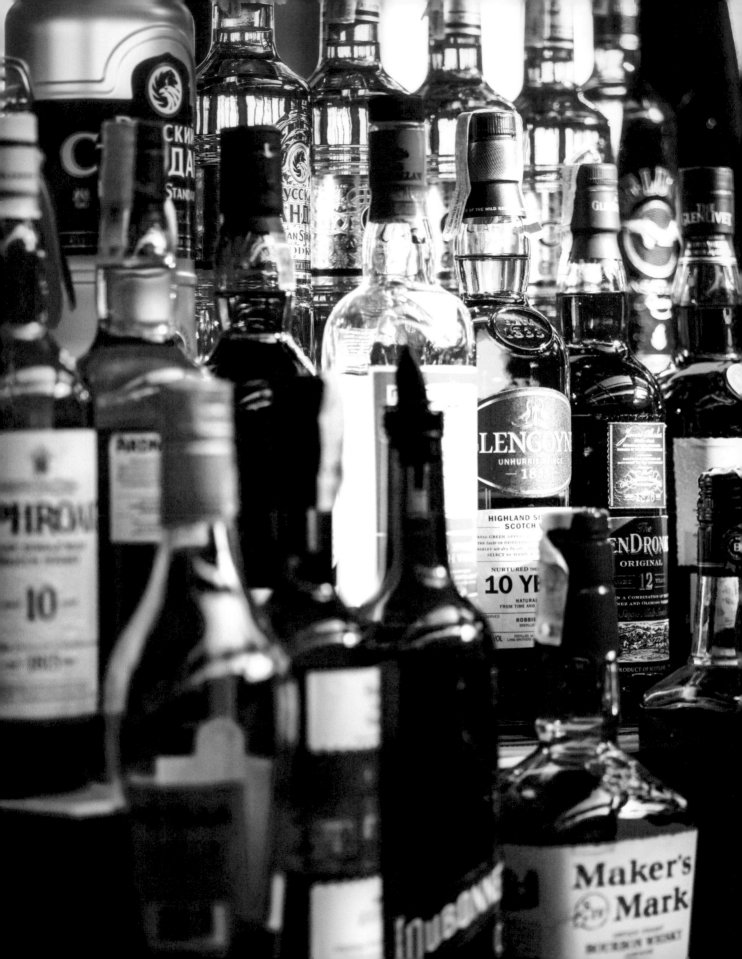

Navigating Alcohol on a Low-Carb Diet

So it's Friday night and you're feeling all right. You're ready to dance the night away with a cocktail in your hand. Or, if you are more like me, you want to have a cocktail at home with friends. You might be saying to yourself, "But wait! I can't! I'm low-carb!" You are *not* low-carb. You are a person following a low-carb lifestyle. Do not be defined by your dietary decisions. Doing so will lead to a life of restriction, and feeling restricted often causes us to stray from our intended path.

If you want a drink, have a drink, but be smart about it. Don't go overboard, and be sure to make the best choices possible. If you put the same conscious effort into your drink choices as you do into your food choices, you can enjoy that evening cocktail without derailing your weight-loss, health, and fitness goals.

Alcohol on a low-carb ketogenic lifestyle can seem like a real no-go. I've read countless articles on the subject, and there are strong cases made on both sides. Ultimately, it boils down to a matter of personal preference. If it works for you, great. If it doesn't work for you, that's fine, too.

But my goal throughout this book is to give you as many tools as possible to help you achieve your goals. Sometimes figuring out exactly what works for your body is more a matter of trial-and-error than a matter of science. There is no one-size-fits-all approach to life, and there is no one-size-fits-all approach to keto.

As you review this guide, please note that nutritional information can vary from brand to brand. However, these are great general guidelines to follow.

LIQUOR

Not all liquors are gluten-free. Refer to each brand individually to obtain product-specific information.

LIQUOR (UNFLAVORED)	Carb Count in 1½ Fluid Ounces
Vodka	0 g
Gin	0 g
Rum	0 g
Dark rum	0 g
Tequila	0 g
Whiskey/Bourbon	0 to 0.3 g (varies by brand)
Spiced rum	0.5 g
Brandy	0 to 3 g (varies by brand)

SPIKED SELTZER WATER	Carb Count in a 12-Fluid-Ounce Can
Truly Spiked and Sparkling	2 g
White Claw	4 g
Spiked Seltzer	5 g

tips.

- Drink in moderation. Overconsumption of alcohol often leads to poor food choices.

- Don't be afraid to ask questions. Talk to your server. Talk to the bartender. Research anything you are unsure of. Not to sound cliché, but the only stupid questions are the ones that go unasked.

- Be in control of your environment. If going out for drinks leads to poor food and drink choices, plan to indulge only at home.

- Be sure to drink a lot of water while drinking alcohol. Alcohol is dehydrating, which can lead to a hangover the next day.

- Don't be afraid to say no! I can't stress this point enough. It can be really easy to cave to peer pressure if the people around you are less than supportive of your lifestyle. Don't hesitate to simply say no and move on.

MIXERS

ACCEPTABLE MIXERS

Plain sparkling water

Naturally flavored sparkling water

Citrus essential oil–infused water

Zevia colas and naturally flavored sodas

Unsweetened cranberry juice

Sugar-free bitters

Kombucha

Flavored stevia drops

DRINK GARNISHES AND FLAVOR ENHANCERS

Citrus essential oils

Fresh fruit slices

Fresh herbs

Fruit extracts

Powdered erythritol

MIXERS TO AVOID

The complete list of mixers to avoid would be really long. Here are some of the main ones to watch for, especially when you are out for a night on the town:

- Daiquiri mix
- Grenadine
- Margarita mix
- Piña colada mix
- Pop
- Simple syrup
- Sweet-and-sour mix
- Triple sec

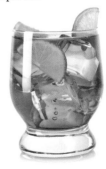
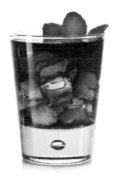

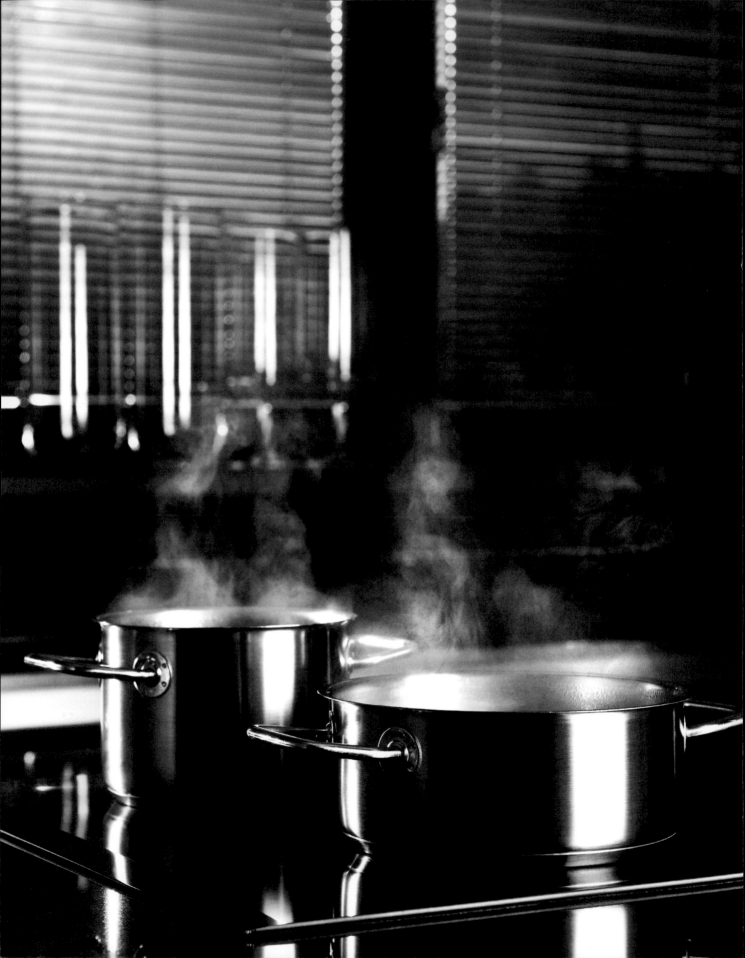

Cooking Terms Defined

Al dente: An Italian term meaning "to the tooth," usually used to describe pasta that is cooked until it is just firm and offers a slight resistance when you bite into it. This term typically refers to pasta, but in the low-carb world, it can also be applied to low-carb replacements for pasta, like zucchini noodles.

Bake: To cook food in an oven, surrounded by dry heat. Often referred to as *roasting* when applied to meat, poultry, or vegetables and done at a higher temperature.

Barbecue: See *Grill*.

Bard: To secure an additional type of fat, such as bacon, around a food to prevent it from drying out during dry-heat cooking. This is a great option for really lean meats, not only for flavor but also to boost the ketogenic value of the meat by adding more healthy fat.

Baste: To repeatedly spoon a liquid such as pan drippings, stock, or butter over food to moisten it during cooking.

Batter: An uncooked, pourable mixture typically made up of some sort of flour or meal, liquid, and other ingredients.

Beat: To use a whisk, spoon, or electric mixer to make a mixture smooth and light by rapidly incorporating air.

Blanch: To briefly cook food in boiling water to seal in the flavor while maintaining the food's vibrant color; typically used for vegetables.

Blend: To combine two or more ingredients thoroughly, either by hand, with a whisk or spoon, or with an electric mixer, blender, or food processor.

Boil: To cook a food in water that has reached 212°F and is rapidly bubbling.

Bone: To remove the bones from meat, poultry, or fish.

Braise: To gently simmer food, covered, for a long time in a small amount of liquid. Braising is usually done after meat or vegetables have been browned in fat.

Bread: To coat food with a breading mixture prior to cooking.

Broil: To cook food on a grill, a spit, or the top rack of the oven under intense direct heat.

Brown: To cook food quickly over high heat, typically on the stovetop, in order to brown the surface.

Caramelize: To melt the sugar within a food by cooking it over low heat until its natural sugars break down and turn caramel colored.

Chiffonade: A French term for a specific type of knife cut whereby herbs or greens are stacked and rolled and then cut into thin strips.

Chop: To cut food with a knife or food processor into bite-sized or smaller pieces. For finely chopped, the pieces should be very small. For roughly chopped, the pieces can be larger and less uniform.

Core: To remove the seeds and/or tougher fleshy material from the center of a fruit or vegetable.

Cream: To beat ingredients, usually sugar or eggs and a fat, until they form a smooth, thick mixture.

Crisp-tender: A term that describes the state of vegetables that have been cooked all the way through but still have some snap to them. At this stage, a fork can be inserted with light pressure.

Crush: To press or smash food into smaller pieces, generally using hands, a mortar and pestle, a rolling pin, or a mallet. Crushing dried herbs helps release their flavors and aromas.

Cube: To cut food into about ½-inch cubes.

Dash: A term that often refers to a small amount of seasoning, generally between ¹⁄₁₆ and ⅛ teaspoon. Also refers to a few drops of a liquid ingredient, such as hot sauce.

Deep-fry: To cook food by completely immersing it in hot fat.

Deglaze: To loosen browned bits from the bottom of a pan by adding a liquid, then heating while stirring and scraping the pan. Deglazing helps enhance the flavors of pan sauces.

Dice: To cut food into very small (⅛- to ¼-inch) cubes.

Dollop: A small mound of a soft food, such as whipped cream or sour cream, placed as a topping.

Double boiler: A two-pan/bowl arrangement in which one pan or bowl nests partway inside the other. The lower pan contains a small amount of simmering water that gently cooks heat-sensitive food in the upper pan or bowl without touching it.

Dough: A mixture that consists primarily of flour or meal and a liquid (such as milk or water) and is stiff enough to knead or roll. In many low-carb recipes, doughs are comprised of ingredients like almond flour, coconut flour, and many times even melted cheeses.

Dredge: To coat uncooked food, usually with some sort of breading mixture, before frying.

Dress: To coat a food such as salad with a sauce. Also, to clean fish, poultry, or game in preparation for cooking.

Drippings: The fats and juices rendered by meat or poultry during cooking.

Drizzle: To pour liquid back and forth over food in a fine stream.

Dust: To lightly sprinkle a fine layer of a powdered ingredient onto food.

Emulsify: To combine two liquid or semi-liquid ingredients, such as oil and vinegar, that don't ordinarily mix easily. One way to do so is to gradually add one ingredient to the other while whisking rapidly and continuously.

Fillet: A flat piece of boneless meat, poultry, or fish. Also, to cut out the bones from a piece of meat, poultry, or fish.

Flambé: To add alcohol to a hot pan so that it ignites.

Fold: To gently combine delicate ingredients such as whipped cream or beaten egg whites with a heavier mixture using a rubber spatula in an over-and-under motion.

Glaze: To coat food with a glossy mixture, often sweet but sometimes savory.

Grate: To rub a firm food against a grating instrument to produce shredded or fine bits.

Grease: To rub the interior surface of a baking dish or pan with a cooking fat to prevent food from sticking to it.

Grill: To cook food on a rack, grill, or spit over hot coals or gas heat. (Outside the United States, the term *barbecue* is synonymous with *grill*.)

Grind: To break solid a food into smaller particles using a grinder or food processor.

Herb bouquet: A bundle of tied herbs that is used to flavor soups, stews, and sauces but is removed before serving. Also known as a *bouquet garni*.

Julienne: To cut food into long, thin matchstick-like strips.

Knead: To combine dough ingredients with hands or in a stand mixer using a dough hook attachment. Kneading is usually used for wheat-based, yeast-risen doughs, but in the low-carb world, the same technique is used to mix a mozzarella cheese–based dough (such as for the bagels on page 130).

Macerate: To use a liquid to soften or break down food. Macerating is typically done with fruits and vegetables.

Marinate: To soak food in a seasoned, flavored, and often acidic liquid.

Mince: To cut food into tiny pieces, usually with a knife or food processor.

Par-bake: To partially bake something that will be baked again later, either after being frozen or during a later stage in a recipe.

Parboil: To partially cook by boiling. Parboiling is typically done to prepare food for final cooking by another means or at a later time.

Pinch: A dry ingredient in an amount small enough that it can be pinched between the forefinger and thumb.

Poach: A type of moist-heat cooking that involves cooking food submerged in a liquid, such as water, milk, or stock.

Puree: To mash or grind food until it is completely smooth, with the consistency of a creamy paste or thick liquid, usually done in a food processor, blender, sieve, or food mill.

Reduce: To thicken a liquid and intensify its flavor by simmering.

Render: To cook the fat out of a food in order to retain the drippings.

Roast: To cook meat or vegetables uncovered in a hot oven surrounded by dry heat. A large piece of meat cooked in this manner is often called a roast.

Sauté: To cook food quickly in a small amount of fat over relatively high heat.

Scald: To heat a liquid until it is just about to reach the boiling point.

Sear: To brown the surface of meat by quick-cooking it over high heat until a caramelized crust forms.

Shred: To cut food into narrow strips with a sharp knife, food processor, or grater.

Simmer: To cook food in a hot liquid that is just below the boiling point (212°F). Bubbles begin to form but do not burst on the surface of the liquid.

Skim: To remove the foamy surface or fat from a liquid.

Steam: To cook food in the hot steam provided by boiling water without the food actually making contact with the water.

Steep: To soak an ingredient in a liquid that is just below the boiling point to extract flavor.

Stew: To cook food by simmering or gently boiling it in a liquid.

Stir-fry: To quickly cook small pieces of food over high heat, stirring constantly.

Whip: To beat ingredients with a whisk or an electric mixer to incorporate air and increase volume.

Whisk: To beat ingredients with a fork or whisk to blend them together or incorporate air.

Zest: The outer, colorful part of the skin of an unwaxed citrus fruit.

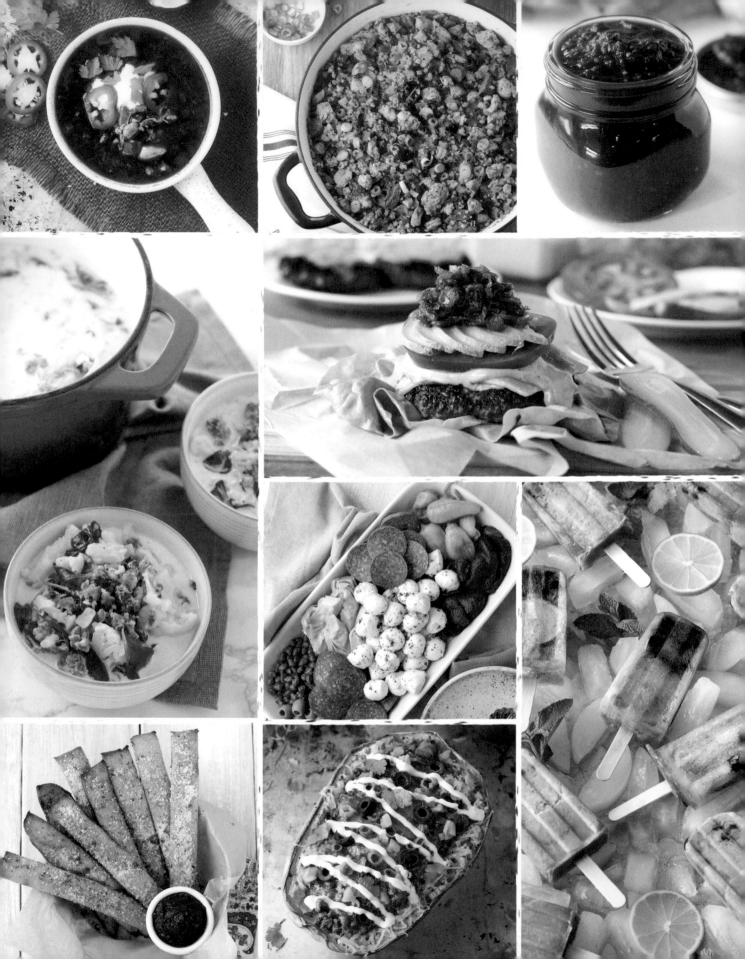

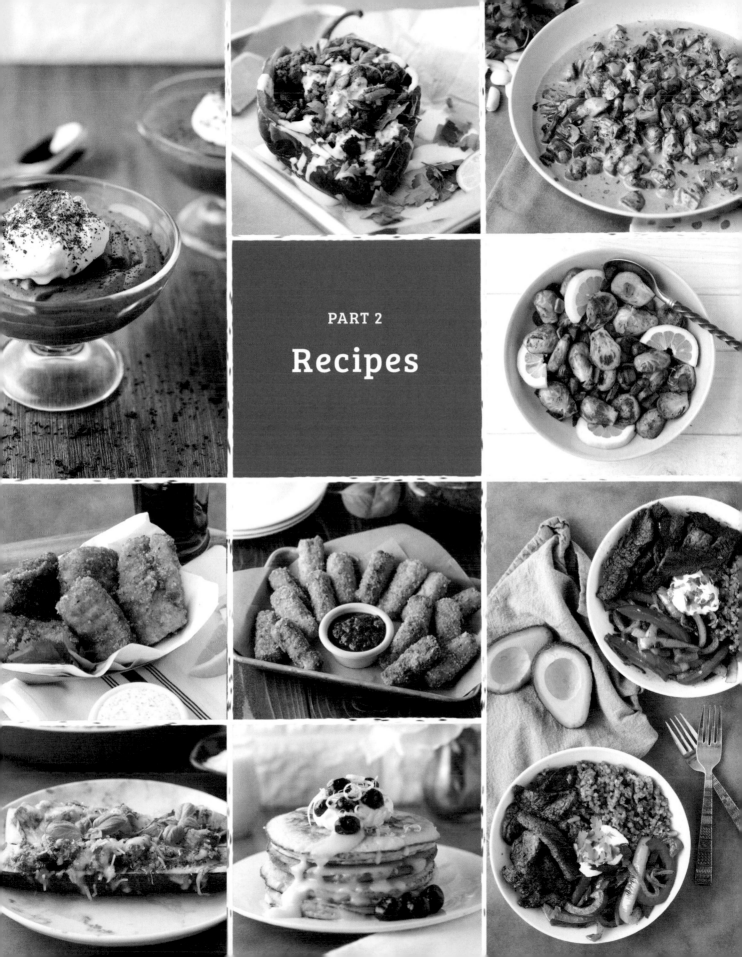

PART 2

Recipes

HOW TO USE THE RECIPES

1 TITLE OF THE RECIPE

2 NET CARBS PER SERVING

3 DIETARY AND ALLERGEN KEY—THESE ICONS PROVIDE A QUICK AND EASY WAY TO IDENTIFY WHICH RECIPES ARE DAIRY-FREE, EGG-FREE, NUT-FREE, OR PALEO.

4 SERVINGS, PREP TIME, AND COOK TIME—THIS SECTION TELLS YOU HOW MANY SERVINGS THE RECIPE PROVIDES, AS WELL AS HOW LONG IT WILL TAKE YOU TO PREP AND COOK THE RECIPE.

5 INGREDIENT LIST—EVERYTHING YOU NEED, AND IN THE EXACT PROPORTIONS TO PREPARE THE RECIPE.

6 DIRECTIONS—THIS SECTION TAKES YOU THROUGH THE STEP-BY-STEP PREPARATION OF THE RECIPE.

7 TIPS—THIS IS WHERE YOU WILL FIND HELPFUL HINTS, TIPS, AND TRICKS, AS WELL AS SUBSTITUTION RECOMMENDATIONS.

8 NUTRITIONAL ANALYSIS—AT THE BOTTOM OF EACH RECIPE YOU WILL FIND THE CALORIES, FAT, PROTEIN, TOTAL CARBS, DIETARY FIBER, AND NET CARBS PER SERVING.

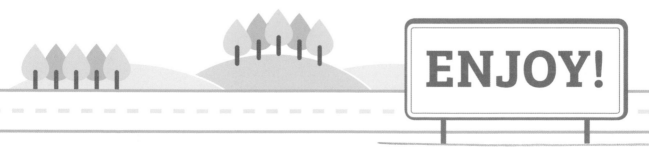

ENJOY!

Garlic Dill Quick Pickled Brussels Sprouts

NET CARBS
2.8g

 DAIRY-FREE EGG-FREE NUT-FREE PALEO makes 10 servings · prep time: 15 minutes, plus at least 48 hours to brine
cook time: 5 minutes

Everyone has tried regular pickles. Many people have tried pickled green beans or pickled asparagus, but have you ever tried pickled Brussels sprouts? These tiny cabbage-shaped vegetables have an almost cultlike following, and here is one more way to enjoy them.

 ## ingredients

12 ounces Brussels sprouts, trimmed and halved

1½ cups apple cider vinegar

1 cup water

1½ teaspoons sea salt

10 whole black peppercorns

2 bay leaves

½ teaspoon yellow mustard seeds

Pinch of red pepper flakes

6 cloves garlic, peeled

6 large sprigs fresh dill weed

1 small shallot, thinly sliced

directions

1. In a large saucepan over medium-high heat, combine the Brussels sprouts, vinegar, water, salt, peppercorns, bay leaves, mustard seeds, and red pepper flakes. Bring to a boil. Blanch the Brussels sprouts in the brine for 4 minutes, then use a slotted spoon to transfer them to an ice bath to shock them and stop the cooking process.

2. Once the brine has cooled, pour it into a 32-ounce mason jar. Add the Brussels sprouts, garlic cloves, dill sprigs, and sliced shallot to the jar. Cap the jar and put it in the refrigerator for 48 hours to a week before eating.

3. Store in the refrigerator for up to 3 months.

 tip: For extra-crunchy pickled Brussels sprouts, skip the step of boiling them in the liquid. Instead, pack the Brussels sprouts, garlic cloves, dill, and shallot slices into the jar. Bring the vinegar, water, and seasonings to a boil, then pour the hot liquid over the ingredients in the jar. Allow to cool to room temperature, then seal and place the jar in the refrigerator. You may need to let the Brussels sprouts sit in the refrigerator longer in order to adequately pickle them.

CALORIES: 20 · FAT: 0 · PROTEIN: 1.6g · TOTAL CARBS: 4.4g · DIETARY FIBER: 1.6g · NET CARBS: 2.8g

156   Snacks & Starters

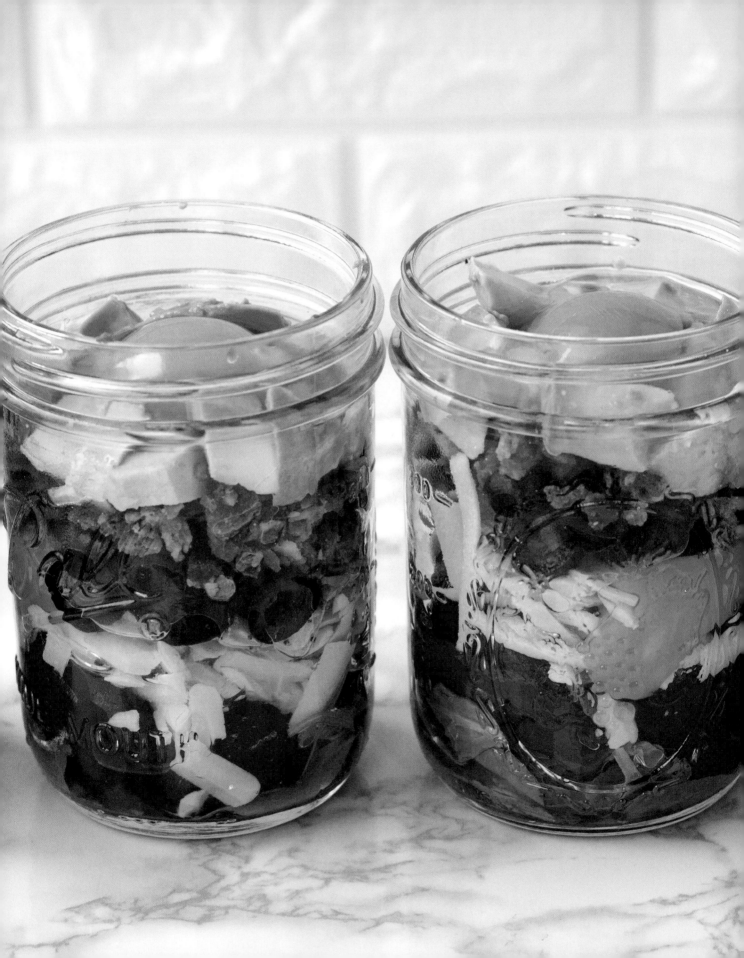

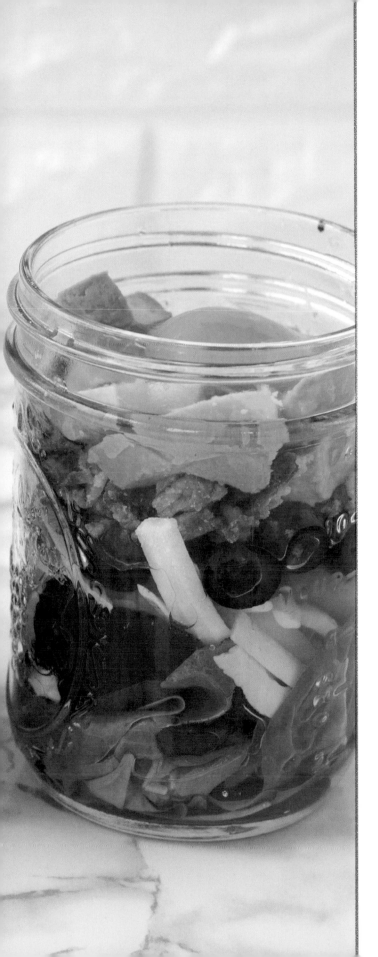

Breakfast

Sausage, Egg, and Cheese Pinwheels

NET CARBS
3g

makes 12 pinwheels (2 per serving) · prep time: 15 minutes · cook time: 25 minutes

This is one of those dishes that you can easily change up to your liking. Try making it with bacon or ham or replacing the cheddar cheese with one of your favorite cheeses. Add some vegetables to help boost the nutritional content.

ingredients

For the dough:

¼ cup blanched almond flour

3 tablespoons coconut flour

1 teaspoon garlic powder

1 teaspoon onion powder

1½ cups shredded low-moisture, part-skim mozzarella cheese

2 tablespoons butter

1 ounce full-fat cream cheese (2 tablespoons)

1 large egg

For the filling:

1 cup shredded sharp cheddar cheese

5 large eggs, soft-scrambled

8 ounces bulk Italian sausage, cooked and crumbled

Tips: To save time, you can make the roll-up ahead of time and freeze it. When you are ready to eat it, just slice and bake.

You can also bake the roll-up slices in a 12-cup muffin pan. This will keep them from spreading and sticking together.

directions

1. Preheat the oven to 375°F.

2. In a small mixing bowl, whisk together the almond flour, coconut flour, garlic powder, and onion powder. Set aside.

3. In a separate microwave-safe bowl, combine the mozzarella cheese, butter, and cream cheese. Microwave for 1 minute 30 seconds to soften. Mix until everything is well combined. If the mixture gets stringy or is not quite melted enough, put the bowl back in the microwave for another 30 seconds.

4. Add the dry ingredients and the egg to the cheese mixture. Using your hands, mix until the ingredients are well incorporated. If you are having a hard time mixing the ingredients together, put the bowl back in the microwave for another 20 to 30 seconds to soften. If the dough starts sticking to your hands, wet your hands slightly and continue working the dough.

5. Once the ingredients are well combined, place the dough on a silicone baking mat or large sheet of parchment paper (about 14 inches long). Using your hands, spread the dough into a thin, even rectangle about 13 by 9 inches.

6. Sprinkle the cheddar cheese over the top, covering all of the dough.

7. Layer the scrambled eggs on top of the cheese, then layer the sausage on top of the scrambled eggs.

8. Roll the dough up tightly lengthwise. Turn the roll-up so that the seam is facing down.

9. Cut the ends off each side of the roll-up to even it out. Then cut the roll-up into 1-inch slices.

10. Place the roll-up slices cut side down in a 10-inch square baking dish. Make sure that they are crowded together so that they do not spread out and flatten.

11. Bake for 20 to 25 minutes, until they are fluffy and golden brown.

12. Store leftovers in the refrigerator for up to 1 week, or freeze for later use. Reheat in the oven or microwave.

CALORIES: 454 · FAT: 38g · PROTEIN: 23g · TOTAL CARBS: 5g · DIETARY FIBER: 2g · NET CARBS: 3g

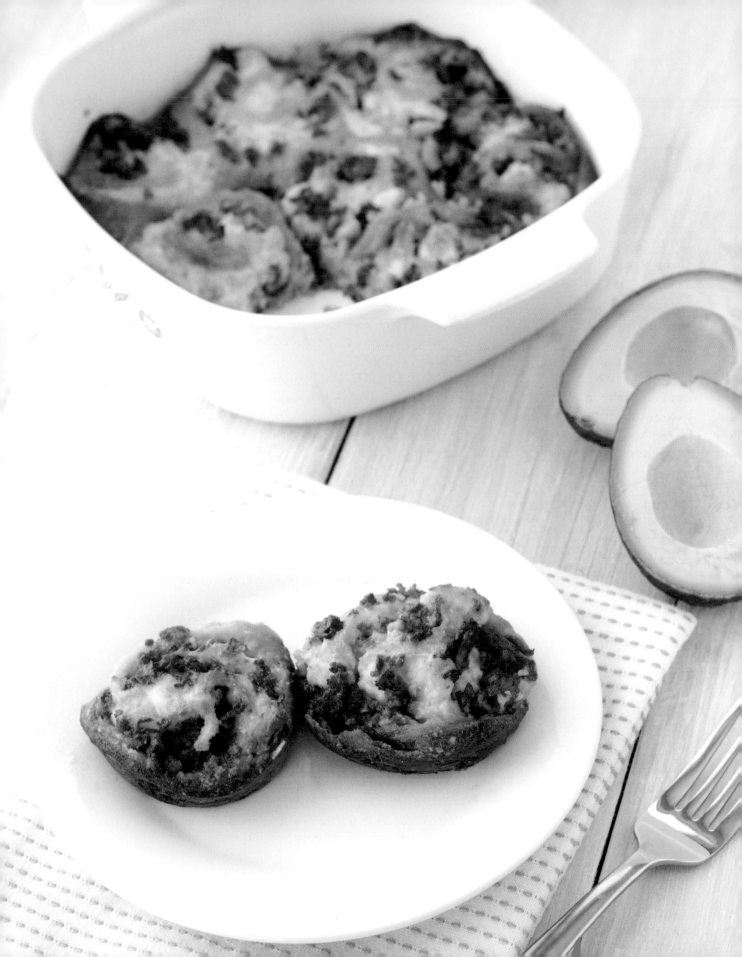

Cheesy Chorizo Breakfast Bake

 makes 6 servings · prep time: 15 minutes · cook time: 1 hour

I love to top this dish with a little sour cream and green onions. The cool creaminess of the sour cream perfectly complements the spiciness of the chorizo.

ingredients

2 tablespoons butter

1 small onion, thinly sliced

2 large cloves garlic, minced

½ teaspoon sea salt

¼ teaspoon ground black pepper

9 ounces bulk Mexican-style fresh chorizo

4 ounces cremini mushrooms, sliced

4 ounces full-fat cream cheese (½ cup)

6 large eggs

⅔ cup shredded sharp cheddar cheese

½ cup grated Parmesan cheese

directions

1. Melt the butter in a large skillet over medium-low heat. When the butter is hot, add the onion, garlic, salt, and pepper and cook until the onions are nice and caramelized, about 20 minutes.

2. Add the chorizo and mushrooms to the skillet and increase the heat to medium. Sauté until the chorizo is cooked all the way through and the mushrooms are tender and have released their liquid.

3. Drain the excess grease from the pan, then reduce the heat to low and stir in the cream cheese until the ingredients are well combined. Pour the chorizo mixture into an 8-inch square casserole dish.

4. Preheat the oven to 350°F.

5. Crack the eggs into a large mixing bowl and whisk with a fork. Mix in the cheddar and Parmesan cheeses.

6. Pour the egg and cheese mixture over the top of the chorizo. Mix just slightly until some of the chorizo shows through the egg layer.

7. Bake for 30 minutes, until the top is golden brown and the eggs are cooked through.

CALORIES: 452 · FAT: 37g · PROTEIN: 24g · TOTAL CARBS: 5g · DIETARY FIBER: 0 · NET CARBS: 5g

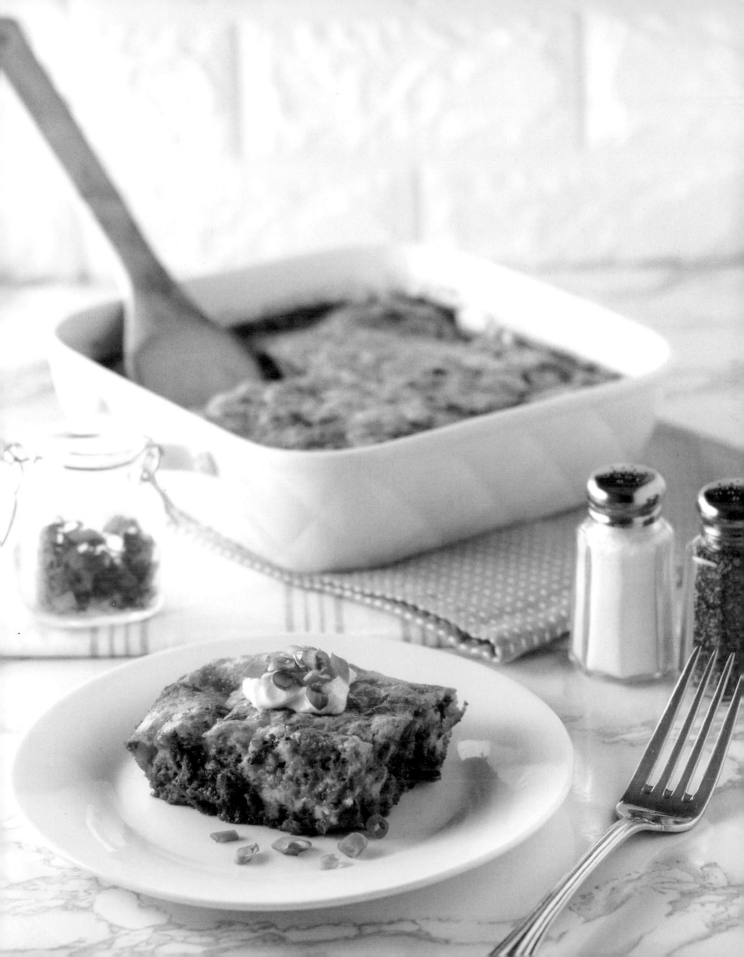

Breakfast Pizza

 makes 8 servings · prep time: 15 minutes · cook time: 20 minutes

I am definitely a fan of the "put an egg on it" culture. I think just about any savory meal can be made better by topping it with a perfectly yolky egg. I'll also take any excuse to eat pizza for breakfast!

ingredients

1 baked Nut-Free Pizza Crust (page 358)

⅓ cup Pizza Sauce (page 343)

¼ cup shredded Romano cheese

5 slices Canadian bacon

2 cremini mushrooms, thinly sliced

3 slices bacon, cooked crisp and crumbled

2 ounces full-fat ricotta cheese (¼ cup)

2 large eggs

5 fresh basil leaves, sliced into chiffonade

directions

1. Preheat the oven to 375°F. Lightly grease a pizza pan or rimmed baking sheet.

2. Place the baked pizza crust on the greased pan. Top the crust with the pizza sauce and spread it around until it evenly covers the crust. Sprinkle the Romano cheese over the sauce.

3. Place the Canadian bacon on top of the cheese, then layer on the mushrooms and bacon. Top the pizza with dollops of ricotta cheese. Crack the eggs on top of the pizza.

4. Bake the pizza for 20 minutes or until the eggs are set.

5. Sprinkle the fresh basil over the pizza, then cut it into 8 slices and serve.

CALORIES: 220 · FAT: 60g · PROTEIN: 16g · TOTAL CARBS: 3.7g · DIETARY FIBER: 0.4g · NET CARBS: 3.3g

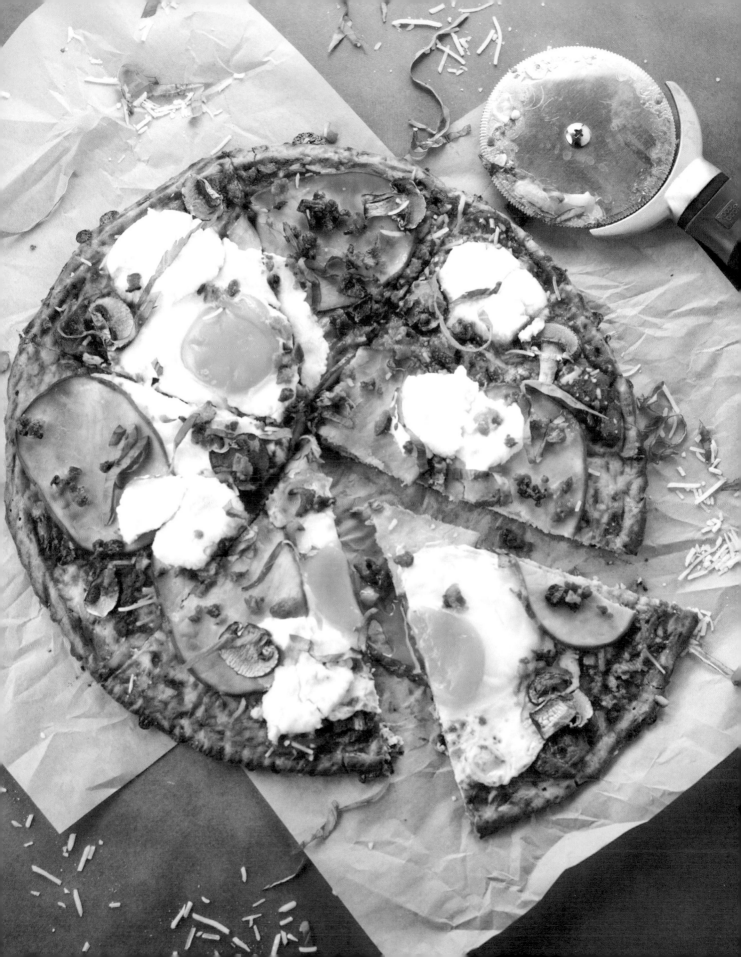

Baked Eggs with Chorizo and Ricotta

 NUT-FREE · makes 6 servings · prep time: 15 minutes · cook time: 35 minutes

One of my favorite things to do in the kitchen is to combine a bunch of random ingredients and come up with different breakfast creations. A lot of low-carbers get stuck in a breakfast rut and wear themselves out on eggs. Well, not this girl. To me, each morning is like a blank canvas that I get to paint. Breakfast should be amazing. After all, it is the most important meal of the day.

ingredients

2 tablespoons olive oil

2 tablespoons butter or ghee

1 pound bulk Mexican-style fresh chorizo

¾ cup diced mixed bell peppers

1 small onion, diced (about ½ cup)

1 (14½-ounce) can fire-roasted tomatoes

3 packed cups fresh spinach

4 cloves garlic, minced

1 teaspoon dried oregano leaves

½ teaspoon chili powder

½ teaspoon smoked paprika

Sea salt and black pepper (optional)

12 large eggs

4 ounces full-fat ricotta cheese (½ cup)

¼ cup shredded Asiago cheese

6 sprigs fresh thyme

1 tablespoon chopped fresh flat-leaf parsley

directions

1. Heat the olive oil and butter in a large skillet over medium heat. Add the chorizo and sauté until it is almost cooked through.

2. Add the bell peppers, onion, tomatoes, spinach, garlic, oregano, chili powder, and smoked paprika to the skillet. Cook until the vegetables are tender and the spinach is wilted. Taste and add salt and pepper, if desired.

3. Preheat the oven to 350°F.

4. Divide the chorizo and veggie mixture among six 10-ounce baking dishes. Alternatively, you can use one large baking dish, about 10 inches square.

5. Use a spoon to make 4 wells in each dish. Crack an egg into two of the wells and put a dollop of ricotta cheese in each of the other two wells. Top each dish with Asiago cheese, a sprig of fresh thyme, and some parsley.

6. Bake until the whites are set and the yolks have reached the desired level of doneness. (About 10 minutes of baking time will provide runny yolks; bake longer if you prefer set yolks.)

CALORIES: 623 · FAT: 49g · PROTEIN: 34g · TOTAL CARBS: 9g · DIETARY FIBER: 3g · NET CARBS: 6g

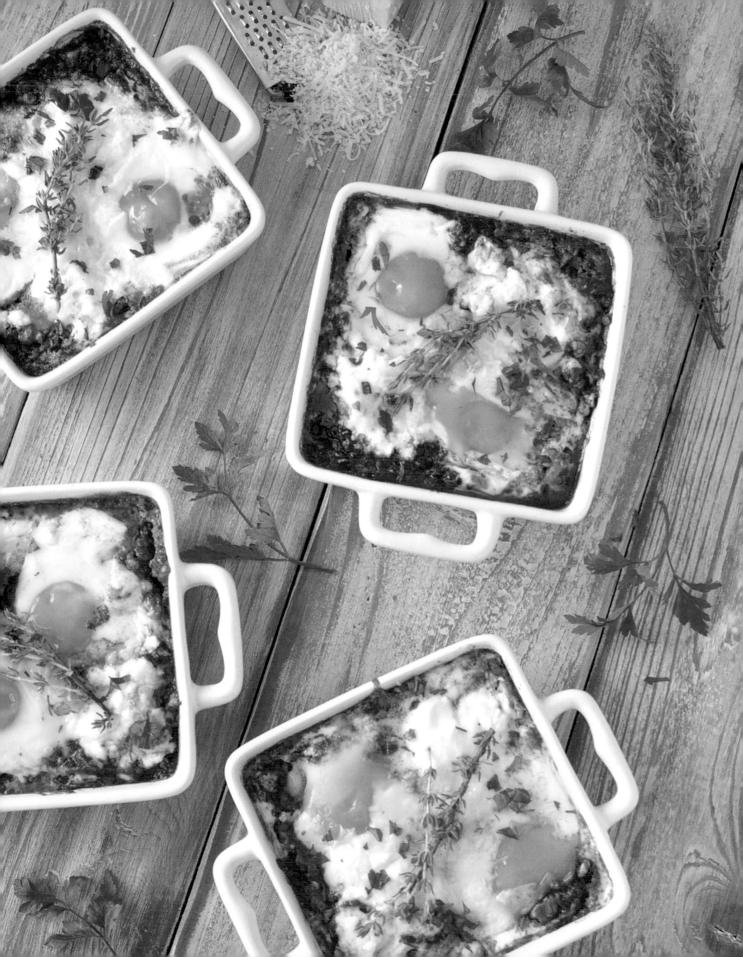

Baked Egg Jars

NUT-FREE *makes 4 servings · prep time: 10 minutes · cook time: 30 minutes*

My favorite thing about these egg jars is that there are no rules. You can use any meats and vegetables you have on hand, and they will taste delicious every time. They are perfect for quick-and-easy meal prep. We bake them all at once and then eat them throughout the week. With these on hand, you will find that there is always time for breakfast, even on those rushed mornings—just heat and eat. You can even take them with you!

ingredients

1 packed cup fresh spinach

8 ounces roasted red peppers, cut into large chunks

1 cup shredded sharp cheddar cheese

8 large eggs

Sea salt and black pepper

⅓ cup sliced black olives

8 slices bacon, cooked crisp and crumbled

1 medium avocado, peeled, pitted, and cubed

tip: Mix all of the ingredients together in a bowl before pouring into the jars for a more omelet-like texture.

directions

1. Preheat the oven to 350°F.

2. Divide the spinach among 4 wide-mouthed pint-sized mason jars. Add the red peppers and cheese, dividing them equally among the jars.

3. Crack an egg into each jar and sprinkle with a little salt and pepper. Sprinkle the black olives on top of the eggs, then add the bacon and avocado to the jars. Top each jar with another egg.

4. Bake for 30 minutes or until the eggs are set and have reached the desired level of doneness.

CALORIES: 581 · FAT: 49g · PROTEIN: 26g · TOTAL CARBS: 11g · DIETARY FIBER: 5g · NET CARBS: 6g

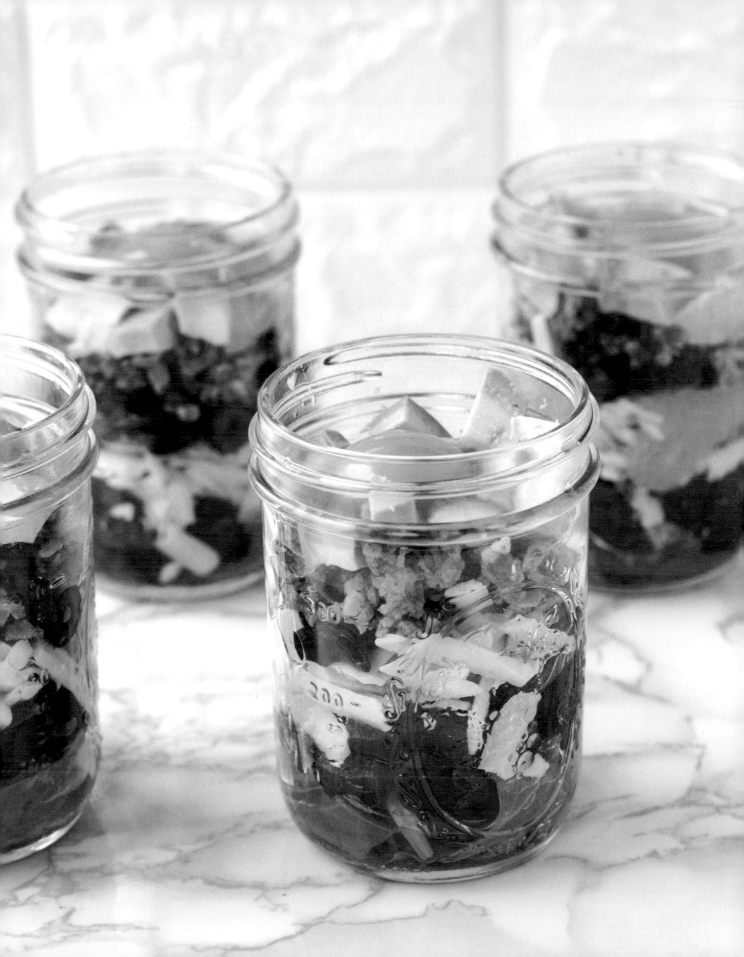

13 Jon's Special

makes 6 servings · prep time: 10 minutes · cook time: 20 minutes

This might be one of my very favorite recipes in this book because of the meaning behind it. For many years, I worked at an iconic Seattle restaurant called 13 Coins. It is an institution in the Seattle area and has been in business since 1967. One spring evening in 2008, a handsome gentleman sat in my section and ordered a steak—a New York steak, cooked medium-rare, to be exact. There was just something about him. I found myself fumbling over my words and blushing whenever I had to talk to him. That was definitely not me; I was never the type to lose my head over a guy. But, like I said, there was just something about him. I immediately ran over to the manager on duty and pointed at him and said, "See that guy? He doesn't know it yet, but I'm going to marry him." And marry him I did. Our first date was the very next night, and we got married on the two-year anniversary of our first date. That was more than nine years ago. He is the best partner in crime a girl could ever ask for. What does any of this have to do with this recipe, you might ask? Well, 13 Coins was known for a dish called the Joe's Special. This is my take on a classic, but I decided to call mine 13 Jon's Special because he is clearly the most special thing that came from my time there.

ingredients

2 tablespoons butter or ghee

1 medium onion, diced (about 1 cup)

3 cloves garlic, minced

½ teaspoon sea salt

¼ teaspoon ground black pepper

1 pound ground beef

10 cremini mushrooms, thinly sliced

2 packed cups fresh spinach

6 large eggs

¼ cup shredded Parmesan cheese

¼ cup shredded Asiago cheese

¼ cup full-fat sour cream

2 green onions, sliced

directions

1. Heat the butter in a large skillet over medium-low heat. Add the onion, garlic, salt, and pepper and cook until the onion is translucent and the garlic is fragrant.

2. Add the ground beef to the skillet, increase the heat to medium, and cook until it is browned.

3. Add the mushrooms and spinach and sauté until the mushrooms have released their liquid and the spinach is wilted.

4. Crack the eggs into a mixing bowl and whisk with a fork. Pour the eggs into the skillet and mix them into the meat mixture. Cook until the eggs are set. Taste and add more salt and pepper, if desired.

5. Top with the cheeses, sour cream, and green onions before serving.

CALORIES: 307 · FAT: 21g · PROTEIN: 25.5g · TOTAL CARBS: 4.3g · DIETARY FIBER: 1.3g · NET CARBS: 3g

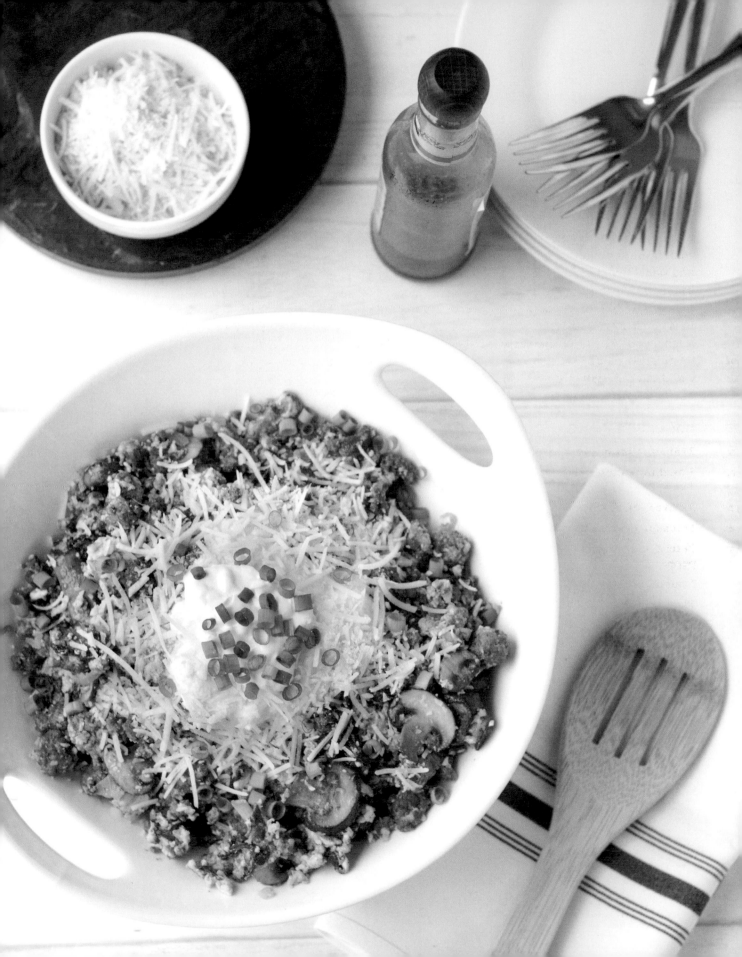

Sausage and Egg Breakfast Sandwich

 makes 1 serving · prep time: 10 minutes · cook time: 10 minutes

Who needs fast food when you can make dishes like this in the comfort of your own kitchen and save money in the process? There are a lot of clean sausage brands on the market, but I like to make this sandwich with the Maple Chicken Sausage Patties from my website. You can find the recipe at peaceloveandlowcarb.com.

ingredients

1 tablespoon butter or ghee

2 large eggs

1 tablespoon mayonnaise, store-bought or homemade (page 336)

2 sausage patties, cooked

2 slices sharp cheddar cheese

2 avocado slices

directions

1. Heat the butter in a large skillet over medium heat. Place two lightly oiled mason jar rings or silicone egg molds in the skillet.

2. Crack an egg into each ring and use a fork to break the yolks and gently whisk. Cover and cook for 3 to 4 minutes, until the eggs are cooked through. Remove the eggs from the rings.

3. Place one of the eggs on a plate and top it with half of the mayonnaise. Then place a sausage patty on the mayo-topped egg. Top the sausage with a slice of cheese and 2 avocado slices.

4. Put the second sausage patty on top of the avocado and top it with the remaining cheese slice.

5. Spread the remaining mayonnaise on the second cooked egg and place it on top of the sandwich.

CALORIES: 880 · FAT: 82g · PROTEIN: 32g · TOTAL CARBS: 5g · DIETARY FIBER: 2g · NET CARBS: 3g

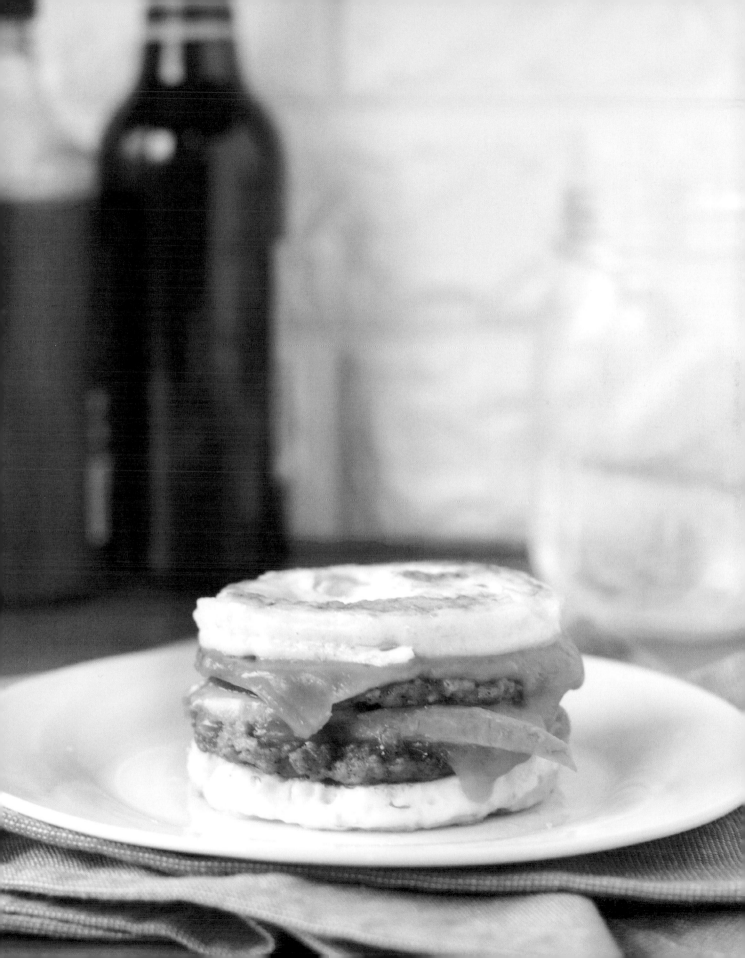

Reuben Frittata

NET CARBS
1.5g

 makes 8 servings · prep time: 10 minutes · cook time: 40 minutes

I just love the classic flavors of a Reuben sandwich. When I made the Reuben Biscuit Sandwiches on page 226 and had leftover ingredients, I immediately knew that I wanted to make something breakfast themed. But I must say, the Thousand Island dressing takes this dish to a whole new level. Have your favorite classic sandwich for breakfast. Who needs the bread, anyway?

ingredients

12 ounces deli corned beef, chopped

½ cup sauerkraut

8 large eggs

¼ cup heavy cream

1 cup shredded Swiss cheese

½ teaspoon caraway seeds

½ cup shredded Parmesan cheese

¼ cup Thousand Island Dressing (page 330)

2 tablespoons chopped fresh chives

directions

1. Preheat the oven to 350°F.

2. Heat a large ovenproof skillet over medium heat. Add the corned beef and sauerkraut and cook for 5 minutes.

3. Meanwhile, crack the eggs into a mixing bowl and whisk with a fork. Add the cream and whisk to combine. Stir in the Swiss cheese.

4. Pour the egg mixture over the corned beef and sauerkraut in the skillet. Mix just slightly. Cook, without stirring, until the sides and bottom begin to set. Top the frittata with the caraway seeds.

5. Transfer the skillet to the oven and bake for 20 to 30 minutes, until the eggs are firm.

6. Top the frittata with the Parmesan cheese, Thousand Island dressing, and chives before serving.

CALORIES: 261 · FAT: 18g · PROTEIN: 21g · TOTAL CARBS: 2g · DIETARY FIBER: 0.5g · NET CARBS: 1.5g

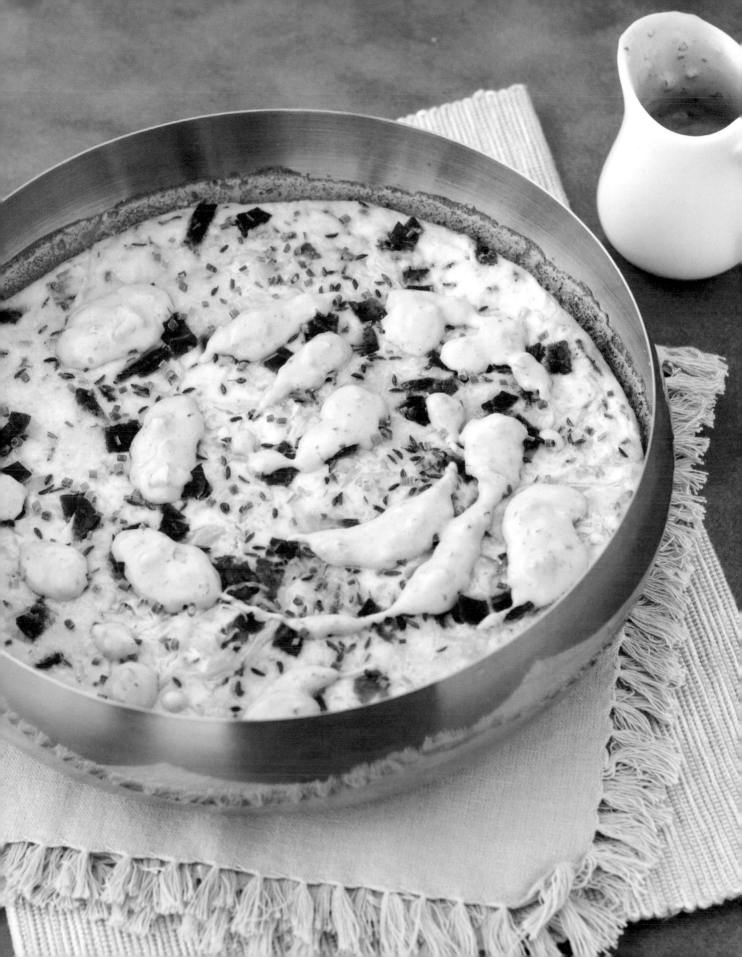

Radishes O'Brien

makes 6 servings · prep time: 15 minutes · cook time: 20 minutes

When I was growing up, we ate those frozen bags of potatoes O'Brien. They were always a sad, mushy mess. But I still really liked them because I didn't know what I was missing. When I started cooking my own meals, I began making this same breakfast, but with fresh potatoes, peppers, and onions. It became an instant favorite. When I switched to a low-carb lifestyle, I knew that I wasn't going to want to give up this dish, so I had to get creative. When cooked correctly, radishes make an excellent stand-in for potatoes.

ingredients

1 pound radishes (about 2 pounds with greens)

2 tablespoons butter or ghee

2 cloves garlic, minced

1 small green bell pepper, seeded and diced

1 small orange bell pepper, seeded and diced

1 small onion, diced (about ½ cup)

Sea salt and ground black pepper

tip: To make this dish dairy-free and Paleo compliant, use ghee rather than butter.

directions

1. Slice the greens off the tops of the radishes, if still attached, and trim any roots. Thoroughly rinse the radishes, then quarter them.

2. Heat the butter in a large skillet over medium heat. Add the radishes, garlic, bell peppers, and onion to the pan. Sauté until the vegetables are tender, 15 to 20 minutes. Taste and add salt and pepper to your liking.

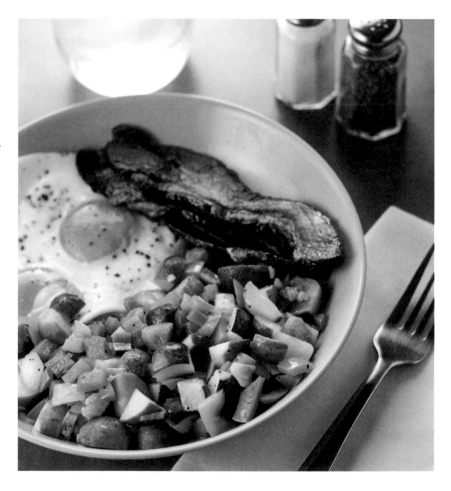

CALORIES: 58 · FAT: 4g · PROTEIN: 1g · TOTAL CARBS: 5g · DIETARY FIBER: 2g · NET CARBS: 3g

Pastrami Breakfast Hash

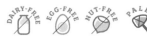 makes 4 servings · prep time: 15 minutes · cook time: 20 minutes

Quick, easy, and flavorful—exactly what breakfast should be! I like to top my breakfast hash with a sunny-side-up egg and some fresh herbs.

ingredients

2 tablespoons butter or ghee

1 medium onion, diced (about 1 cup)

3 cloves garlic, minced

3 cups riced cauliflower (see page 76)

12 ounces deli-style pastrami, chopped

¼ cup chopped fresh flat-leaf parsley

Sea salt and black pepper (optional)

tips: To make this dish dairy-free and Paleo compliant, use ghee rather than butter.

You can also make this recipe with corned beef.

directions

1. Heat the butter in a large skillet over medium heat. Add the onion and garlic and sauté until the onion is translucent and the garlic is fragrant.

2. Add the cauliflower to the skillet and sauté until it is cooked through and slightly caramelized.

3. Add the pastrami to the skillet. Sauté, stirring often, until the pastrami is crispy on the edges.

4. Stir in the parsley. Taste and add salt and pepper, if desired.

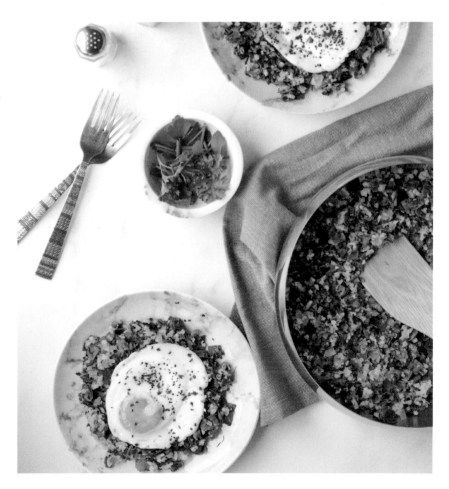

CALORIES: 212 · FAT: 11g · PROTEIN: 21g · TOTAL CARBS: 8g · DIETARY FIBER: 2g · NET CARBS: 6g

Pizza Eggs

NET CARBS
3g

 makes 1 serving · prep time: 5 minutes · cook time: 10 minutes

This recipe pretty much sums up my low-carb mission in life: to get creative and re-create my favorite comfort foods in as many versions as possible. I am all about easy and flavorful in one dish. The less time spent in the kitchen, the better. I'm sure you agree! The secret to getting perfectly gooey yolks and still getting crispy pepperoni is to take your time and cook it low and slow. And get creative with it! Use any cheese and pizza toppings you prefer.

ingredients

1 tablespoon butter or ghee

2 large eggs

2 tablespoons Pizza Sauce (page 343)

2 tablespoons crumbled feta cheese

5 slices pepperoni

2 tablespoons shredded mozzarella cheese

1 tablespoon grated Parmesan cheese

Pinch of Italian seasoning

directions

1. Heat the butter in a small skillet over medium-low heat. When the butter is melted and the skillet is hot, crack the eggs into the pan.

2. Once the whites just barely start to set and turn white, reduce the heat to low, spoon the pizza sauce over the eggs, and sprinkle the feta over the top.

3. Continue cooking and, when the whites are almost completely set, add the pepperoni, mozzarella, Parmesan, and Italian seasoning on top.

4. Continue cooking over low heat until the whites are completely set, the pepperoni is cooked, and the cheese is melted.

CALORIES: 512 · FAT: 41g · PROTEIN: 30g · TOTAL CARBS: 3g · DIETARY FIBER: 0 · NET CARBS: 3g

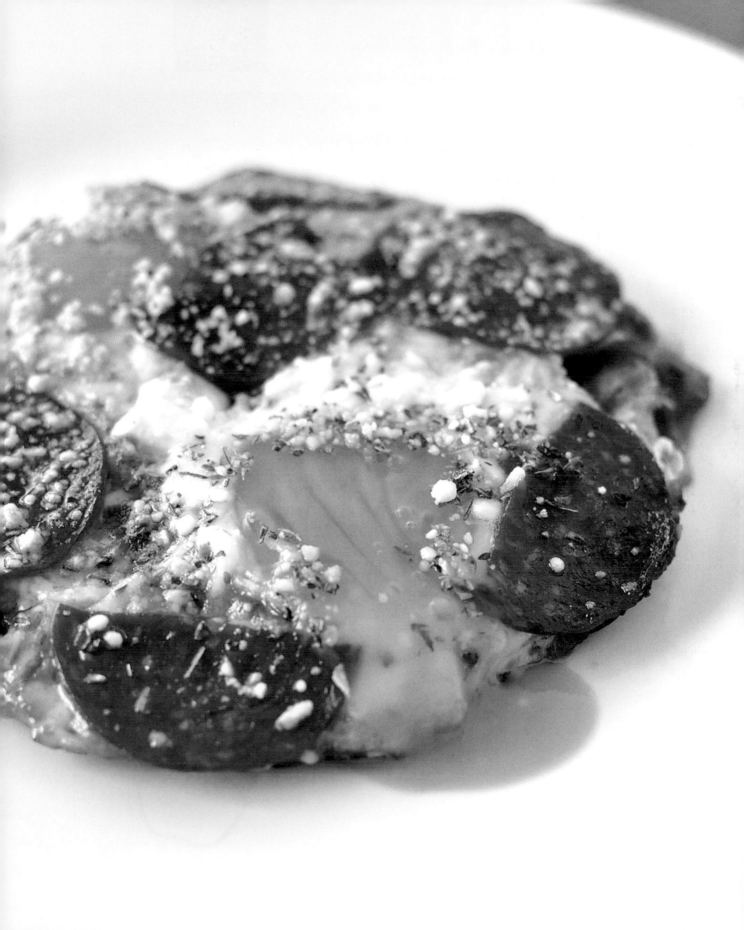

Pancetta, White Cheddar, and Spinach Frittata

makes 8 servings · prep time: 15 minutes · cook time: 40 minutes

Frittatas are my favorite way to use up the last of the groceries in my fridge. I call it a fridge dump breakfast. Frittatas are also a great way to repurpose leftovers. I can't even tell you how many times last night's dinner has become today's breakfast.

ingredients

2 tablespoons butter or ghee

1 shallot, minced

2 cloves garlic, minced

¼ teaspoon sea salt

⅛ teaspoon ground black pepper

5 ounces thinly sliced pancetta

6 cremini mushrooms, sliced

2 packed cups fresh spinach

8 large eggs

½ cup heavy cream

¾ cup shredded white cheddar cheese

Pinch of red pepper flakes

tip: If you can't find pancetta for this dish or you just want to save a few dollars, you can substitute bacon.

directions

1. Heat the butter in a large ovenproof skillet over medium heat. Add the shallot, garlic, salt, and pepper and sauté until the shallot is translucent and the garlic is fragrant.

2. Chop the pancetta, reserving 4 or 5 slices for the top of the frittata. Add the chopped pancetta to the skillet and cook until it is crispy.

3. Add the mushrooms and spinach to the skillet, reserving a few of each for the top of the frittata, and cook until the mushrooms are tender and the spinach is wilted.

4. Preheat the oven to 350°F.

5. Crack the eggs into a mixing bowl and whisk with a fork. Whisk in the cream and cheese.

6. Pour the egg mixture into the skillet over the top of the pancetta and vegetables. Mix just slightly.

7. Cook, without stirring, until the sides and bottom begin to set. Top the frittata with the remaining pancetta slices, mushrooms, and spinach and the red pepper flakes.

8. Transfer the skillet to the oven and bake for 20 to 30 minutes, until the eggs are firm.

CALORIES: 276 · FAT: 24g · PROTEIN: 12g · TOTAL CARBS: 3g · DIETARY FIBER: 1g · NET CARBS: 2g

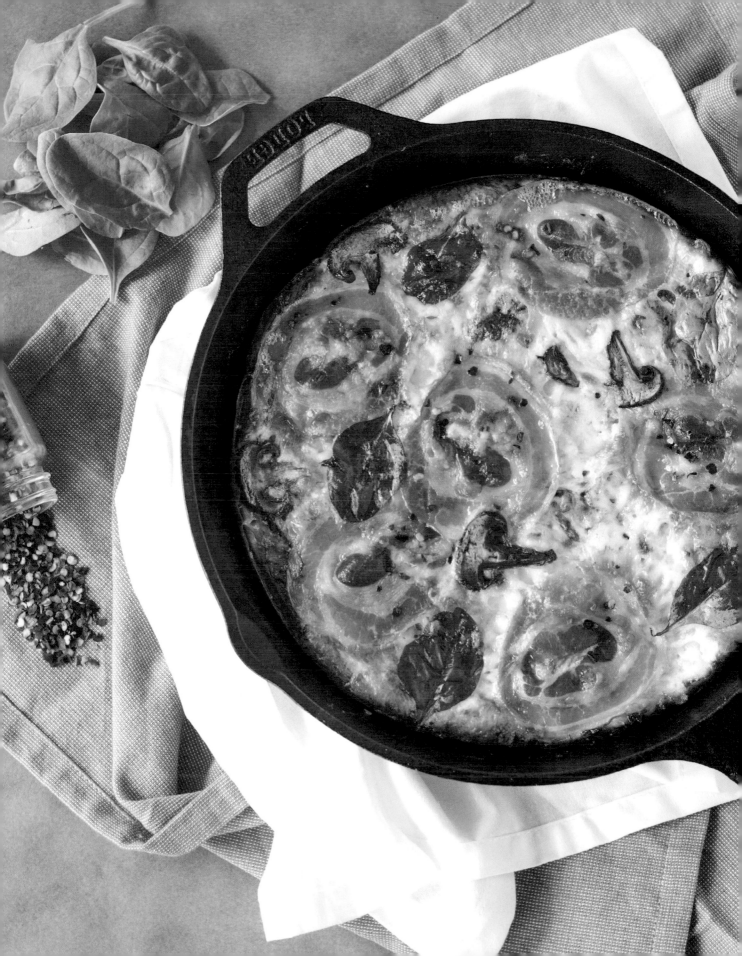

Oven-Roasted Garlic and Herb Home Fries

makes 6 servings · prep time: 15 minutes · cook time: 30 minutes

Before you scream, "WHAT?! This isn't keto," let's talk about how you could work this dish into a day of keto eating and still hit your macros for the day. A little root vegetable food for thought, if you will. What if you looked at your ratios for the day as a whole and not just for one single meal? You could easily eat a serving of these home fries with bacon and eggs for breakfast, the Deviled Ham and Egg Salad Wraps on page 204 for lunch, and the Seared Scallops with Sherry Beurre Blanc on page 222 for dinner. You would still be under twenty net carbs for the day and could easily hit your fat and protein goals, too. Sometimes the key to staying on track is thinking outside the strict keto box.

ingredients

2 medium turnips (about 10 ounces)

2 parsnips (about 1½ pounds)

1 pound radishes (about 2 pounds with greens)

Leaves from 1 sprig fresh rosemary, finely chopped

2 tablespoons chopped fresh flat-leaf parsley, divided

1 teaspoon sea salt

½ teaspoon black ground pepper

½ teaspoon smoked paprika

4 tablespoons (½ stick) butter or ghee, melted, divided

2 tablespoons olive oil

4 cloves garlic, minced

2 tablespoons chopped fresh chives

directions

1. Clean and trim the turnips, parsnips, and radishes. Cut into ½-inch cubes.

2. Preheat the oven to 425°F.

3. In a large mixing bowl, combine the turnips, parsnips, radishes, rosemary leaves, 1 tablespoon of the parsley, salt, pepper, and smoked paprika. Toss the vegetables with 2 tablespoons of the melted butter and the olive oil until they are evenly coated.

4. Spread the vegetables in a single layer on a rimmed baking sheet. Roast on the bottom rack of the oven for 15 minutes.

5. Remove the baking sheet from the oven and toss the vegetables with the garlic and the remaining 2 tablespoons of butter. Roast for an additional 15 minutes, until the vegetables are golden brown and crispy.

6. Top with the remaining parsley and the chives before serving.

tip: To make this dish dairy-free and Paleo compliant, use ghee rather than butter.

CALORIES: 166 · FAT: 10g · PROTEIN: 2g · TOTAL CARBS: 20g · DIETARY FIBER: 6g · NET CARBS: 14g

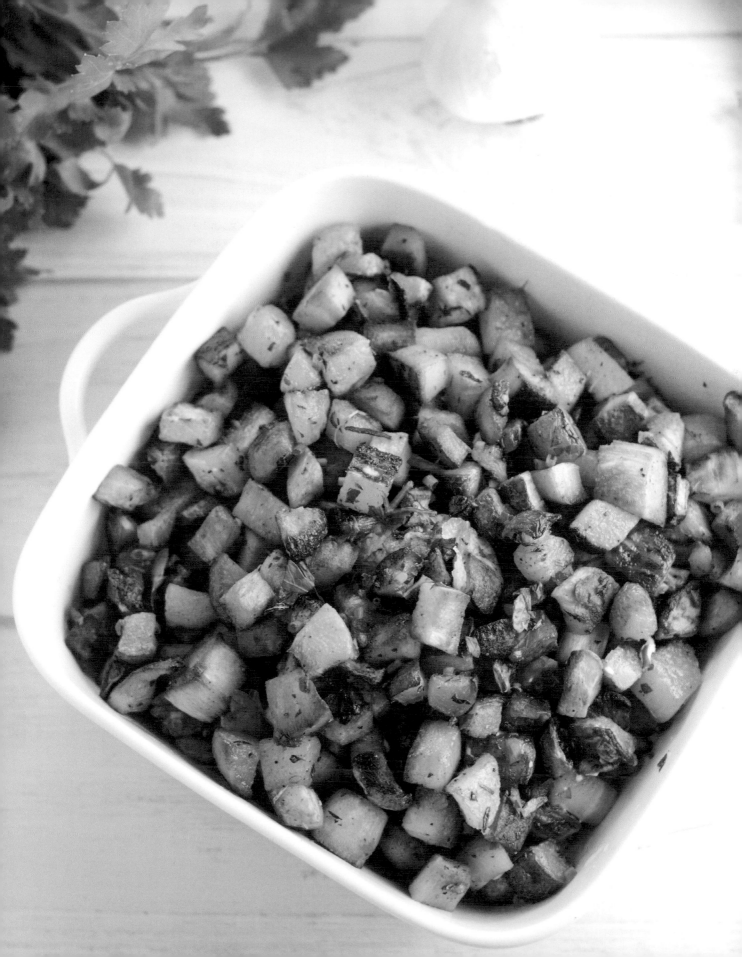

Lemon Ricotta Pancakes

NET CARBS
2g

makes eight 5- to 6-inch pancakes (1 per serving)
prep time: 10 minutes · cook time: 20 minutes

Have I mentioned my deep love of all things lemon flavored? Lemon is such a fresh and bright taste. Putting lemon curd on these pancakes is like having breakfast and dessert all in one. They are decadent enough to make you feel like you are doing something naughty, but low enough in carbs to remind you that you aren't. That's a win in my book. Now go be naughty and eat your pancake for dessert.

ingredients

4 ounces full-fat ricotta cheese (½ cup)

4 large eggs

¼ cup coconut flour

2 tablespoons powdered erythritol

2 teaspoons baking powder

2 teaspoons pure vanilla extract

1 teaspoon lemon extract

Butter or ghee, for the pan

For serving (optional):

½ cup Lemon Curd (page 310)

½ cup Fresh Whipped Cream (page 327)

½ cup fresh blueberries

Fine strips of lemon zest or grated lemon zest, for garnish (optional)

directions

1. In a blender, combine the ricotta cheese and eggs. Pulse until smooth.

2. Add the coconut flour, erythritol, baking powder, vanilla extract, and lemon extract to the blender and pulse until the ingredients are well combined and the batter is smooth.

3. Brush a large nonstick skillet or griddle pan with butter and heat over medium-low heat. Once the pan is hot, add ¼ cup of the batter and cook until it is bubbly on the top and golden brown on the bottom, about 3 minutes. Flip and cook the other side until it is golden brown, 2 to 3 minutes. Repeat this process until all of the batter is gone, regreasing the skillet between batches.

4. Top each pancake with 1 tablespoon of lemon curd, 1 tablespoon of whipped cream, and a few blueberries, if using. Garnish with lemon zest, if desired.

5. Store leftovers in a resealable plastic bag in the fridge for up to 5 days, or freeze for later use. Reheat in a preheated 200°F oven until warmed through.

CALORIES: 74 · FAT: 4g · PROTEIN: 5g · TOTAL CARBS: 3g · DIETARY FIBER: 1g · NET CARBS: 2g

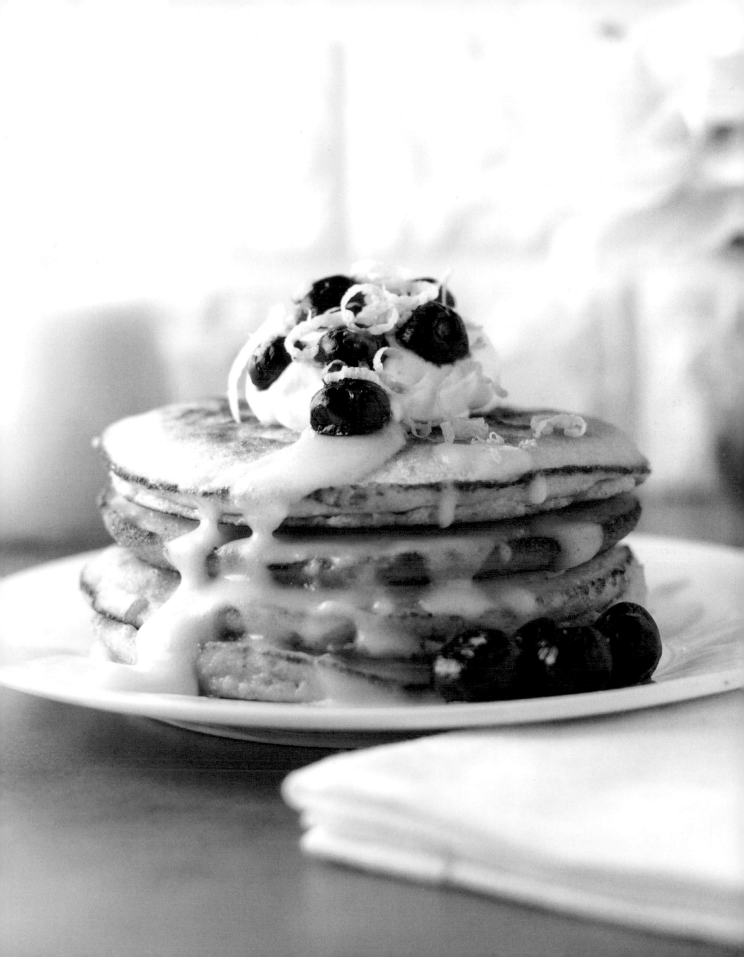

Kyndra's Favorite Buttery Herbed Eggs

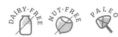

makes 1 serving · prep time: 5 minutes · cook time: 10 minutes

If there were a video camera in my kitchen, breakfast might look a lot like the movie *Groundhog Day*. I eat these eggs probably five times a week. I have been asked countless times on my various social media accounts how I make them, so it seemed only fitting that they should make it into this book. My secret to perfect sunny-side-up eggs is to cook them low and slow. I keep the heat really low and give them time to do their thing. They come out with perfectly set whites and deliciously runny yolks every time.

ingredients

1 tablespoon butter or ghee

3 large eggs

1 teaspoon Everything Bagel Seasoning (page 352)

½ teaspoon chopped fresh chives

½ teaspoon chopped fresh dill weed

¼ teaspoon chopped fresh flat-leaf parsley

directions

1. Heat the butter in a small skillet over medium-low heat. When the butter is melted and the pan is hot, crack the eggs into the skillet.

2. Once the egg whites just barely start to set and turn white, reduce the heat to low and top the eggs with the bagel seasoning and herbs.

3. Continue cooking on low until the whites are completely set but the yolks are still runny.

tip: To make this dish dairy-free and Paleo compliant, use ghee rather than butter.

CALORIES: 328 · FAT: 26g · PROTEIN: 19g · TOTAL CARBS: 1.5g · DIETARY FIBER: 0.2g · NET CARBS: 1.3g

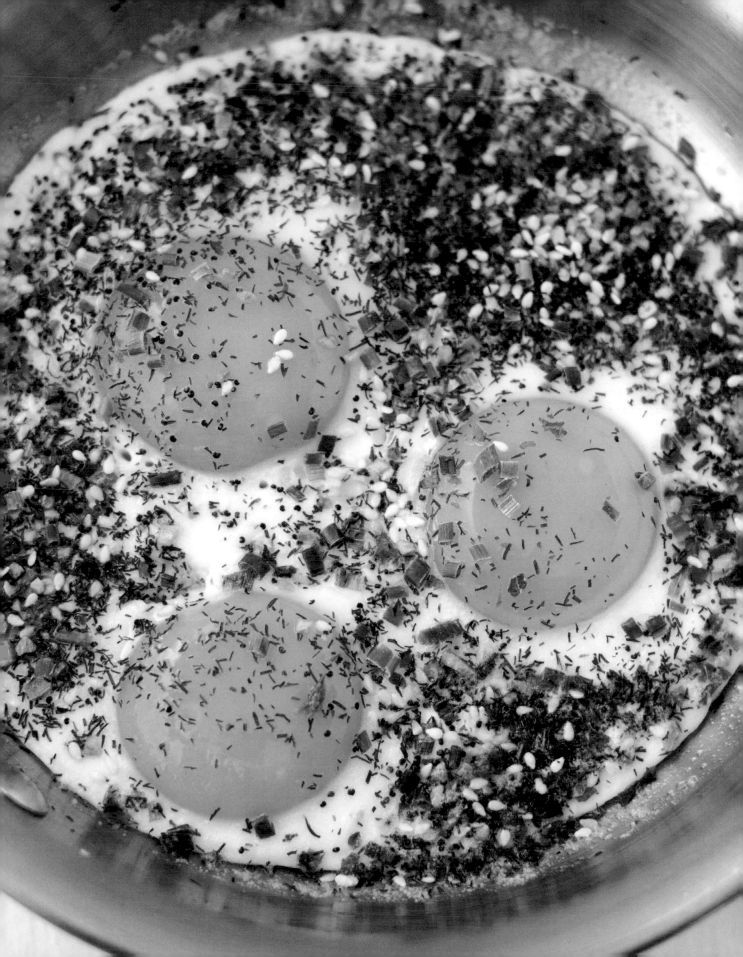

French Toast Egg Puffs

 makes 12 egg puffs (2 per serving) · prep time: 5 minutes · cook time: 30 minutes

It doesn't get much easier than throwing ingredients into a blender and turning it on. This is a recipe the whole family will love—perfect for those lazy Saturday mornings when you just don't feel like putting a lot of work into cooking. These egg puffs are also great for make-ahead meals. Make a batch on the weekend and eat them throughout the week. We like to enjoy them with sugar-free maple syrup.

ingredients

8 large eggs

1 (8-ounce) package full-fat cream cheese, softened

2 tablespoons heavy cream

1 teaspoon pure vanilla extract

¼ cup coconut flour

2 tablespoons granular erythritol

1 teaspoon baking soda

½ teaspoon ground cinnamon

1 tablespoon powdered erythritol, for dusting (optional)

tips: If you do not have a blender, you can make the batter using a hand mixer.

These egg puffs are amazing topped with sugar-free maple syrup.

directions

1. Preheat the oven to 350°F. Use a silicone muffin pan or lightly grease a 12-well muffin pan.

2. Combine the eggs, cream cheese, cream, vanilla extract, coconut flour, granular erythritol, ground cinnamon, and baking soda in a blender. Blend until the ingredients are well incorporated. You may need to use a rubber spatula to scrape down the sides of the blender.

3. Pour the batter into the wells of the muffin pan, filling each well nearly to the top.

4. Bake for 25 minutes, or until the egg puffs have risen and are no longer runny. Remove from the oven and let rest in the pan for 5 minutes. Use a rubber spatula to slide each puff out of the pan.

5. Before serving, dust each puff with powdered erythritol, if using.

6. Store leftovers in an airtight container in the refrigerator for up to 1 week. Reheat in the oven or microwave.

CALORIES: 256 · FAT: 21g · PROTEIN: 11.5g · TOTAL CARBS: 3.3g · DIETARY FIBER: 0.8g · NET CARBS: 2.5g · ERYTHRITOL: 4g

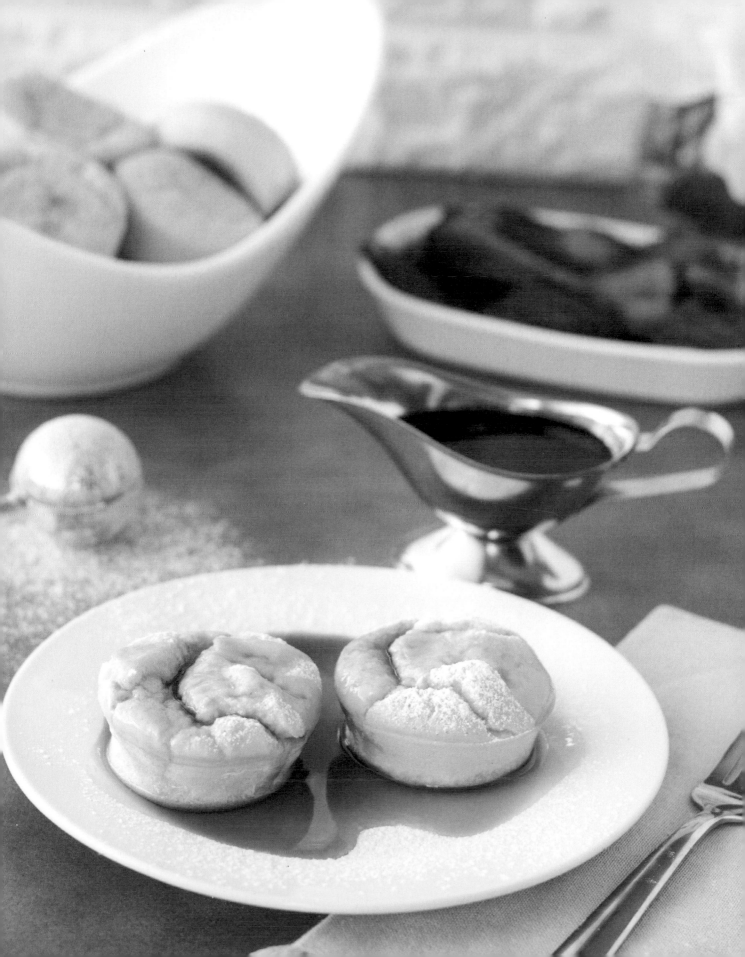

Keto Everything Bagels

NET CARBS
6g

makes 6 bagels (1 per serving) · prep time: 15 minutes · cook time: 14 minutes

Oh, how I miss the days of going to Starbucks for a mocha and a toasted Chonga bagel with cream cheese. The Chonga bagel is their version of an everything bagel—sinfully delicious. There are not a lot of things that I miss from my old lifestyle, but those comforting morning trips to Starbucks are one of them. But these days, I'm not missing out on anything. I'm making my Boosted Coffee (page 140) and low-carb bagels at home instead.

ingredients

2 cups blanched almond flour

1 tablespoon baking powder

1 teaspoon garlic powder

1 teaspoon onion powder

1 teaspoon Italian seasoning

3 cups shredded low-moisture, part-skim mozzarella cheese

2½ ounces full-fat cream cheese (5 tablespoons)

3 large eggs, divided

3 tablespoons Everything Bagel Seasoning (page 352)

tip: If everything bagels aren't your thing, you can always omit the bagel seasoning and make a seriously delicious plain bagel.

directions

1. Preheat the oven to 425°F. Line a rimmed baking sheet with parchment paper or a silicone baking mat.

2. In a medium mixing bowl, combine the almond flour, baking powder, garlic powder, onion powder, and Italian seasoning. Mix until well combined. I like to put the mixture through a flour sifter to ensure that all of the baking powder gets mixed in with the rest of the ingredients.

3. In a large microwave-safe mixing bowl, combine the mozzarella and cream cheese. Microwave for 1 minute 30 seconds. Remove from the microwave and stir to combine. Return to the microwave for 1 additional minute. Mix until well combined.

4. To the large mixing bowl, add two of the eggs and the almond flour mixture. Using your hands, mix until the ingredients are well incorporated. If you are having a hard time mixing the ingredients together, put the bowl back in the microwave for another 20 to 30 seconds to soften. If the dough starts sticking to your hands, wet your hands slightly and continue working the dough.

5. Divide the dough into 6 equal portions. Using your hands, roll each portion into a ball. Gently press your finger into the center of each dough ball to form a ring. Stretch the ring to make a small hole, about the size of a quarter, in the center and form it into a bagel shape.

6. Make the egg wash: Crack the remaining egg into a small bowl and whisk with a fork.

7. Brush each bagel with the egg wash. Sprinkle the top of each bagel with 1½ teaspoons of the bagel seasoning.

8. Bake on the middle rack for 12 to 14 minutes, until golden brown.

9. Store in a resealable plastic bag in the refrigerator for up to 5 days. Reheat in the oven or toaster.

CALORIES: 449 · FAT: 35.5g · PROTEIN: 27.8g · TOTAL CARBS: 10g · DIETARY FIBER: 4g · NET CARBS: 6g

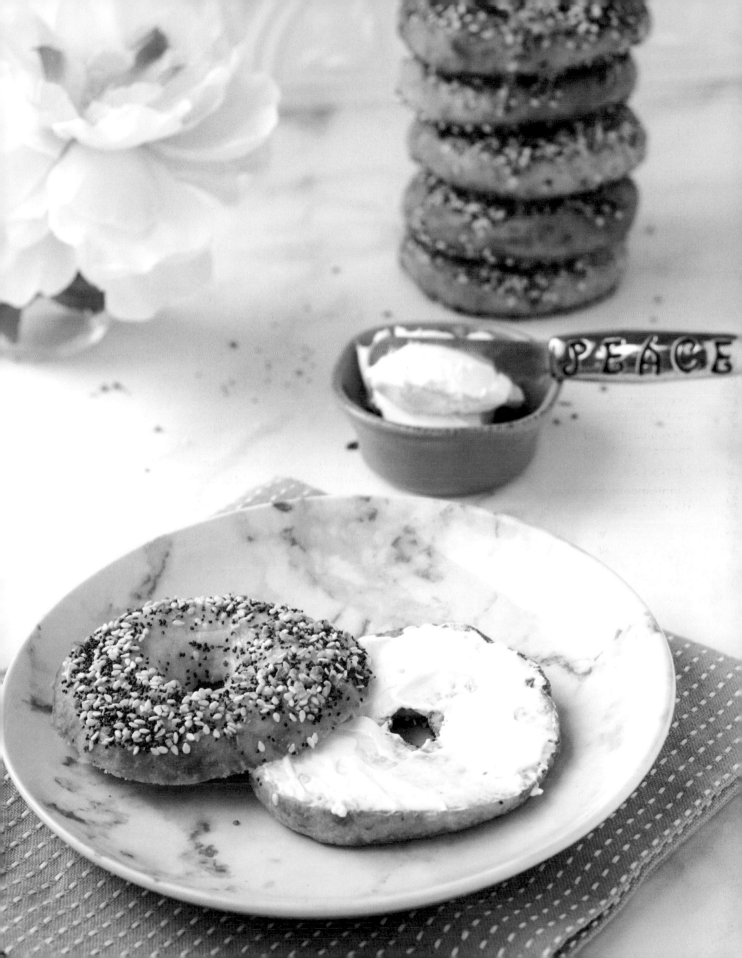

Creamy Herbed
Bacon and Egg Skillet

NET CARBS
3.8g

 makes 4 servings · prep time: 10 minutes · cook time: 15 minutes

Cooking breakfast really doesn't get much simpler than this. If you can stir, you can make this dish. I have played around with different cheeses—be sure to try it with goat cheese! Breakfast doesn't have to be boring, and a delicious breakfast doesn't have to be time-consuming. This recipe is ready and on the table in less than thirty minutes.

ingredients

½ cup heavy cream

¼ cup full-fat sour cream

2 tablespoons chopped fresh chives

2 tablespoons chopped fresh flat-leaf parsley

1 tablespoon chopped fresh dill weed

1 teaspoon garlic powder

1 teaspoon onion powder

¼ teaspoon sea salt

¼ teaspoon ground black pepper

8 large eggs

6 slices bacon, cooked crisp and crumbled

¼ cup crumbled feta cheese

directions

1. Preheat the oven to 425°F.

2. In a large ovenproof skillet, combine the heavy cream, sour cream, chives, parsley, dill, garlic powder, onion powder, salt, and pepper. Whisk to combine and bring to a low boil over medium-low heat.

3. Crack the eggs into the skillet. Transfer the skillet to the oven. Bake until the whites are set and the yolks have reached the desired level of doneness. (About 10 minutes of baking time will give you runny yolks; bake longer if you prefer set yolks.)

4. Remove the skillet from the oven and sprinkle the bacon and feta over the top.

CALORIES: 321 · FAT: 25g · PROTEIN: 20g · TOTAL CARBS: 4.3g · DIETARY FIBER: 0.5g · NET CARBS: 3.8g

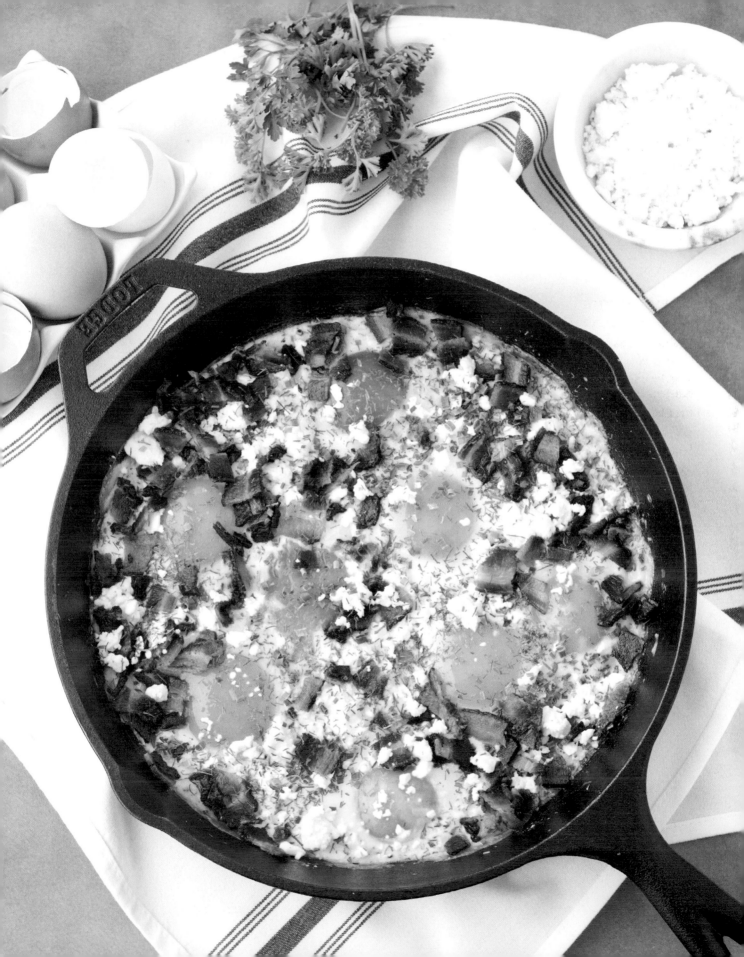

Easy Peasy Maple Blender Pancakes

makes eight 5- to 6-inch pancakes (2 per serving)
prep time: 10 minutes · cook time: 20 minutes

These pancakes are so easy that even your kids can make them—that is, if they are old enough to use the stove. This is one of our favorite Saturday morning family breakfasts: it is guilt-free comfort food at its finest. We like to top the pancakes with a little salted grass-fed butter and sugar-free maple syrup.

ingredients

2 ounces full-fat cream cheese (¼ cup), softened

2 ounces full-fat ricotta cheese (¼ cup)

4 large eggs

2 tablespoons granular erythritol

2 teaspoons sugar-free maple extract

1 teaspoon pure vanilla extract

¼ cup coconut flour

2 teaspoons baking powder

½ teaspoon ground cinnamon

Butter or ghee, for the pan

directions

1. In a blender, combine the cream cheese, ricotta cheese, and eggs. Pulse until smooth.

2. To the blender, add the erythritol, maple extract, vanilla extract, coconut flour, baking powder, and cinnamon. Pulse until the ingredients are well combined and the batter is smooth.

3. Brush a large nonstick skillet or griddle pan with butter and heat over medium-low heat. When the pan is hot, add ¼ cup of the batter and cook until bubbly on the top and golden brown on the bottom, about 3 minutes. Flip and cook the other side until golden brown, 2 to 3 minutes. Repeat this process until all of the batter is gone, regreasing the skillet between pancakes.

4. Store leftovers in a resealable plastic bag in the fridge for up to 5 days. Reheat in a preheated 200°F oven until warmed through.

CALORIES: 177 · FAT: 12g · PROTEIN: 10g · TOTAL CARBS: 5.5g · DIETARY FIBER: 2.8g · NET CARBS: 2.8g · ERYTHRITOL: 6g

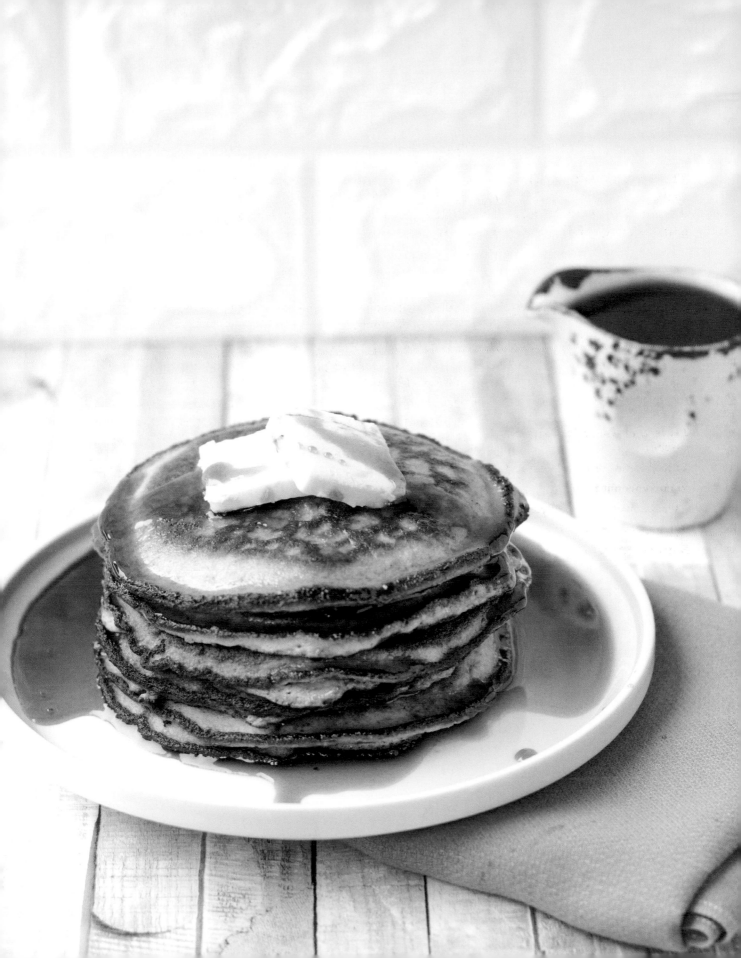

Cranberry Cream Cheese Spread

 EGG-FREE NUT-FREE makes 2 cups (2 tablespoons per serving)
prep time: 5 minutes · cook time: 25 minutes

I love to serve this cream cheese spread on Keto Everything Bagels (page 130). I enjoy the strong contrast of sweet and savory. If you do not wish to use orange juice or zest, you can substitute a teaspoon of pure orange extract. This substitution will lower the overall carb count even further, and the spread will taste just as great.

ingredients

1 cup fresh cranberries

¼ cup granular erythritol

1 tablespoon grated orange zest

2 tablespoons fresh orange juice

1 (8-ounce) package full-fat cream cheese

Leaves from a few fresh mint sprigs, chopped, for garnish (optional)

directions

1. In a small saucepan over medium-high heat, combine the cranberries, erythritol, orange zest, and orange juice. Simmer until the berries begin to pop and the sauce begins to thicken. You can speed things along by smashing the berries with a fork as they pop.

2. Once the berries start to pop, reduce the heat to low and simmer gently, stirring occasionally, for 10 minutes.

3. Let the berries cool, then mix in the cream cheese. Garnish with fresh mint before serving, if desired. Store in the refrigerator for up to 2 weeks.

CALORIES: 55 · FAT: 4.5g · PROTEIN: 1g · TOTAL CARBS: 1.7g · DIETARY FIBER: 0.3g · NET CARBS: 1.4g · ERYTHRITOL: 3g

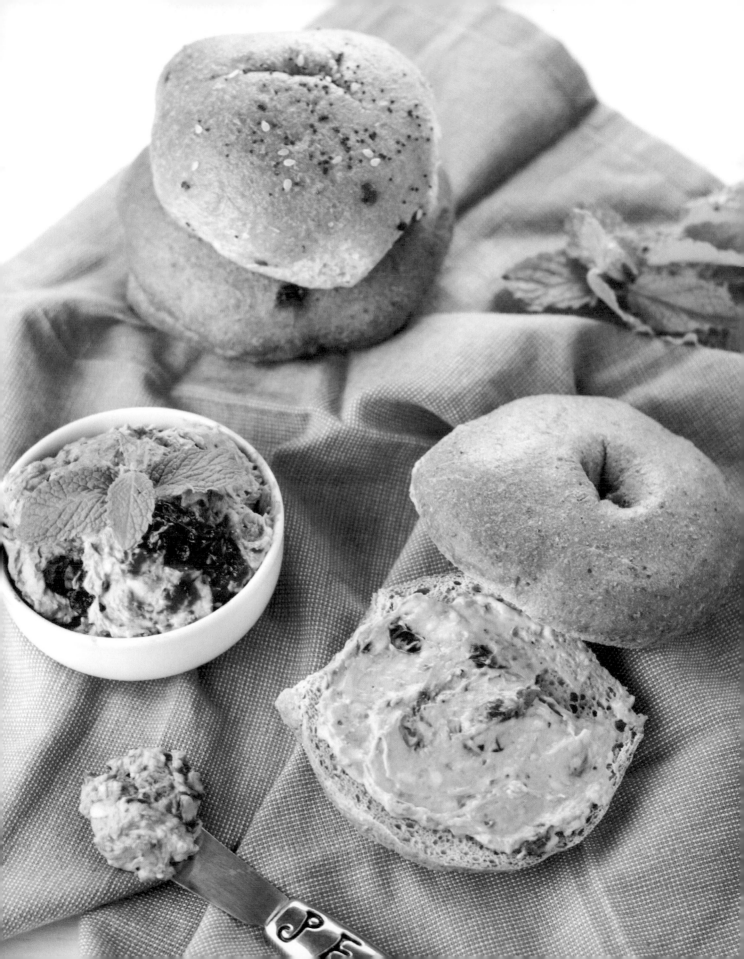

Chocolate Peanut Butter Waffles

makes 6 Belgian-style waffles (1 per serving)
prep time: 15 minutes · cook time: 30 minutes

These waffles pack so much flavor that they are great even without syrup. They also freeze and reheat well. I like to make a double batch, freeze them, and then reheat them in the toaster. It makes those hectic weekday mornings just a little bit easier—and I can have a weekend-style breakfast all week long.

ingredients

5 large eggs

1 cup reduced-sugar creamy peanut butter

¾ cup powdered erythritol

2 teaspoons pure vanilla extract

¾ cup water

¼ cup coconut flour

¼ cup unsweetened cocoa powder

½ teaspoon baking soda

Butter or coconut oil, for the waffle iron

tips: For a crispier waffle, try toasting it after cooking it in the waffle iron.

To lower the carb count even further, substitute unsalted almond butter for the peanut butter.

directions

1. Preheat a waffle iron.

2. Put the eggs, peanut butter, erythritol, vanilla extract, and water in a large mixing bowl. Using a hand mixer, beat until the ingredients are well combined.

3. In a separate mixing bowl, whisk together the coconut flour, cocoa powder, and baking soda until well combined.

4. Use a rubber spatula to fold the dry ingredients into the wet ingredients. Mix until the ingredients are well incorporated and the batter is smooth.

5. Lightly grease the waffle iron. Ladle the batter onto the center of the waffle iron; the amount will vary by waffle iron. Consult the manufacturer's directions for the recommended amount of batter.

6. Cook for 5 minutes or until the waffle iron stops steaming. Repeat this process until all of the batter is gone, regreasing the iron between waffles.

CALORIES: 368 · FAT: 28g · PROTEIN: 17g · TOTAL CARBS: 13g · DIETARY FIBER: 5.7g · NET CARBS: 7.3g · ERYTHRITOL: 24g

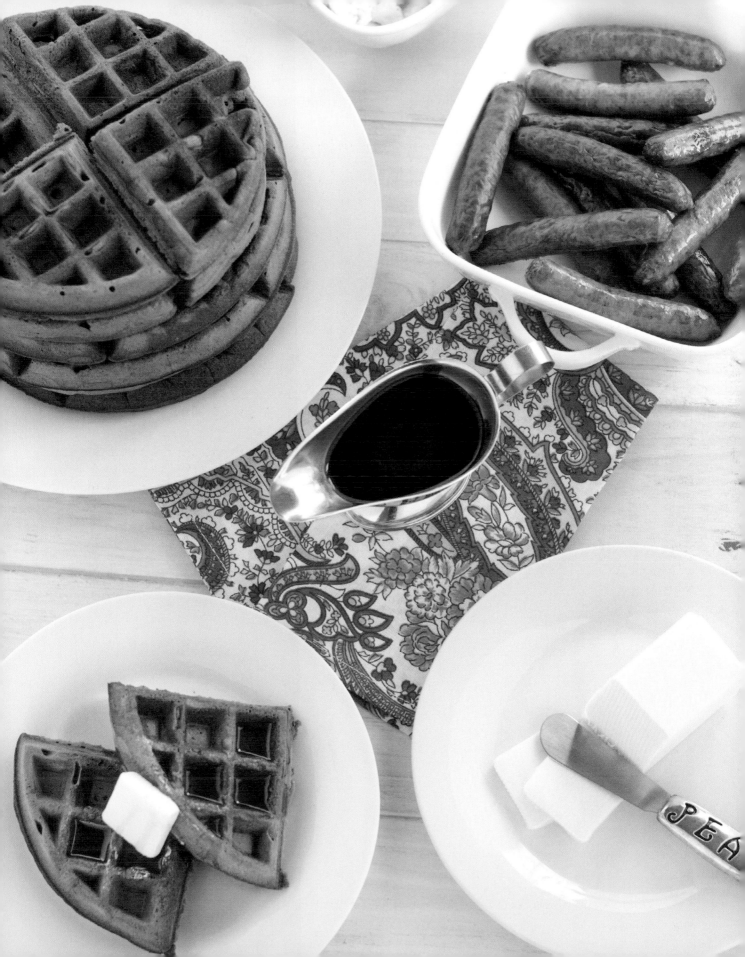

Boosted Coffee

   makes 1 serving · prep time: 5 minutes

Drinking boosted coffee is a great way to start your day with healthy fats and an extra hit of energy. It really helps curb my hunger and keep cravings at bay. It keeps me feeling satiated for hours. When I drink boosted coffee for breakfast, I am typically not hungry until well into the afternoon. Not to mention that it just tastes really great.

ingredients

8 ounces hot dark-roast coffee

1 tablespoon butter or ghee

1 tablespoon heavy cream

1 tablespoon coconut oil or MCT oil powder

1 tablespoon grass-fed collagen peptides

1 tablespoon powdered erythritol, or more to taste (optional)

directions

Combine all of the ingredients in a milk frother or blender. Blend until frothy and creamy.

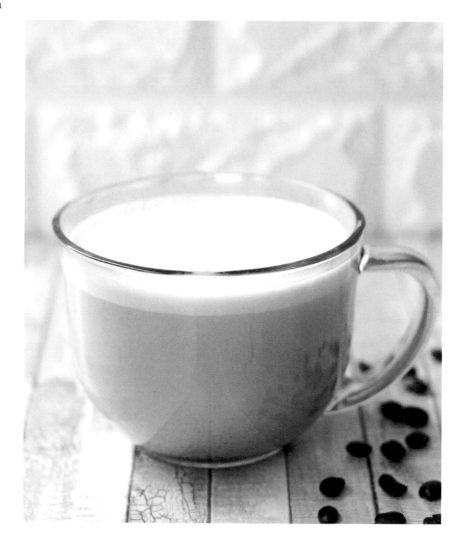

CALORIES: 299 · FAT: 31g · PROTEIN: 7g · TOTAL CARBS: 0 · DIETARY FIBER: 0 · NET CARBS: 0

Vanilla Coffee Creamer

  makes 2½ cups (2 tablespoons per serving)
prep time: 5 minutes · cook time: 15 minutes

Is a sweet coffee creamer something you have been missing in your low-carb lifestyle? Well, now you don't have to miss it any longer. This creamer is super easy to make and is free of all the nasty chemicals and synthetic ingredients in store-bought coffee creamers.

ingredients

1½ cups heavy cream

1 (14½-ounce) can coconut cream

¼ cup powdered erythritol

1 tablespoon vanilla bean paste

1 teaspoon pure vanilla extract

Pinch of sea salt

tips: Don't have vanilla bean paste? You can use a freshly scraped vanilla bean or extra vanilla extract.

Try changing up the flavor by using different sugar-free pure extracts.

To make a dairy-free version, substitute almond milk, coconut milk, or cashew milk for the heavy cream.

directions

1. In a medium saucepan, combine all of the ingredients. Bring to a boil over medium-high heat, whisking continuously, then reduce the heat to low and simmer for 10 to 15 minutes.

2. Let cool, then transfer to a 32-ounce mason jar. Store in the refrigerator for up to 2 weeks. Shake before using.

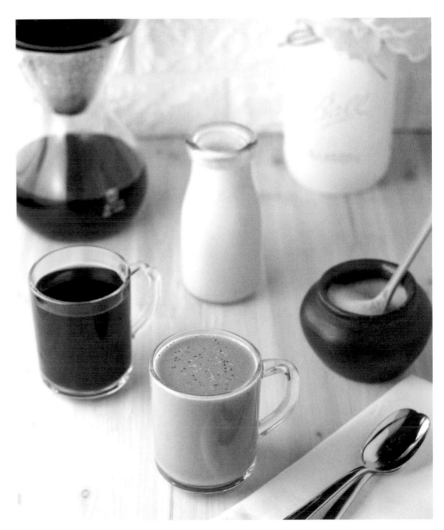

CALORIES: 121 · FAT: 12.5g · PROTEIN: 1g · TOTAL CARBS: 1.4g · DIETARY FIBER: 0.7g · NET CARBS: 0.7g · ERYTHRITOL: 2.4g

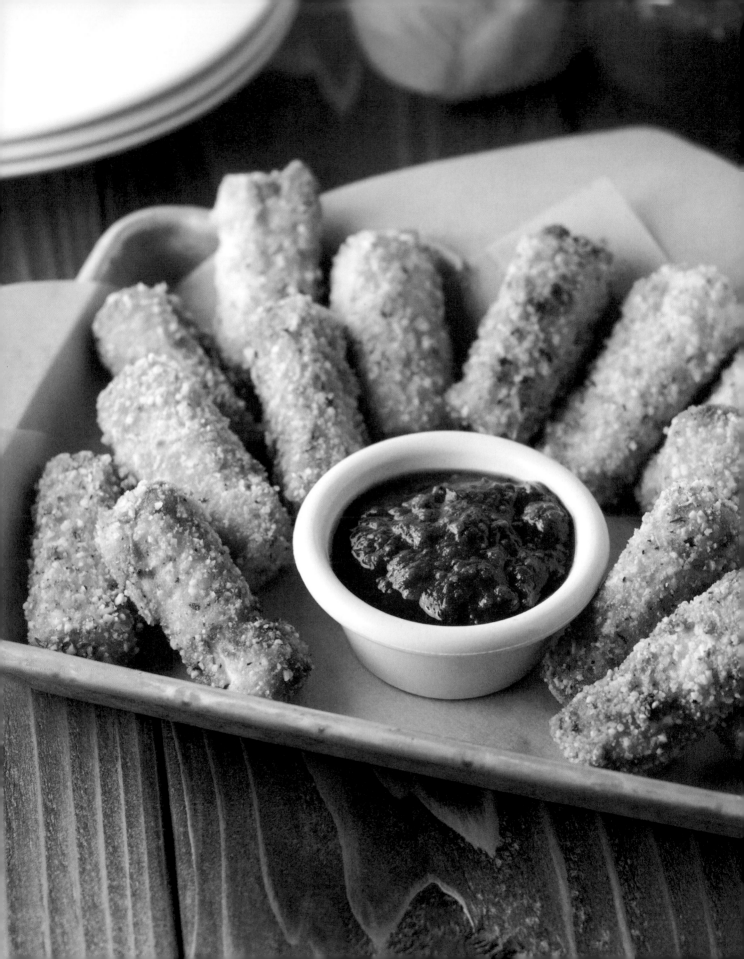

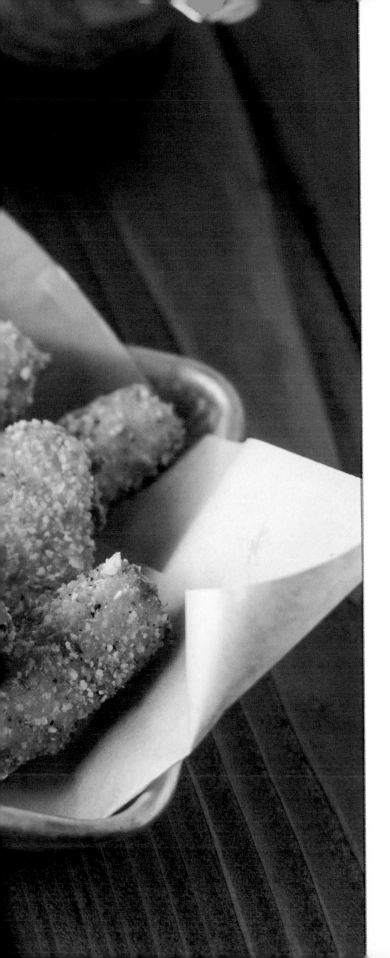

Snacks & Starters

Parmesan Italian Breadsticks

makes 10 breadsticks (1 per serving) · prep time: 10 minutes · cook time: 12 minutes

These breadsticks are the perfect accompaniment to just about any dinner. But when I think of breadsticks, my mind instantly goes to pasta. I love to serve these breadsticks with the Chicken Zoodle Alfredo on page 252 or with a monstrous amount of Pizza Sauce (page 343) for dipping. Sometimes I swear that what I am eating is just a vessel for delivering the sauce. Sauce and breadstick lovers unite!

ingredients

¼ cup blanched almond flour

3 tablespoons coconut flour

1½ teaspoons Italian seasoning, divided

1 teaspoon baking powder

1 teaspoon garlic powder

1 teaspoon onion powder

½ teaspoon sea salt

1½ cups shredded low-moisture, part-skim mozzarella cheese

1 ounce full-fat cream cheese (2 tablespoons)

1 large egg

2 tablespoons butter or ghee, melted

3 tablespoons grated Parmesan cheese

Finely chopped fresh flat-leaf parsley, for garnish (optional)

tip: I recommend reheating the breadsticks in a preheated 275°F oven and then brushing a little melted butter over the top.

directions

1. Preheat the oven to 400°F. Line a rimmed baking sheet with parchment paper or a silicone baking mat.

2. In a small mixing bowl, combine the almond flour, coconut flour, ½ teaspoon of the Italian seasoning, baking powder, garlic powder, onion powder, and salt.

3. In a separate mixing bowl, combine the mozzarella and cream cheese. Microwave for 1 minute 30 seconds to soften. Mix the cheeses together until they are well combined. If the mixture gets stringy or is not quite melted enough, put the bowl back in the microwave for another 30 seconds.

4. Add the dry ingredients and the egg to the cheese mixture. Using your hands, mix until the ingredients are well incorporated. If you are having a hard time mixing the ingredients together, put the bowl back in the microwave for another 20 to 30 seconds to soften. If the dough starts sticking to your hands, wet your hands slightly and continue working the dough.

5. Use your hands to spread the dough on the prepared baking sheet in a thin, even rectangle about 12 by 9 inches.

6. Using a pizza cutter, cut the dough crosswise into 10 even breadsticks, about 1⅛ inches wide. Pull the breadsticks apart just slightly and sprinkle the remaining 1 teaspoon of Italian seasoning over the top.

7. Bake for 12 minutes, until golden brown.

8. Before serving, but while still warm, brush the melted butter over the breadsticks, then sprinkle them with the Parmesan cheese and some chopped parsley, if using.

9. Store leftovers in an airtight container in the refrigerator for up to 1 week.

CALORIES: 120 · FAT: 9g · PROTEIN: 7.3g · TOTAL CARBS: 3g · DIETARY FIBER: 1.1g · NET CARBS: 1.9g

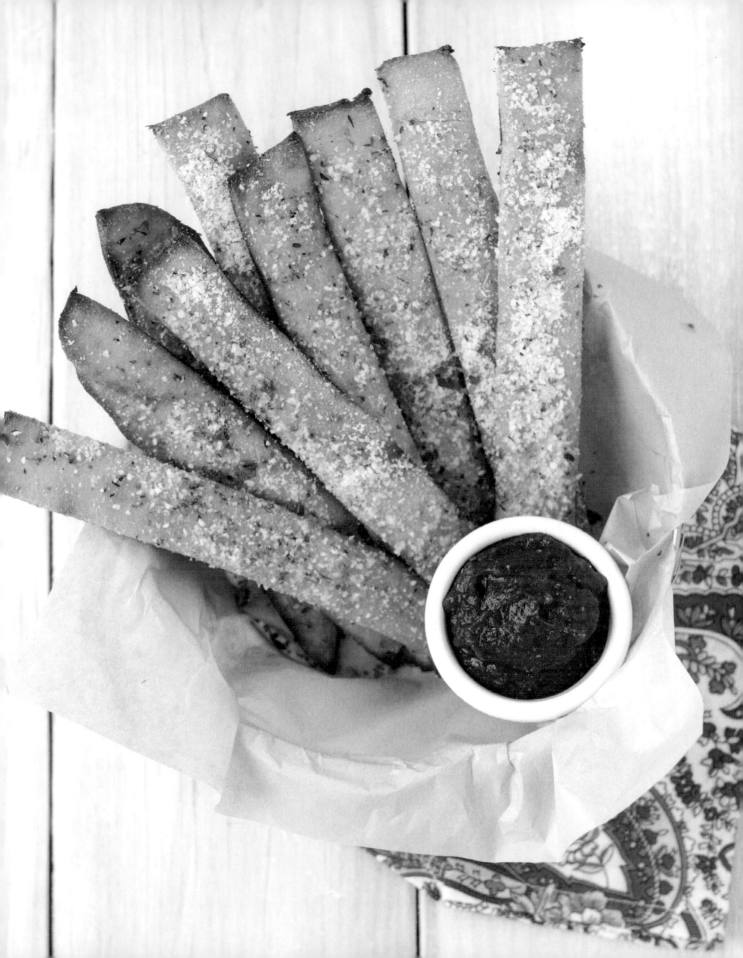

Warm Mediterranean Goat Cheese Dip

  makes 2 cups (¼ cup per serving) · prep time: 15 minutes · cook time: 20 minutes

I love to serve this dip with crispy salami chips (see tips below) and crunchy mini seedless cucumber slices.

ingredients

8 ounces fresh (soft) goat cheese

4 ounces full-fat cream cheese (½ cup), softened

¼ cup crumbled feta cheese, divided

2 tablespoons chopped Kalamata olives

2 tablespoons chopped sun-dried tomatoes

2 tablespoons chopped fresh chives, plus more for garnish

2 cloves garlic, minced

1 tablespoon diced red onions

1 tablespoon capers

4 canned artichoke hearts, roughly chopped

1 tablespoon chopped fresh basil, plus more for garnish

1 tablespoon chopped fresh flat-leaf parsley

Pinch of red pepper flakes

Ground black pepper

directions

1. Preheat the oven to 350°F.

2. In a 6-inch baking dish, combine the goat cheese, cream cheese, 2 tablespoons of the feta, olives, sun-dried tomatoes, chives, garlic, red onions, capers, artichoke hearts, basil, parsley, red pepper flakes, and black pepper to taste. Mix until the ingredients are well incorporated.

3. Bake for 20 minutes, until bubbling. Garnish with the remaining feta and more fresh basil and chives.

tips: If you aren't a fan of goat cheese, try making this dip with all cream cheese.

Making your own crispy salami chips for dipping is easy. Simply lay salami slices in a single layer on a rimmed baking sheet lined with parchment paper. Bake in a preheated 325°F oven for 20 minutes or until the salami is crispy and starts to brown just slightly.

CALORIES: 145 · FAT: 11g · PROTEIN: 7g · TOTAL CARBS: 1.9g · DIETARY FIBER: 0.2g · NET CARBS: 1.7g

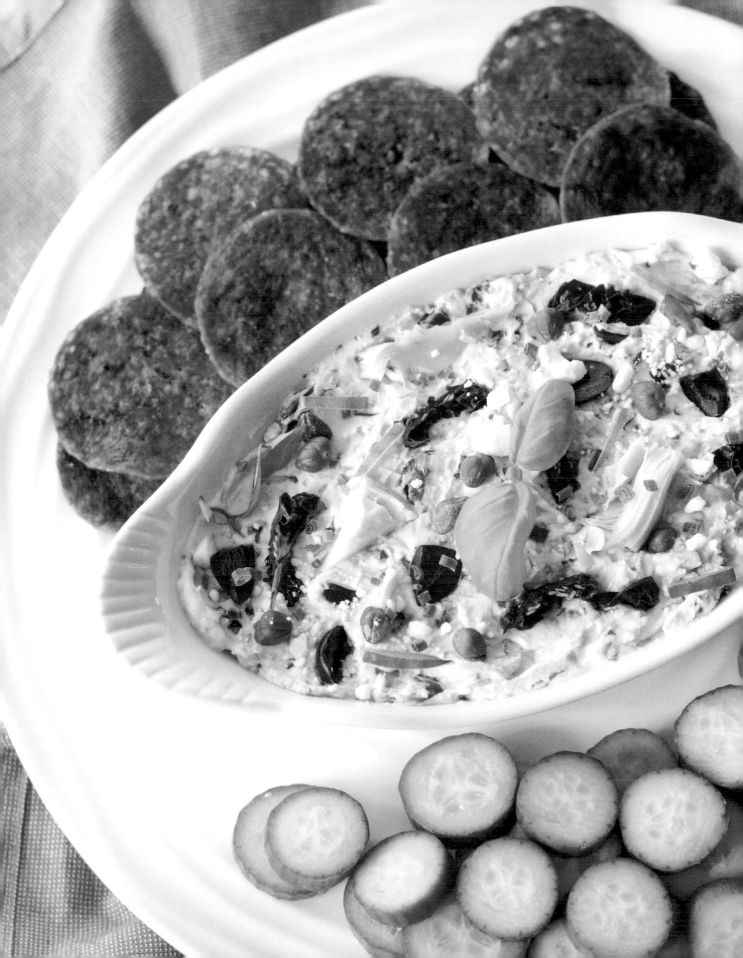

Tuna Salad Pickle Boats

    makes 10 pickle boats (2 per serving) · prep time: 15 minutes

This is one of my favorite lazy lunches. Not only does it have me eating within fifteen minutes, but it consists of ingredients I always have on hand. Quick and easy is the name of the game with these pickle boats.

ingredients

5 large dill pickles, halved

2 (5-ounce) cans sustainably caught albacore tuna, drained

½ cup mayonnaise, store-bought or homemade (page 336), or more to taste

1 tablespoon spicy brown mustard

1 rib celery, finely chopped

1 teaspoon dried minced onions

1 teaspoon garlic powder

2 tablespoons Everything Bagel Seasoning (page 352)

1 tablespoon chopped fresh chives

directions

1. Use a spoon to gently scrape the seeds out of the center of each pickle, creating a well in which to stuff the tuna salad. Put the scrapings in a large mixing bowl.

2. Add the tuna, mayonnaise, mustard, celery, dried minced onions, and garlic powder to the bowl. Mix until the ingredients are well combined.

3. Divide the tuna mixture evenly among the pickles. Sprinkle them with the bagel seasoning and chives before serving.

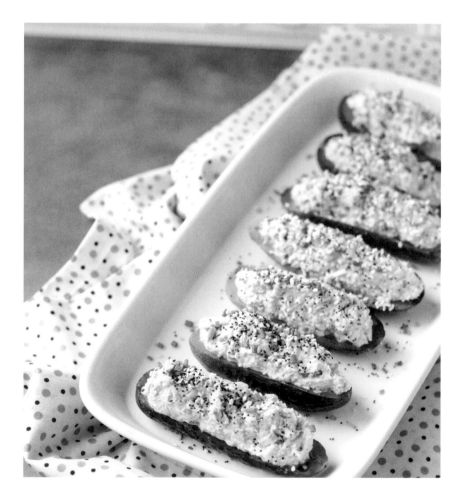

CALORIES: 279 · FAT: 23g · PROTEIN: 14g · TOTAL CARBS: 2.5g · DIETARY FIBER: 0.4g · NET CARBS: 2.1g

Avocado Feta Salsa

  makes 6 servings · prep time: 15 minutes, plus 1 to 2 hours to refrigerate

I love how fresh and light this salsa is. It enhances so many different dishes and pairs perfectly with any Mexican-inspired dish. I even love it on my morning eggs. But perhaps my favorite way to serve it is alongside the Steak Fajita Bowls on page 210.

ingredients

1 large avocado, peeled, pitted, and cubed

1 Roma tomato, diced

3 cloves garlic, minced

¼ cup chopped red onions

¼ cup chopped canned artichoke hearts

¼ cup capers

¼ cup crumbled feta cheese

2 tablespoons olive oil

Juice of ½ lime

Sea salt and ground black pepper, to taste

1 tablespoon chopped fresh cilantro (optional)

directions

Combine all of the ingredients in a large mixing bowl and toss to combine. Refrigerate for 1 to 2 hours before serving. This salsa is best the day it is made.

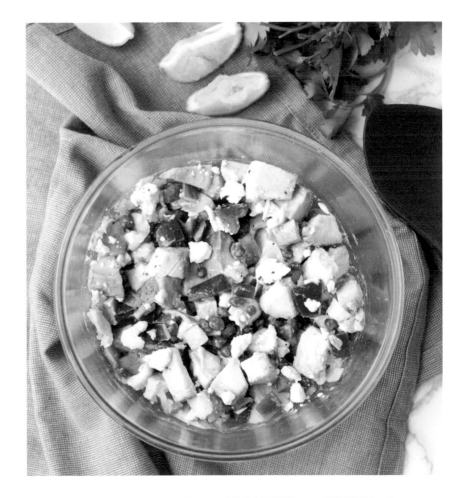

CALORIES: 133 · FAT: 10.5g · PROTEIN: 3.4g · TOTAL CARBS: 6.8g · DIETARY FIBER: 3g · NET CARBS: 3.8g

Marinated Mozzarella Balls

NET CARBS
2.5g

  makes 8 servings · prep time: 10 minutes, plus up to 24 hours to refrigerate

These mozzarella balls are beautiful as the centerpiece of an antipasto tray. When I entertain, I always make these, and they are usually the first thing to go. Another fun way to serve them is to skewer them with different meats and vegetables and make antipasto kebabs. For this recipe, I use avocado oil over the traditional olive oil because it is lighter and more mild-flavored. It really allows the flavors of the other ingredients to shine.

ingredients

16 ounces fresh mozzarella cheese balls (cherry sized), drained

2 cloves garlic, minced

¾ cup avocado oil

1 teaspoon Italian seasoning

½ teaspoon onion powder

½ teaspoon red pepper flakes

¼ teaspoon sea salt, or more to taste

¼ teaspoon ground black pepper

directions

Combine all of the ingredients in a large mixing bowl with a lid. Refrigerate for up to 24 hours before serving to allow the flavors to fully come together. Store leftovers in the fridge for up to 1 week.

CALORIES: 328 · FAT: 31g · PROTEIN: 10g · TOTAL CARBS: 2.5g · DIETARY FIBER: 0 · NET CARBS: 2.5g

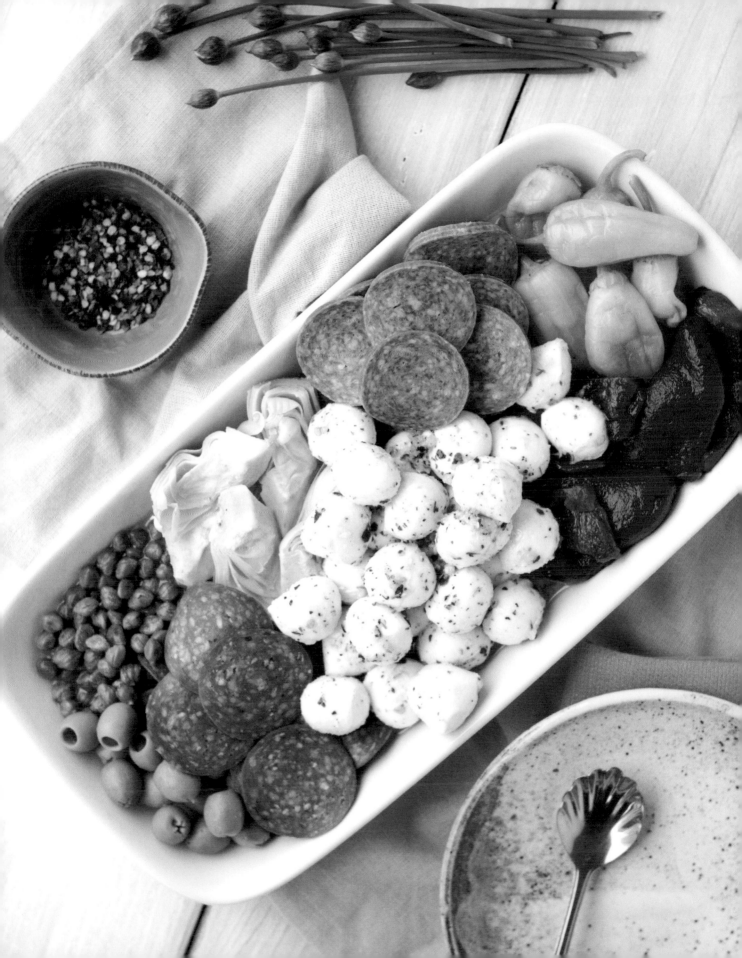

Sour Lemon Gummy Snacks

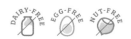

makes 110 gummy snacks (10 per serving)
prep time: 10 minutes, plus 1 hour to set · cook time: 5 minutes

Not only are these gummy snacks super quick and easy to make, but they also pack a great health punch. Grass-fed gelatin is amazing for healthy hair, skin, and nails. It helps improve joint health, reduce inflammation, and improve gut health and overall digestive strength. It also helps improve your quality of sleep while supporting healthy adrenal function. You've got to love any snack that is delicious *and* loaded with health benefits.

ingredients

3 tablespoons grass-fed gelatin collagen protein

2 tablespoons powdered erythritol

¼ cup plus 2 tablespoons fresh lemon juice

¼ cup water

Special equipment:

Silicone gummy molds with 110 cavities

directions

1. Combine the gelatin, erythritol, lemon juice, and water in a small saucepan over low heat. Heat, while whisking, to dissolve the gelatin and combine the ingredients. They will form a thick paste. Heat until the mixture is warm and pourable.

2. Transfer the mixture to a measuring cup or bowl with a pour spout, then quickly pour it into the silicone gummy molds.

3. Transfer the molds to the refrigerator to cool and solidify the gummy snacks, about 1 hour. Pop the gummy snacks out of the molds and enjoy!

4. Store leftovers in a sealed jar in the refrigerator for up to 2 weeks.

CALORIES: 8.5 · FAT: 0 · PROTEIN: 1.7g · TOTAL CARBS: 0.5g · DIETARY FIBER: 0 · NET CARBS: 0.5g · ERYTHRITOL: 2g

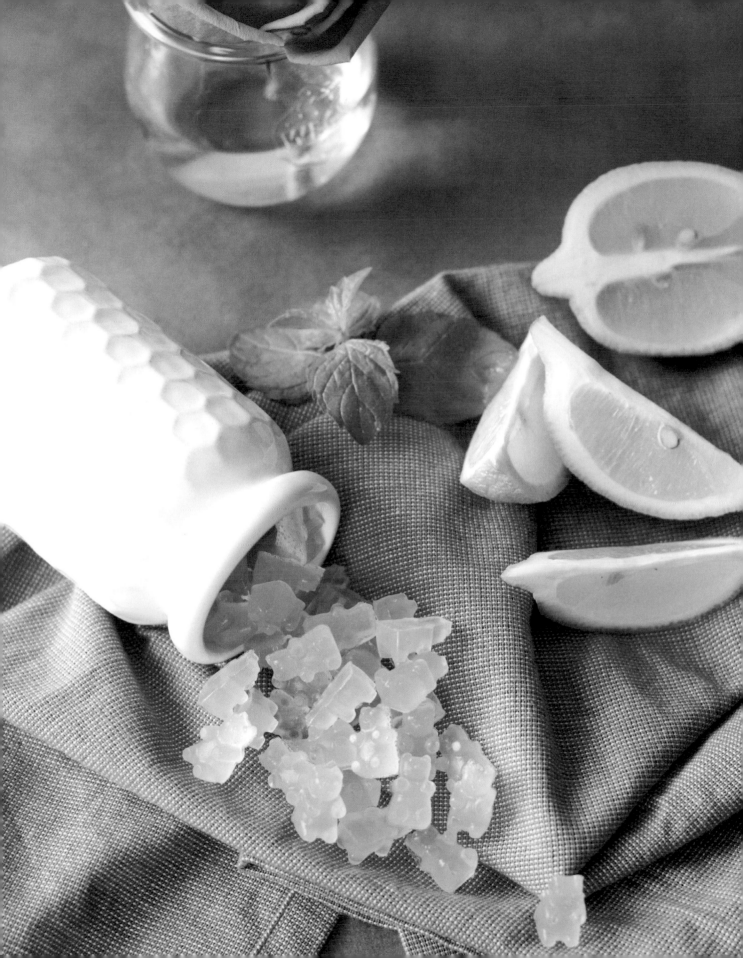

Green Goddess Chicken Dip

NUT-FREE · makes 10 servings · prep time: 15 minutes · cook time: 15 minutes

This dip is terrific when you need something quick and easy to whip up for a potluck or get-together. It is also amazing served warm. I like to heat it in a preheated 275°F oven for about 20 minutes. Serve it with your favorite low-carb dippers. I love it with fresh veggies, cheese crisps, and pork rinds.

ingredients

2 tablespoons butter or ghee

1 pound boneless, skinless chicken breasts or thighs, cut into small pieces

1 (8-ounce) package full-fat cream cheese, softened

½ cup Avocado Green Goddess Dressing (page 333)

1 tablespoon hot sauce, such as Cholula or Tapatio

2 tablespoons diced red onions, plus more for garnish

1 green onion, chopped

1 teaspoon chopped fresh dill weed, plus more for garnish

1 teaspoon fresh lemon juice

2 cloves garlic, minced

6 slices bacon, diced and cooked crisp

Sea salt and ground black pepper (optional)

directions

1. Heat the butter in a large skillet over medium heat. Add the chicken and sear until it is golden brown and cooked all the way through. Set aside.

2. In a large mixing bowl, combine the cream cheese, dressing, hot sauce, red onions, green onion, dill, lemon juice, garlic, and most of the bacon (reserve some for garnish). Mix until the ingredients are well combined.

3. Mix the cooked chicken into the cream cheese mixture. Taste and add salt and pepper, if desired. Garnish with fresh dill, diced red onions, and the reserved bacon before serving.

4. Store leftovers in the refrigerator for up to 1 week. Reheat in the oven or microwave.

CALORIES: 213 · FAT: 17g · PROTEIN: 11g · TOTAL CARBS: 1.9g · DIETARY FIBER: 0.3g · NET CARBS: 1.6g

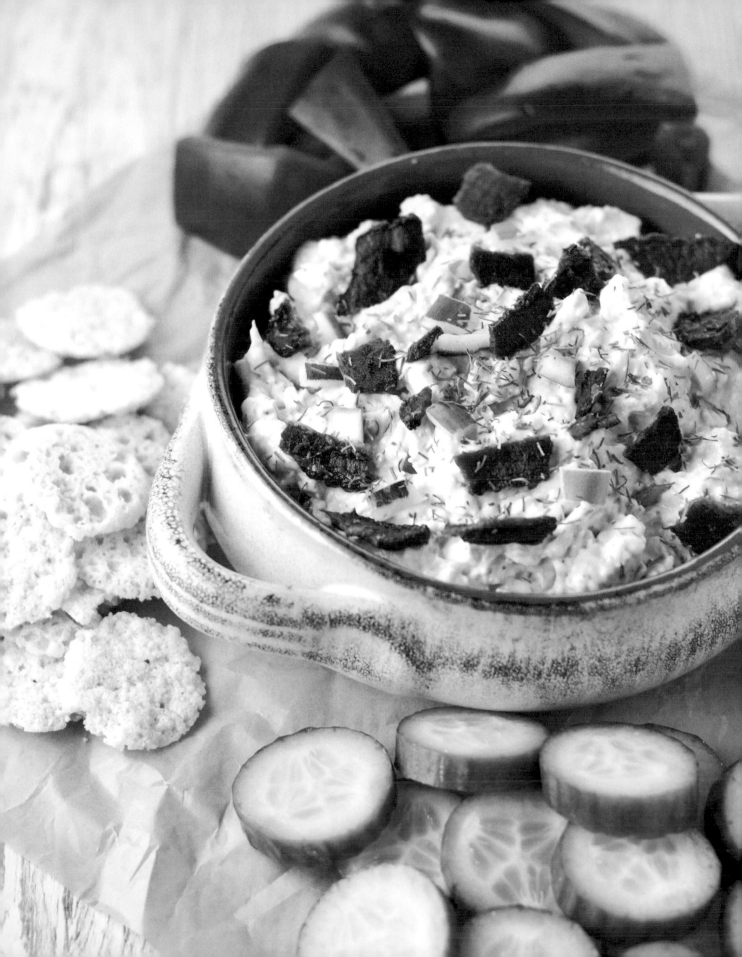

Garlic Dill Quick Pickled Brussels Sprouts

    makes 10 servings · prep time: 15 minutes, plus at least 48 hours to brine
cook time: 5 minutes

Everyone has tried regular pickles. Many people have tried pickled green beans or pickled asparagus, but have you ever tried pickled Brussels sprouts? These tiny cabbage-shaped vegetables have an almost cultlike following, and here is one more way to enjoy them.

ingredients

12 ounces Brussels sprouts, trimmed and halved

1½ cups apple cider vinegar

1 cup water

1½ teaspoons sea salt

10 whole black peppercorns

2 bay leaves

½ teaspoon yellow mustard seeds

Pinch of red pepper flakes

6 cloves garlic, peeled

6 large sprigs fresh dill weed

1 small shallot, thinly sliced

directions

1. In a large saucepan over medium-high heat, combine the Brussels sprouts, vinegar, water, salt, peppercorns, bay leaves, mustard seeds, and red pepper flakes. Bring to a boil. Blanch the Brussels sprouts in the brine for 4 minutes, then use a slotted spoon to transfer them to an ice bath to shock them and stop the cooking process.

2. Once the brine has cooled, pour it into a 32-ounce mason jar. Add the Brussels sprouts, garlic cloves, dill sprigs, and sliced shallot to the jar. Cap the jar and put it in the refrigerator for 48 hours to a week before eating.

3. Store in the refrigerator for up to 3 months.

tip: For extra-crunchy pickled Brussels sprouts, skip the step of boiling them in the liquid. Instead, pack the Brussels sprouts, garlic cloves, dill, and shallot slices into the jar. Bring the vinegar, water, and seasonings to a boil, then pour the hot liquid over the ingredients in the jar. Allow to cool to room temperature, then seal and place the jar in the refrigerator. You may need to let the Brussels sprouts sit in the refrigerator longer in order to adequately pickle them.

CALORIES: 20 · FAT: 0 · PROTEIN: 1.6g · TOTAL CARBS: 4.4g · DIETARY FIBER: 1.6g · NET CARBS: 2.8g

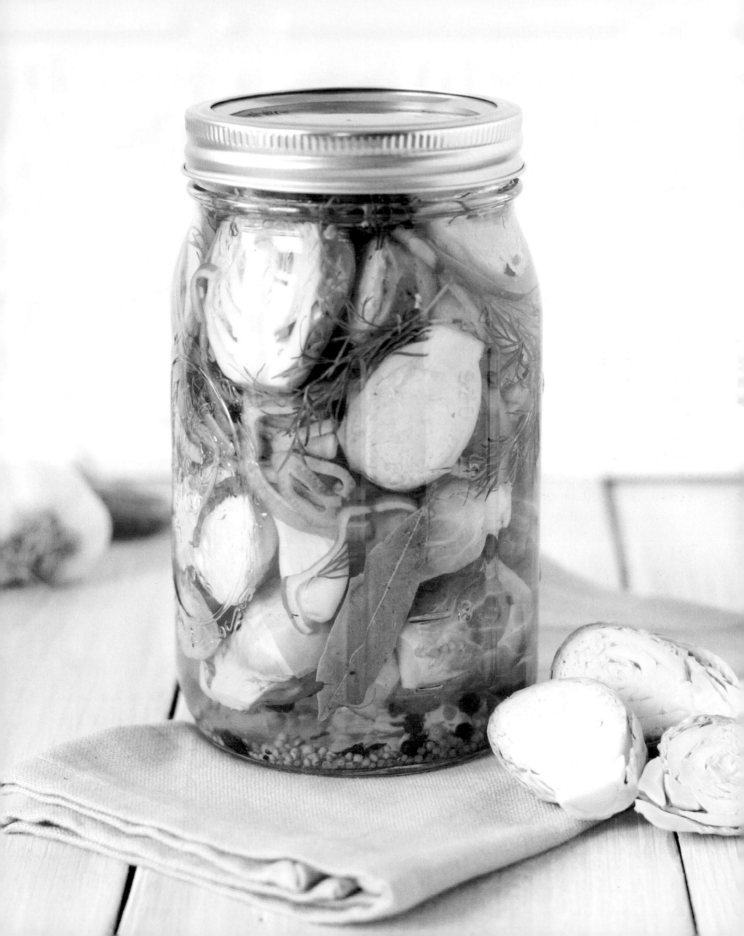

Garlic Dill Baked Cucumber Chips

    makes 6 servings · prep time: 15 minutes · cook time: 3 to 4 hours

Savory, crunchy snacks are my weakness. I used to joke that Doritos were my kryptonite. Put me in front of a plate of sweets, and I will be fine to ignore them. Place me in front of a bowl of chips or crackers, and it is like a tractor beam pulling me in. Salty and crunchy is my jam! So naturally, giving up my favorite savory snacks was one of the harder things for me when I switched over to a real-food, low-carb lifestyle. However, I am a firm believer in the fact that you don't have to sacrifice your favorite flavors and textures to live a healthy and balanced life. Instead, you just have to reframe the way you look at food and get a little creative in the kitchen. Sure, I would rather have potato chips or tortilla chips than cucumber chips. I would be lying if I said otherwise. But I love that there are healthy low-carb options out there. Not to mention that cucumber and dill is one of my all-time favorite flavor pairings. I'm pretty sure that is evident throughout this cookbook. These chips are delicious served with the Ranch Dressing on page 332.

ingredients

2 large seedless cucumbers, 8 to 10 inches long

1 tablespoon dried dill weed

1 teaspoon garlic powder

1 teaspoon onion powder

1 tablespoon apple cider vinegar

Sea salt

tips: The thickness of your cucumber slices and the heat of your oven will determine the exact cook time.

You can get thinner slices by using a mandoline. It is not necessary, but it is definitely recommended.

directions

1. Thinly slice the cucumbers into ⅛-inch slices.

2. In a single layer, line the cucumbers on a paper towel. Place another paper towel on top and press it into the cucumbers to draw out the excess moisture. Repeat this process twice if necessary. The drier the cucumber slices are at this stage, the crisper they will get as they bake.

3. Place the dry cucumber slices in a large mixing bowl.

4. Preheat the oven to 170°F.

5. In a small mixing bowl, combine the dill, garlic powder, onion powder, and vinegar. Spoon the herb mixture over the cucumber slices and toss until each cucumber is saturated.

6. Line two rimmed baking sheets with parchment paper. Lay the cucumber slices on the parchment in a single layer. Sprinkle with a little salt.

7. Bake for 3 to 4 hours, rotating the baking sheets halfway through, until the chips are dried and crispy.

CALORIES: 19 · FAT: 0 · PROTEIN: 0.8g · TOTAL CARBS: 4.5g · DIETARY FIBER: 0.7g · NET CARBS: 3.8g

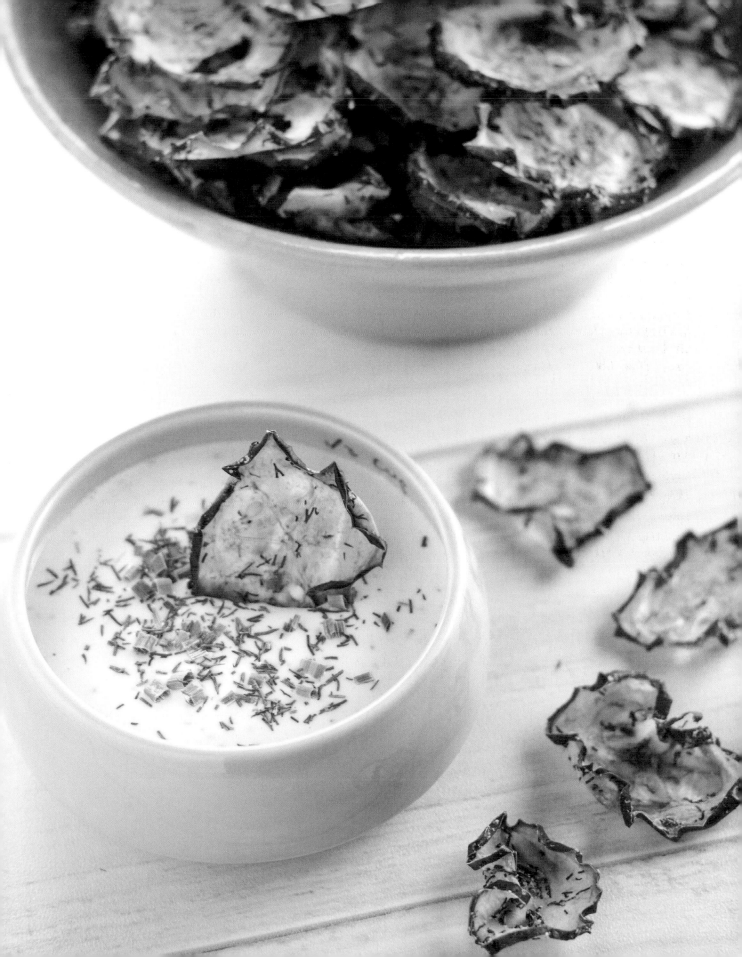

Fried Mozzarella Sticks

makes 16 mozzarella sticks (4 per serving)
prep time: 15 minutes, plus 3 hours to freeze · cook time: 6 minutes

These fried mozzarella sticks are a hot commodity in our house. I have to make a double or triple batch just to ensure that I get to eat a couple of them. They disappear fast—just like your favorite fried bar food, but without the guilt or the upset stomach. I love to serve these with the Garlic and Herb Marinara Sauce on page 344. I like to bread several mozzarella sticks at a time and keep them in the freezer so I always have some prepped and ready to fry.

ingredients

2 tablespoons coconut flour

2 large eggs, whisked

1 batch Savory Breading Mix (page 354)

8 mozzarella string cheese sticks, halved crosswise

Cooking oil, such as avocado oil or tallow

tip: For a nut-free version, use the Nut-Free Keto Breading Mix on page 355.

directions

1. Set up three shallow bowls in a row. Put the coconut flour in the first bowl, the whisked eggs in the second bowl, and the breading mix in the third bowl.

2. Dredge each cheese stick in the coconut flour, then coat it in the egg wash. Finish it off by coating it in the breading mix. Repeat this three-step process with each cheese stick.

3. Freeze the breaded cheese sticks for 3 hours.

4. Heat 1 to 2 inches of oil in a large 4-inch-deep (or deeper) skillet or Dutch oven over medium-high heat. Once the oil is hot and begins to bubble slightly, gently drop the cheese sticks into the oil and fry until they are golden brown and crispy, 2 to 3 minutes on each side.

5. Remove the cheese sticks from the oil and place them on paper towels to absorb the excess oil before serving.

CALORIES: 349 · FAT: 26g · PROTEIN: 26g · TOTAL CARBS: 8.8g · DIETARY FIBER: 3g · NET CARBS: 5.8g

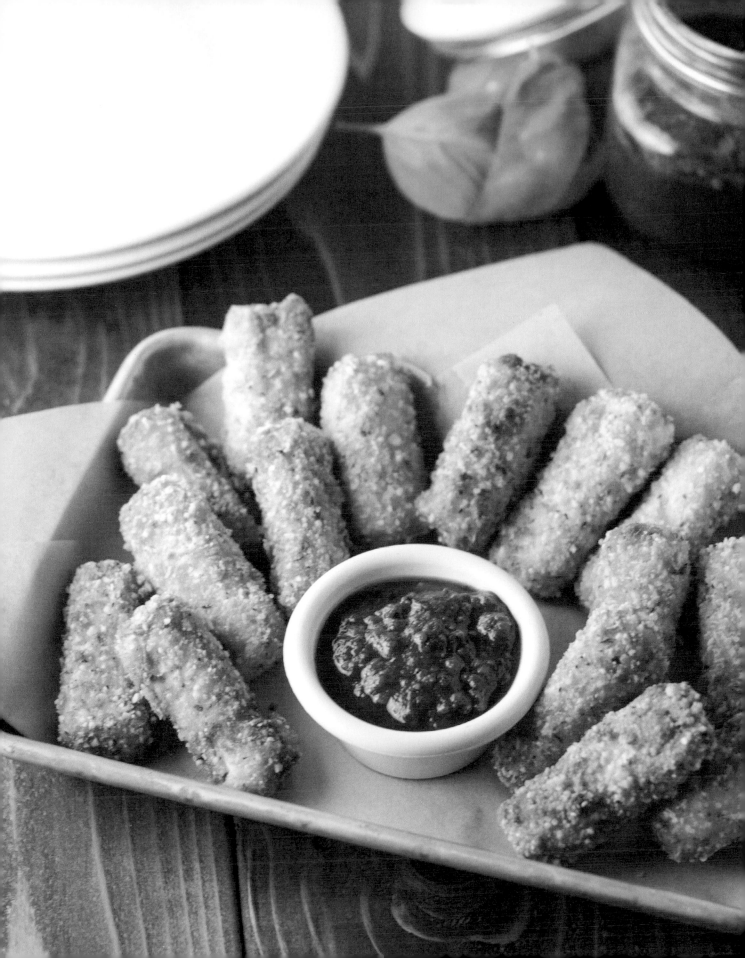

Creamy Avocado Pesto Deviled Eggs

NET CARBS
1.5g

makes 12 deviled eggs (2 per servings) · prep time: 10 minutes

Deviled eggs are easily among my top five favorite foods. I eat them several times a week. Eggs are nature's perfect food! We live about forty-five minutes outside of Seattle and are surrounded by local farms selling fresh pastured eggs. It is amazing to be able to take a short drive down the road and get fresh eggs and support a local farmer at the same time. If you've never had farm-fresh eggs, you are missing out!

ingredients

6 hard-boiled eggs (see tip), peeled

¼ cup mayonnaise, store-bought or homemade (page 336)

3 tablespoons Walnut Avocado Pesto (page 340) or store-bought pesto

3 tablespoons full-fat sour cream

Fresh micro greens, for garnish (optional)

tip: This is how I make the perfect hard-boiled eggs: Place the eggs in large saucepan with cold water. Add enough water so that the eggs are fully submerged. Over high heat, bring the water to a rolling boil. Once the water is boiling, remove the pan from the heat, cover, and let sit for 12 minutes. Submerge the eggs in a cold-water bath before peeling.

directions

1. Slice the eggs in half lengthwise and scoop the yolks into a mixing bowl. Mash the yolks with a fork.

2. To the mixing bowl with the yolks, add the mayonnaise, pesto, and sour cream. Mix until the ingredients are well combined.

3. Transfer the yolk mixture to a pastry bag or resealable plastic bag. If using a resealable plastic bag, snip off a corner of the bag. Pipe the mixture into the egg whites.

4. Top each deviled egg with some fresh micro greens, if desired.

CALORIES: 185 · FAT: 17g · PROTEIN: 7.5g · TOTAL CARBS: 1.7g · DIETARY FIBER: 0.2g · NET CARBS: 1.5g

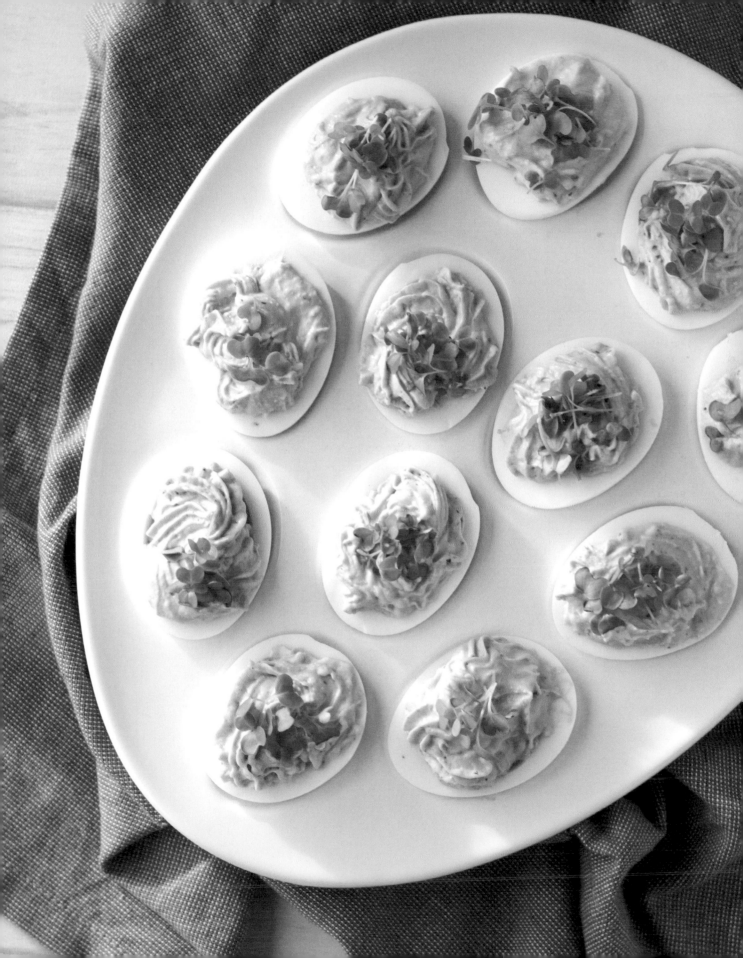

Buffalo Chicken Flatbread

makes 8 servings · prep time: 15 minutes · cook time: 25 minutes

While I was working on this book and I made this recipe, I liked it so much that I immediately made it again, because one batch just wasn't enough. I like to dip this flatbread in Ranch Dressing (page 332). For a nut-free alternative, try using the Nut-Free Pizza Crust on page 358 for the flatbread base.

ingredients

For the crust:

¾ cup blanched almond flour

1 teaspoon garlic powder

1 teaspoon onion powder

1 teaspoon Italian seasoning

½ teaspoon sea salt

¼ teaspoon ground black pepper

1½ cups shredded low-moisture, part-skim mozzarella cheese

1½ ounces full-fat cream cheese (3 tablespoons), softened

1 large egg

⅓ cup Buffalo wing sauce

1 tablespoon butter or ghee, melted

8 ounces boneless, skinless chicken breasts or thighs, cooked and shredded

¼ cup shredded low-moisture, part-skim mozzarella cheese

⅓ cup crumbled blue cheese

A few thin slices red onion

2 green onions, sliced, for garnish

directions

1. Preheat the oven to 425°F. Line a rimmed baking sheet with parchment paper and set aside.

2. In a medium bowl, combine the almond flour, garlic powder, onion powder, Italian seasoning, salt, and pepper. Mix until the ingredients are well incorporated.

3. In a large microwave-safe mixing bowl, combine the mozzarella and cream cheese. Microwave for 1 minute. Remove the bowl from the microwave and stir to combine. Return the bowl to the microwave and heat for 1 additional minute.

4. Add the flour mixture and the egg to the melted cheese and quickly mix with your hands until the ingredients are well incorporated. If you are having a hard time mixing the ingredients, put the bowl back in the microwave for another 20 to 30 seconds to soften. If the dough starts sticking to your hands, wet your hands slightly and continue working the dough.

5. Use your hands to spread the dough into a thin, even rectangle on the lined baking sheet, about 13 by 9 inches.

6. Bake for 10 to 12 minutes, until golden brown. Watch to make sure that it does not bubble up. Use a toothpick to pop any bubbles, if necessary.

7. While the crust is baking, combine the Buffalo sauce and melted butter in a bowl. Toss the shredded chicken in the sauce until the chicken is evenly coated.

8. When the crust is done, remove it from the oven and sprinkle it with the mozzarella cheese.

9. Place the coated chicken on top of the cheese, then top the chicken with the blue cheese and red onion. Return the flatbread to the oven and bake for an additional 10 minutes, or until the cheese is melted and bubbling.

10. Top with the green onions before serving.

CALORIES: 235 · FAT: 16.5g · PROTEIN: 17.6g · TOTAL CARBS: 4.9g · DIETARY FIBER: 1.4g · NET CARBS: 3.5g

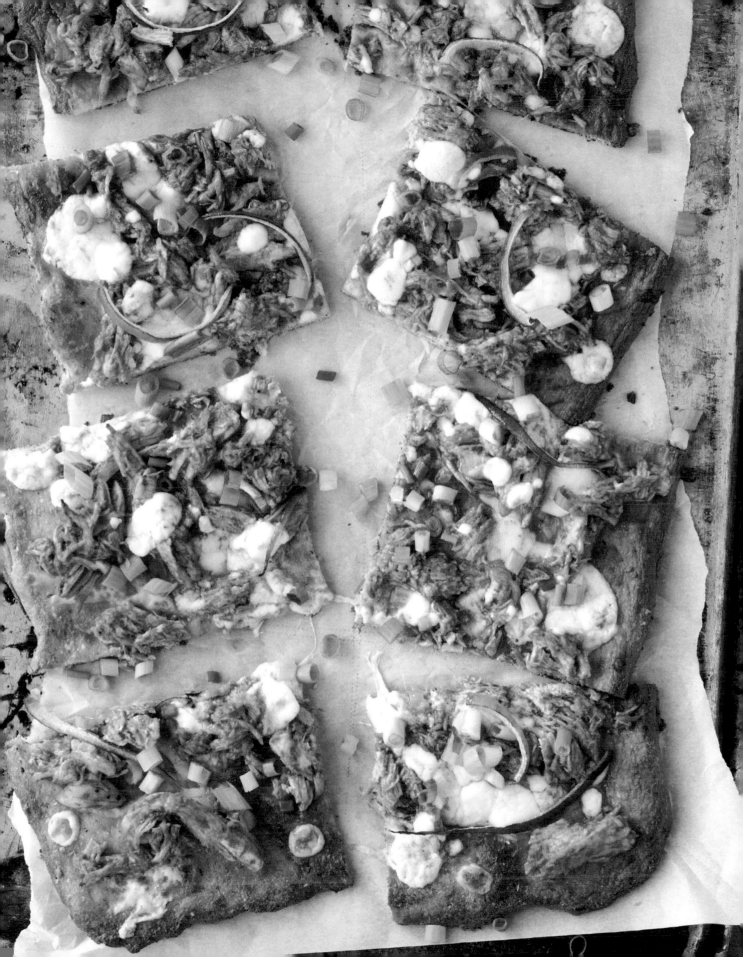

Bloody Mary Deviled Eggs

 makes 12 deviled eggs (2 per serving) · prep time: 15 minutes · cook time: 15 minutes

All of the flavors of your favorite Sunday morning breakfast cocktail in a delicious deviled egg. If you are feeling spicy, try adding a little more horseradish and a sprinkle of Cajun Seasoning (page 351). For a boozy spin, try adding a splash of vodka. I have even been known to serve these as a garnish on an actual Bloody Mary. It makes for an impressive presentation and one that your guests will not see coming.

ingredients

3 slices thick-cut bacon

6 hard-boiled eggs (see page 162), peeled

2 tablespoons mayonnaise, store-bought or homemade (page 336)

2 tablespoons full-fat sour cream

1 tablespoon tomato paste

1½ teaspoons prepared horseradish

1½ teaspoons Worcestershire sauce

1 teaspoon Dijon mustard

1 teaspoon celery salt, or more to taste

¼ teaspoon smoked paprika, plus more for garnish, if desired

¼ teaspoon ground black pepper

12 small pimento-stuffed green olives

1 rib celery, sliced

directions

1. Cook the bacon in a skillet until it is crispy. Cut each slice into fourths and set aside.

2. Slice the eggs in half lengthwise and scoop the yolks into a mixing bowl. Mash the yolks with a fork.

3. To the mixing bowl with the yolks, add the mayonnaise, sour cream, tomato paste, horseradish, Worcestershire sauce, mustard, celery salt, smoked paprika, and pepper. Mix until the ingredients are well combined.

4. Transfer the yolk mixture to a pastry bag or resealable plastic bag. If using a resealable plastic bag, snip off a corner of the bag. Pipe the mixture into the egg whites.

5. Using a toothpick or cocktail skewer, top each deviled egg with an olive, a piece of bacon, and a slice of celery. Garnish with a dusting of smoked paprika, if desired.

CALORIES: 138 · FAT: 11g · PROTEIN: 7.8g · TOTAL CARBS: 1.2g · DIETARY FIBER: 0.2g · NET CARBS: 1g

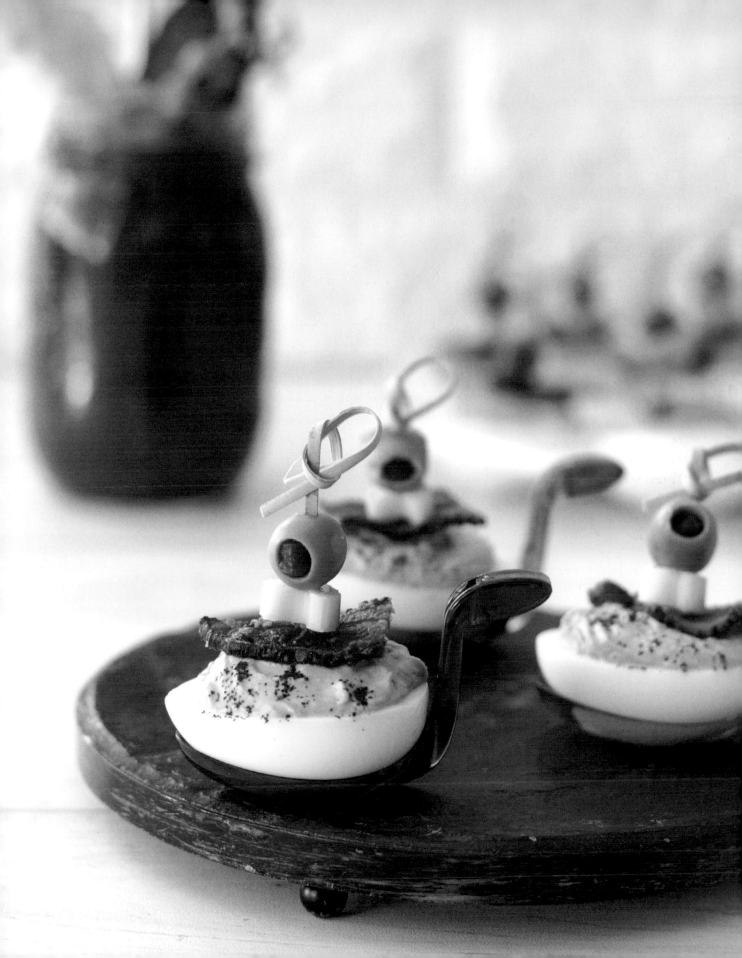

Bacon Chicken Ranch Jalapeño Poppers

 makes 20 jalapeño poppers (4 per serving) · prep time: 20 minutes · cook time: 30 minutes

For this recipe, I took all of the delicious goodness of a traditional jalapeño popper and upped the ante by adding cheddar cheese, chicken, and ranch dressing. You can't really go wrong when you have all of those ingredients in one recipe. I love to serve these poppers with extra ranch dressing on the side.

ingredients

10 large jalapeños, halved and seeded

1 pound boneless, skinless chicken breasts or thighs, cooked and chopped

1 (8-ounce) package full-fat cream cheese, softened

1 cup shredded sharp cheddar cheese, divided

¼ cup Ranch Dressing (page 332)

1 teaspoon garlic powder

1 teaspoon onion powder

6 slices bacon, cooked crisp and crumbled

3 fresh chives, chopped, for garnish

directions

1. Preheat the oven to 350°F. Line a rimmed baking sheet with parchment paper or a silicone baking mat.

2. Spread the jalapeño halves across the prepared baking sheet.

3. In a large mixing bowl, combine the chicken, cream cheese, ½ cup of the cheddar cheese, ranch dressing, garlic powder, and onion powder. Mix until well combined.

4. Fill each jalapeño half with a heaping mound of the chicken and cream cheese mixture. Top each jalapeño half with some of the bacon. Sprinkle the remaining ½ cup of cheddar cheese over the tops of the poppers.

5. Bake for 30 minutes, or until the cheese on top is golden brown and bubbling. Top with fresh chives before serving.

CALORIES: 513 · FAT: 38g · PROTEIN: 35g · TOTAL CARBS: 5.5g · DIETARY FIBER: 1g · NET CARBS: 4.5g

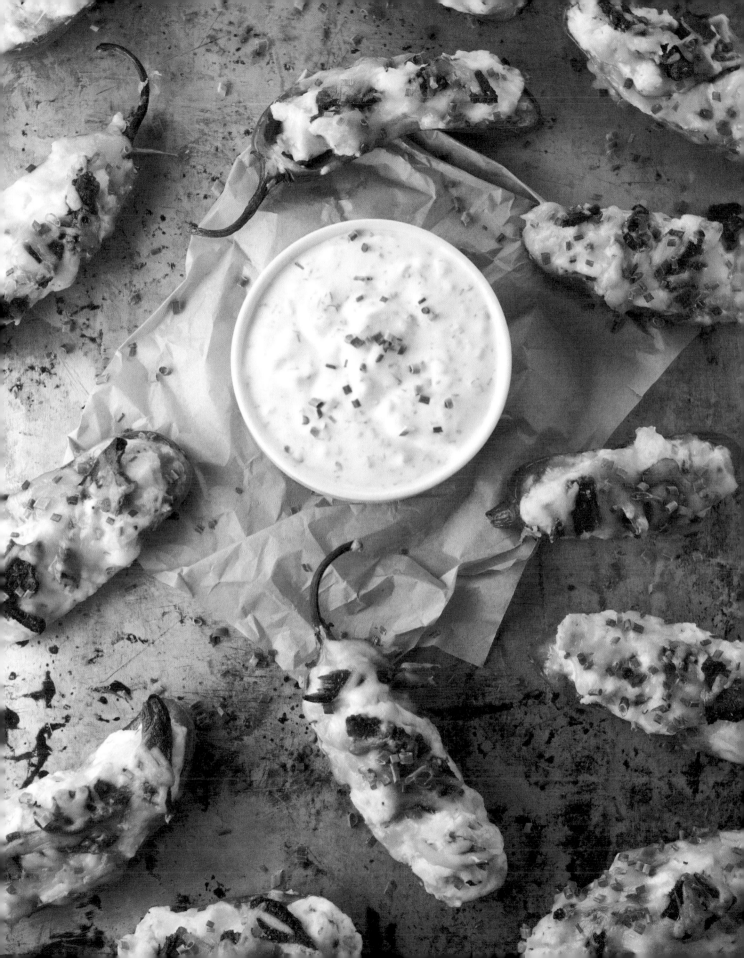

Baked Avocado Fries

NET CARBS
4.1g

makes 5 servings · prep time: 15 minutes · cook time: 15 minutes

It doesn't get much better than delicious, buttery avocado baked in a crispy breading. To make these fries even crispier, you can deep-fry them. I love to serve them with Ranch Dressing (page 332) or Thousand Island Dressing (page 330).

ingredients

2 medium avocados

2 tablespoons coconut flour

2 large eggs, whisked

1 batch Savory Breading Mix (page 354)

directions

1. Preheat the oven to 450°F. Line a rimmed baking sheet with parchment paper or a silicone baking mat.

2. Peel and pit the avocados and slice them lengthwise into ½-inch-thick "fries." Two avocados should yield about 20 slices.

3. Set up three shallow bowls in a row. Put the coconut flour in the first bowl, the whisked eggs in the second bowl, and the breading mix in the third bowl.

4. Dredge an avocado slice in the coconut flour, then coat it in the egg wash. Finish it off by coating it in the breading mix. Repeat this three-step process with each avocado slice, and place them in a single layer on the prepared baking sheet.

5. Bake for 12 minutes or until golden brown.

CALORIES: 247 · FAT: 20g · PROTEIN: 10.5g · TOTAL CARBS: 10.5g · DIETARY FIBER: 6.4g · NET CARBS: 4.1g

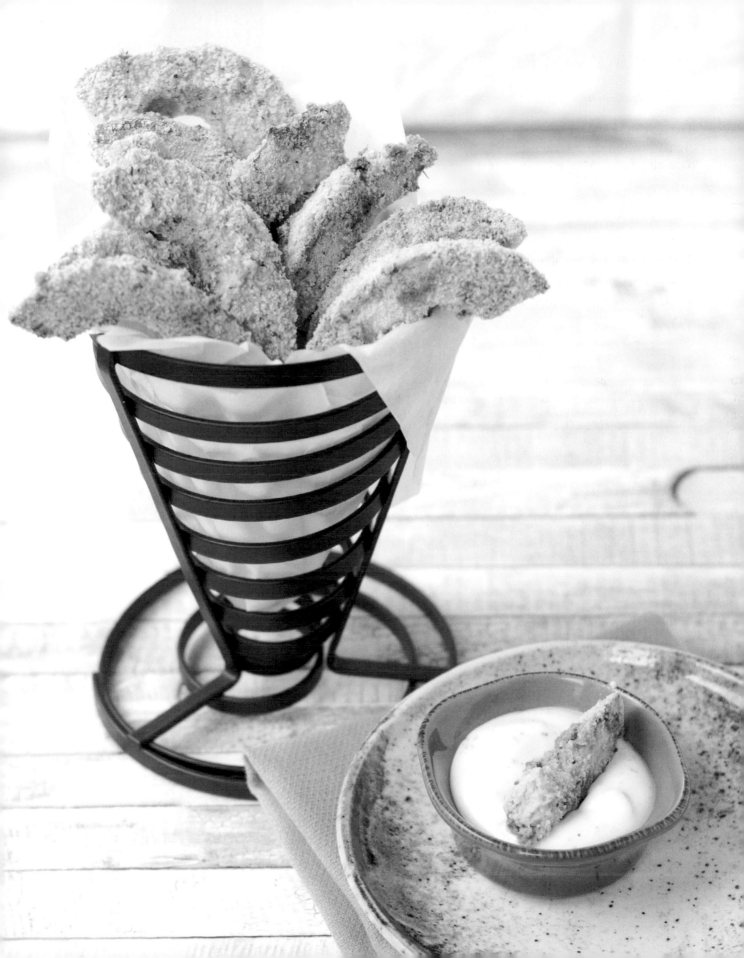

Asiago Rosemary Bacon Biscuits

NET CARBS
3.1g

makes 8 biscuits (1 per serving) · prep time: 15 minutes · cook time: 30 minutes

My favorite thing about these biscuits is their versatility. You can change up the cheeses and herbs and make so many different flavor combinations. Two of my favorites are cheddar and dill and Parmesan and garlic. I even have a breakfast variation on my website, peaceloveandlowcarb.com, that is made with sharp white cheddar and sausage. If you divide the mixture into four biscuits instead of eight, they make great buns for sandwiches and burgers. Let's be honest, aren't we all tired of bunless burgers and lettuce wraps? Have your bun and eat it, too!

ingredients

4 ounces full-fat cream cheese (½ cup), softened

1 large egg

2 cloves garlic, minced

1 tablespoon chopped fresh rosemary

½ teaspoon onion powder

¼ teaspoon sea salt

1¼ cups shredded Asiago cheese, divided

1½ cups blanched almond flour

¼ cup heavy cream

¼ cup water

6 slices bacon, cooked crisp and crumbled

Special equipment:

12-well muffin top pan

directions

1. Preheat the oven to 350°F. Lightly grease 8 wells of a 12-well muffin top pan.

2. In a medium mixing bowl, using a hand mixer, cream the cream cheese and egg together. Add the garlic, rosemary, onion powder, and salt. Mix with the hand mixer until well incorporated.

3. Add 1 cup of the Asiago cheese, the almond flour, cream, and water. Mix until well combined. Using a rubber spatula, fold in the bacon.

4. Using a large spoon or an ice cream scoop, spoon the dough into the muffin top pan in 8 equal-sized heaping mounds. Sprinkle with the remaining ¼ cup of Asiago cheese.

5. Bake for 30 minutes, or until golden brown on top. Place the pan on a cooling rack and allow the biscuits to cool before removing.

6. Store extras in the refrigerator for up to 1 week. Reheat in the oven or toaster.

CALORIES: 256 · FAT: 24g · PROTEIN: 11g · TOTAL CARBS: 5.5g · DIETARY FIBER: 2.4g · NET CARBS: 3.1g

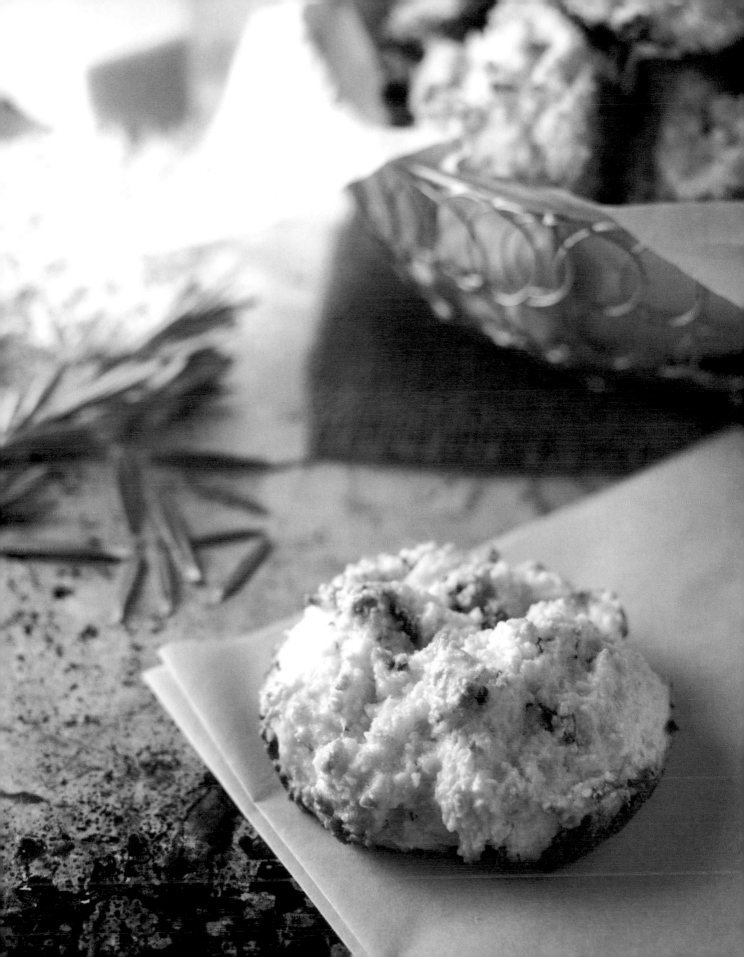

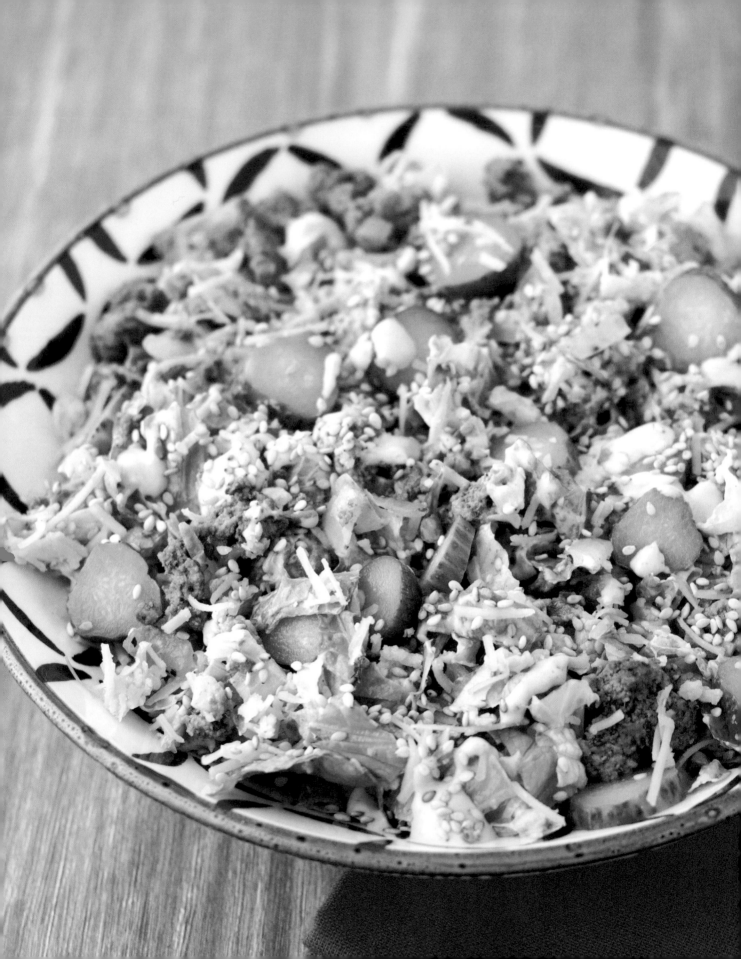

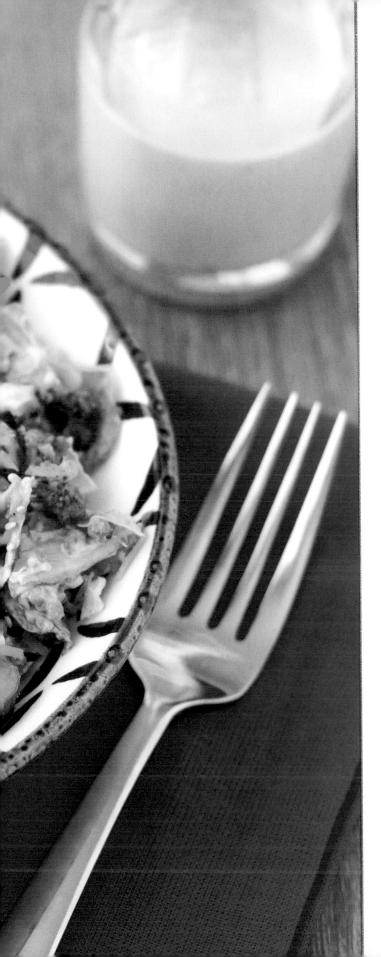

Soups & Salads

Zuppa Toscana

 EGG-FREE NUT-FREE   makes 10 cups (1 cup per serving) · prep time: 15 minutes · cook time: 1 hour

In my late teens and early twenties, I worked at a rib joint. On my breaks between shifts, I frequently went to Olive Garden for their endless soup and salad lunch. I never got tired of it. Every day I ate their Zuppa Toscana. I typically had the same server, and she knew me by name. She also knew that I wasn't the biggest fan of kale, and she would always do her best to pick it out for me. She truly went above and beyond, especially given how busy the lunch rush could be. My love of that soup never left me, so I knew I needed to re-create it as a keto-friendly version. I substituted cauliflower for the potatoes and swapped out the kale for spinach, although you could certainly make it with kale. Radishes also make a great substitution for the potatoes. This soup never lasts long in my house. I've even made two batches in the same day.

ingredients

6 slices bacon, chopped

2 tablespoons butter or ghee

1 medium onion, chopped (about 1 cup)

4 cloves garlic, minced

Sea salt and ground black pepper

1 pound bulk Italian sausage

Pinch of red pepper flakes

6 cups chicken stock

1 small head cauliflower, cored and cut into small florets (about 4 cups)

1 cup heavy cream

2 packed cups fresh spinach

tip: I like to add a little extra cream to the soup when reheating.

directions

1. In a large Dutch oven or stockpot over medium heat, cook the bacon until it is crispy. Using a slotted spoon, remove the bacon from the pot, leaving the drippings in the pot.

2. To the bacon drippings, add the butter, onion, garlic, and a pinch each of salt and pepper. Sauté until the onion is translucent and the garlic is fragrant.

3. Add the Italian sausage and red pepper flakes to the pot. Cook until the sausage is browned, about 10 minutes.

4. Pour the stock into the pot and bring to a boil over medium-high heat. Add the cauliflower.

5. Reduce the heat to low and simmer for 30 minutes, until the cauliflower is crisp-tender.

6. Stir in the cream and spinach and cook for an additional 10 to 15 minutes, until the spinach is wilted and the soup has started to thicken. Add the cooked bacon to the soup. Taste and add more salt and pepper, if needed.

7. Store leftovers in the refrigerator for up to 1 week. Reheat on the stovetop.

CALORIES: 283 · FAT: 22g · PROTEIN: 13g · TOTAL CARBS: 4.5g · DIETARY FIBER: 1.4g · NET CARBS: 3.1g

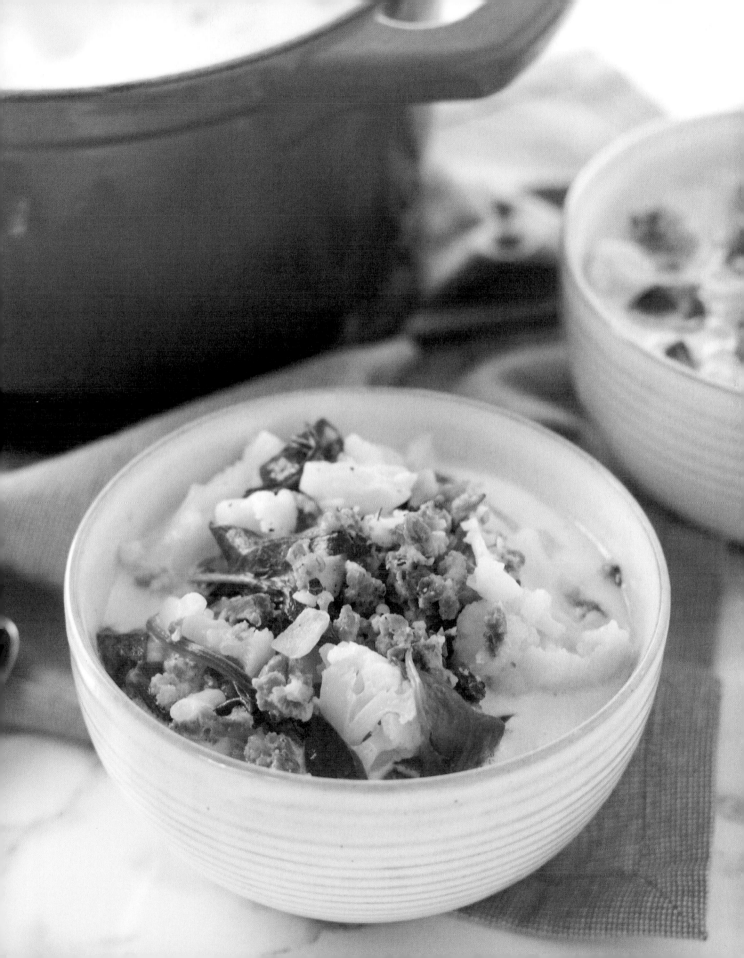

Smoked Sausage and Kale Soup

makes 10 cups (1 cup per serving)
prep time: 15 minutes · cook time: 1 hour

I love when a recipe comes together out of a need to go grocery shopping. Sometimes that is what it takes to get my creative juices flowing. I open the fridge and pretend I am looking at the contents of a *Chopped* basket, and then I get to work. That very same inspiration was at work with this recipe, minus the strange ingredients you might be likely to find in a *Chopped* basket. No sour hard candies in this soup!

ingredients

2 tablespoons butter or ghee

1 medium onion, diced (about 1 cup)

3 cloves garlic, minced

2 bay leaves

½ teaspoon dried oregano leaves

½ teaspoon sea salt

¼ teaspoon ground black pepper

1 pound smoked beef sausage

6 cups beef stock

1 (14½-ounce) can diced tomatoes, with juices

1 bunch radishes, trimmed and halved

3 cups destemmed and torn kale leaves

Red pepper flakes, for garnish (optional)

Shaved Romano cheese, for garnish (optional)

directions

1. Heat the butter in a large Dutch oven or stockpot over medium-low heat. Add the onion, garlic, bay leaves, oregano, salt, and black pepper. Cook until the onion is translucent and the garlic is fragrant.

2. Slice the smoked sausage in half lengthwise, then cut it crosswise into half-moons. Add the sausage to the pot, increase the heat to medium, and cook until the sausage is browned.

3. Remove the bay leaves from the pot and discard. Add the stock and tomatoes and bring to a boil. Add the radishes and kale, reduce the heat to low, and simmer for 30 to 40 minutes, until the kale is wilted and the radishes are tender.

4. Garnish the bowls of soup with red pepper flakes and shaved Romano cheese, if desired. Store leftovers in the refrigerator for up to 1 week. Reheat on the stovetop.

tip: To make this soup dairy-free and Paleo compliant, use ghee rather than butter.

CALORIES: 194 · FAT: 14g · PROTEIN: 10g · TOTAL CARBS: 6.5g · DIETARY FIBER: 1.9g · NET CARBS: 4.6g

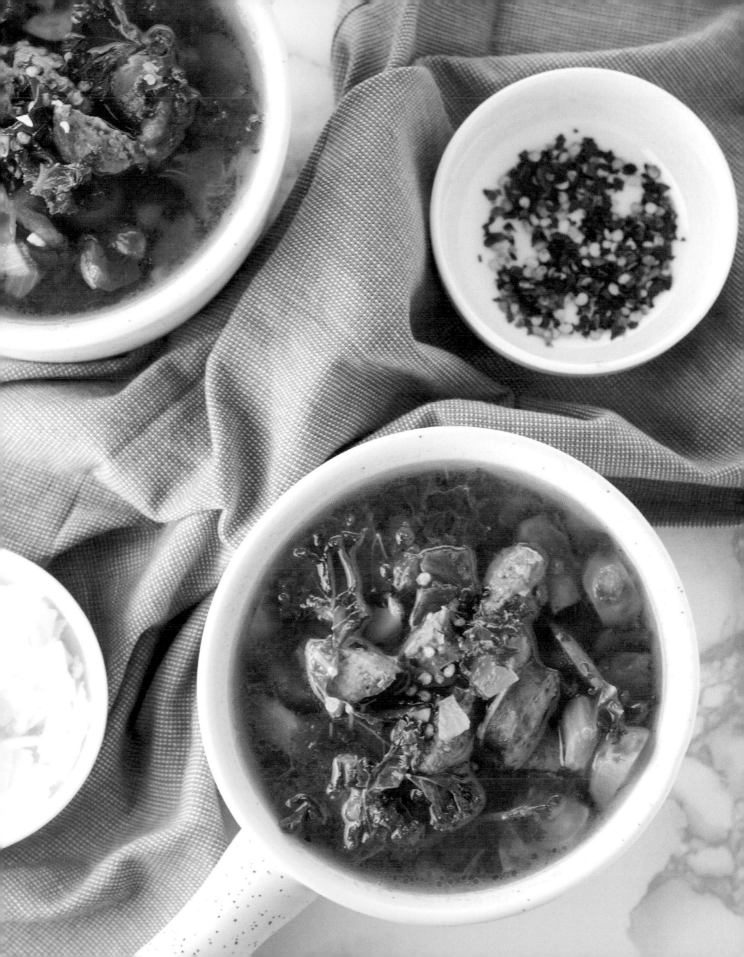

Mexican Chicken Soup

NET CARBS
2.2g

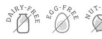

makes 10 cups (1 cup per serving)
prep time: 15 minutes · cook time: 50 minutes

With a short list of ingredients and very little prep work, this is the perfect soup to whip up on a weeknight when you just don't feel like cooking. Have a lonely pack of chicken thighs in the freezer needing to be used up? Well, here you go! Easy peasy. We love to top our bowls of soup with a little sharp cheddar cheese, sour cream, fresh jalapeños, and cilantro, but the soup is equally good just as it is. If you find that the broth is too spicy for you, you can cut some of the spice with a squeeze of fresh lime juice. The citrus also adds a nice burst of freshness.

ingredients

2 tablespoons butter or ghee

1 small onion, diced (about ½ cup)

4 cloves garlic, minced

1½ pounds boneless, skinless chicken thighs, cubed

Sea salt and ground black pepper

2 tablespoons Mexican Seasoning Blend (page 350)

1 (10-ounce) can mild diced tomatoes and green chilies

6 cups chicken stock

Tips: To make this soup dairy-free and Paleo compliant, use ghee rather than butter.

This soup also freezes well.

directions

1. Heat the butter in a large Dutch oven or stockpot over medium-low heat. Add the onion and garlic and cook until the onion is translucent and the garlic is fragrant.

2. Sprinkle the chicken thighs generously with salt and pepper.

3. Increase the heat to medium, add the chicken to the pot, and cook until it is cooked through and slightly browned.

4. Sprinkle the seasoning blend on the chicken, onion, and garlic. Toss until the chicken is completely coated in the seasoning.

5. Add the tomatoes and green chilies and stock to the pot. Bring to a boil, then reduce the heat to low and simmer for 30 minutes, until the broth has reduced just slightly.

6. Taste and add more salt and pepper, if desired.

7. Store leftovers in the refrigerator for up to 1 week. Reheat on the stovetop.

CALORIES: 186 · FAT: 8.5g · PROTEIN: 20g · TOTAL CARBS: 2.9g · DIETARY FIBER: 0.7g · NET CARBS: 2.2g

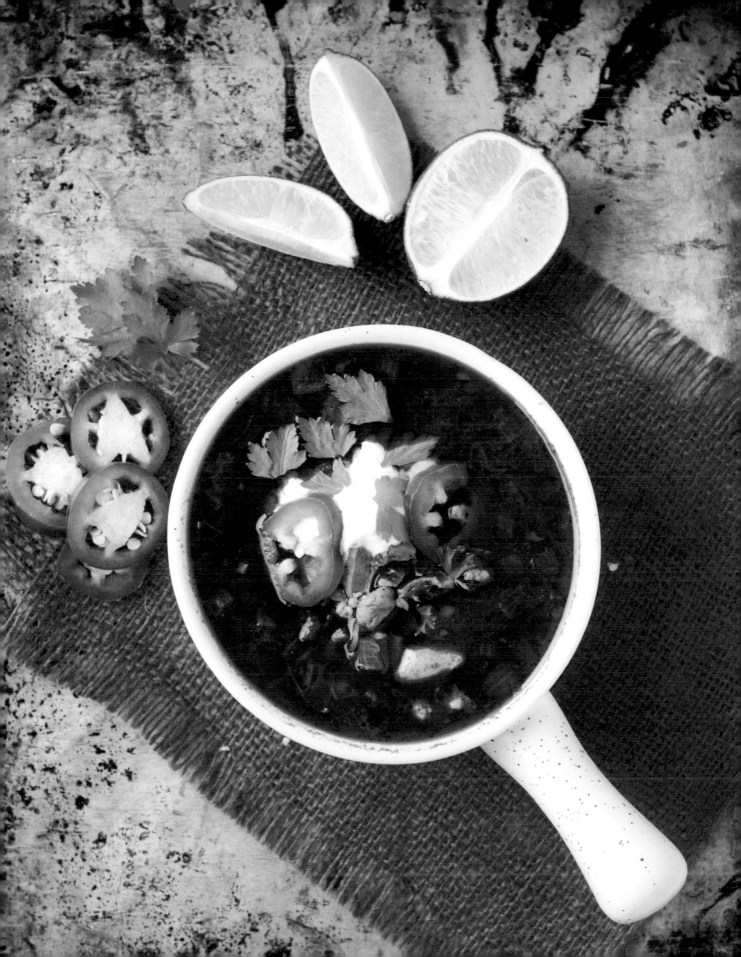

Italian Wedding Soup

 NUT-FREE makes 3 quarts (1 cup per serving) · prep time: 20 minutes · cook time: 1 hour

I think my favorite thing about this soup is how versatile it is. I have made the meatballs with all sorts of different meat combinations. I typically use whatever I have on hand. Feel free to try ground chicken or beef in place of the turkey. Get creative with the vegetables, too. Have some vegetables that need to be used up before they are past their prime? Toss them in! Not a fan of kale? Try subbing escarole or spinach.

ingredients

For the meatballs:

8 ounces ground turkey

8 ounces bulk Italian sausage

½ cup grated Parmesan cheese

2 cloves garlic, minced

1 large egg

2 tablespoons chopped fresh flat-leaf parsley

1 tablespoon Worcestershire sauce

¼ teaspoon sea salt

¼ teaspoon ground black pepper

Pinch of red pepper flakes

1 tablespoon olive oil, for the pot

For the broth:

1 large shallot, chopped

3 cloves garlic, minced

2 ribs celery, sliced

6 cups chicken stock

2 teaspoons chopped fresh dill weed

Pinch of red pepper flakes

3 cups riced cauliflower (see page 76)

3 cups destemmed and torn kale leaves

Shaved Parmesan cheese, for garnish (optional)

directions

1. Make the meatballs: In a large mixing bowl, combine the turkey, sausage, Parmesan, garlic, egg, parsley, Worcestershire sauce, salt, black pepper, and red pepper flakes. Mix until the ingredients are well incorporated. Form the meat mixture into 1-inch meatballs.

2. Heat the olive oil in a large Dutch oven or stockpot over medium-high heat. Add the meatballs and cook in batches until they are seared golden brown, 2 to 3 minutes on each side. Remove the meatballs from the pot and set aside; keep the drippings in the pot.

3. Make the broth: Set the pot with the drippings over medium-low heat. Add the shallot, garlic, and celery to the pot. Deglaze the pot with a splash of the stock, using a rubber spatula to scrape the bottom of the pot to loosen and mix in any stuck-on pieces. Cook the vegetables until they are tender.

4. To the pot, add the remainder of the stock, dill, and red pepper flakes. Increase the heat and bring to a boil.

5. Add the riced cauliflower and reduce the heat to medium. Simmer for 10 minutes, until the cauliflower is tender.

6. Add the meatballs and kale to the pot. Reduce the heat to low and simmer for 30 to 40 minutes, until the meatballs are cooked through and the kale is wilted.

7. Taste and add more salt and pepper, if needed. Garnish the bowls of soup with shaved Parmesan, if desired.

8. Store leftovers in the refrigerator for up to 1 week. Reheat on the stovetop.

tip: Before forming the meat mixture into meatballs, cook a tablespoon-sized portion and taste it. That way you can adjust the seasoning if needed.

CALORIES: 147 · FAT: 7.8g · PROTEIN: 12g · TOTAL CARBS: 3.3g · DIETARY FIBER: 1g · NET CARBS: 2.3g

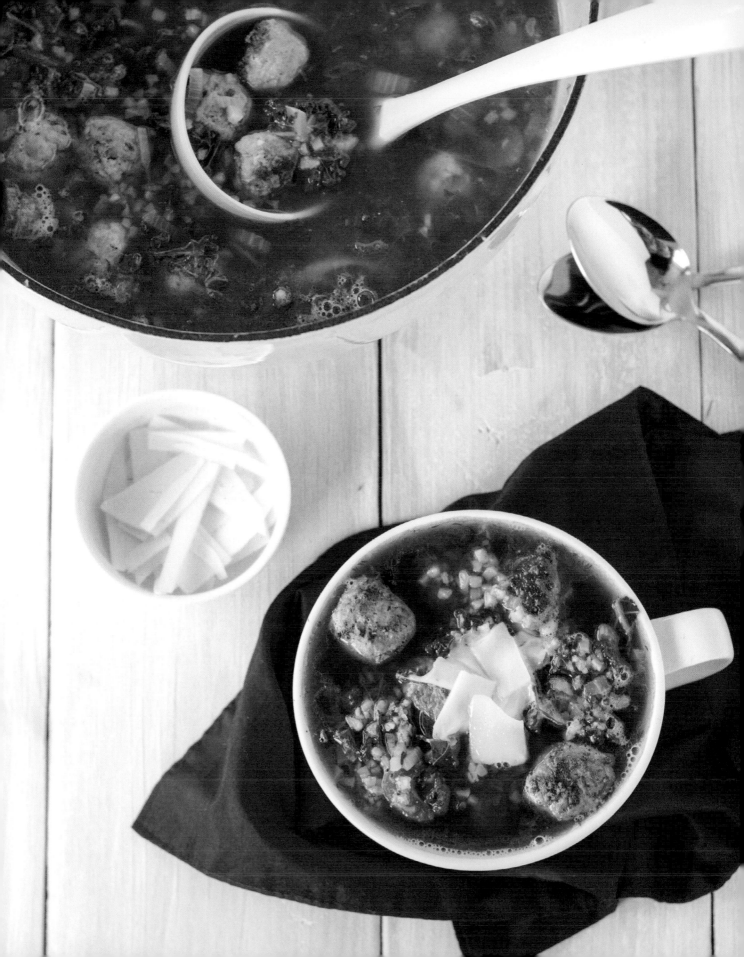

Egg Drop Soup

makes 6 cups (1 cup per serving)
prep time: 10 minutes · cook time: 15 minutes

Quick and easy is the name of the game with this egg drop soup. Don't let the simplicity of the recipe fool you; it really packs a flavor punch. I love loading it up with whatever extra vegetables I have in the fridge at the time. From time to time, I also throw in some shrimp and make a meal out of it.

ingredients

4 cups chicken stock

1 tablespoon toasted sesame oil

2 teaspoons coconut aminos or gluten-free soy sauce

¼ teaspoon ginger powder

5 cremini mushrooms, thinly sliced

4 green onions, sliced on the bias, green and white parts separated

½ teaspoon sea salt

½ teaspoon turmeric powder

4 large eggs, whisked

Red pepper flakes, for garnish (optional)

directions

1. In a stockpot, combine the stock, sesame oil, coconut aminos, ginger, mushrooms, white parts of the green onions, salt, and turmeric. Bring to a boil over high heat, then reduce the heat to low and simmer for 5 minutes.

2. Slowly pour the eggs into the broth, whisking continuously as you pour. The eggs will cook instantly as they hit the hot broth.

3. Mix in the green parts of the onions and top each serving of soup with a pinch of red pepper flakes, if desired.

4. Store leftovers in the refrigerator for up to 1 week. Reheat on the stovetop.

CALORIES: 107 · FAT: 5.5g · PROTEIN: 8g · TOTAL CARBS: 1.3g · DIETARY FIBER: 0.2g · NET CARBS: 1.1g

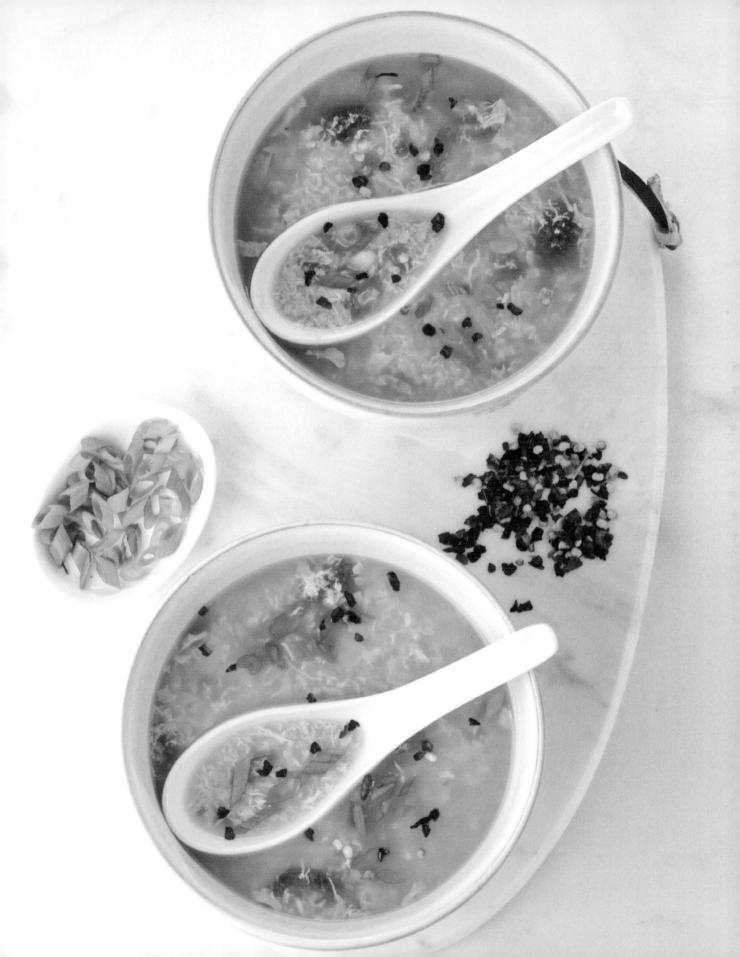

Cheesy Ham and Cauliflower Soup

makes 5 quarts (1 cup per serving) · **prep time: 15 minutes** · **cook time: 1 hour**

Soup is probably my all-time favorite food. I am a year-round soup lover. Through hot and cold weather, I always have soup on the brain. I can't even count the number of times that I have just pulled out a stockpot and started throwing random ingredients into it. Some of my favorite recipes were created this way. I even have an entire soups and stews ebook on my website. Basically, what I am trying to say is that soup is life.

ingredients

3 tablespoons butter or ghee, divided

3 cups diced ham steak, extra for garnish

1 small onion, chopped (about ½ cup)

2 sprigs fresh thyme, plus extra for garnish

1 bay leaf

1 teaspoon garlic powder

1 teaspoon sea salt

½ teaspoon ground black pepper

½ teaspoon mustard powder

½ teaspoon dried rubbed sage

6 cups chicken stock

6 cups cauliflower florets

2 cups heavy cream

2 cups shredded sharp cheddar cheese

½ cup grated Parmesan cheese

directions

1. Heat 2 tablespoons of the butter in a large Dutch oven or stockpot over medium heat. Add the ham and cook until it is browned and slightly crispy on the edges. Using a slotted spoon, remove the ham from the pot and set aside.

2. Reduce the heat to medium-low and add the remaining 1 tablespoon of butter, onion, thyme, bay leaf, garlic powder, salt, pepper, mustard powder, and sage. Cook until the onion is soft and translucent. Remove the bay leaf and thyme sprigs.

3. Deglaze the pot with a splash of the chicken stock. Using a rubber spatula, scrape up and mix in any bits stuck to the bottom of the pot.

4. Add the remaining stock and cauliflower. Increase the heat and bring to a rolling boil. After 5 minutes, reduce the heat to low and simmer for 40 minutes. Using a potato masher, mash the cauliflower florets into smaller pieces.

5. Add the cream and, using an immersion blender, puree the soup until it is thick and creamy.

6. Increase the heat to medium and add the cheeses. Stir to mix in the cheese as it melts. Add the ham back to the pot and mix in.

7. Taste and add additional salt and pepper, if needed.

8. Store leftovers in the refrigerator for up to 1 week. Reheat on the stovetop.

tip: When reheating this soup, I like to add a little heavy cream.

CALORIES: 181 · FAT: 15g · PROTEIN: 8g · TOTAL CARBS: 2.7g · DIETARY FIBER: 0.5g · NET CARBS: 2.2g

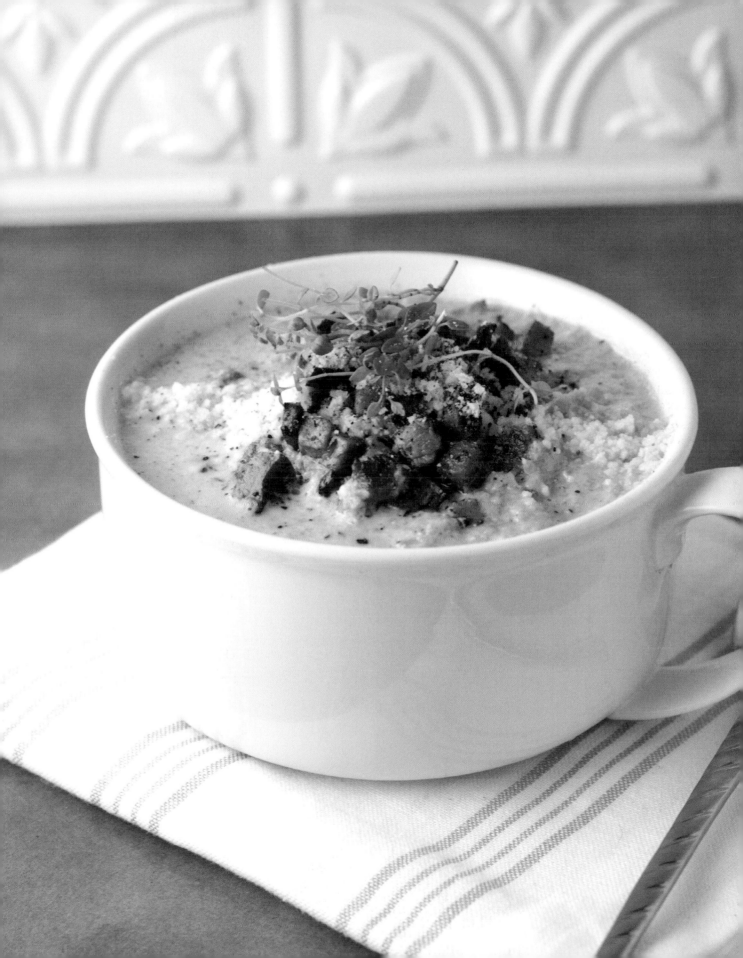

Creamy Lasagna Soup

 EGG-FREE · NUT-FREE · makes 10 cups (1 cup per serving) · prep time: 20 minutes · cook time: 1 hour

Even in my high-carb days, I loved the flavors of a rich and hearty lasagna, but I was never too keen on the thick, gummy lasagna noodles. I typically ate the insides, and what was left on my plate was a pile of limp noodles. This soup has all those same amazing flavors, without the heaviness of the noodles. However, if you want to add something to simulate lasagna noodles, try making the noodles from my "Just Like the Real Thing" Lasagna recipe on page 240.

ingredients

2 tablespoons butter or ghee

1 medium onion, diced (about 1 cup)

2 cloves garlic, minced

Sea salt and ground black pepper

1 pound ground beef

4 cups beef stock

2½ cups Garlic and Herb Marinara Sauce (page 344)

½ cup heavy cream

½ cup full-fat ricotta cheese, plus more for garnish (optional)

½ cup shredded Parmesan cheese, for garnish

¼ cup chopped fresh basil, for garnish

Pinch of smoked paprika, for garnish (optional)

directions

1. Heat the butter in a large Dutch oven or stockpot over medium-low heat. Add the onion, garlic, and a pinch each of salt and pepper. Cook until the onion is translucent and the garlic is fragrant.

2. Increase the heat to medium, add the ground beef to the pot, and cook until browned, breaking up the meat with a spatula as it cooks. Drain the excess grease. You can leave it in for extra fat content, but it will give the soup an oily taste.

3. Add the stock and marinara sauce to the pot. Bring to a boil, then reduce the heat to low to maintain a gentle simmer. Mix in the cream and ricotta cheese.

4. Simmer, stirring occasionally, for 30 to 45 minutes. This is when the flavors really come together. Taste and add additional salt and pepper, if needed, keeping in mind that the Parmesan cheese garnish will add an additional salty component.

5. Before serving, top each bowl of soup with a spoonful of ricotta cheese (if using), a couple teaspoons of Parmesan cheese, some fresh basil, and a sprinkle of smoked paprika, if desired.

6. Store leftovers in the refrigerator for up to 1 week. Reheat on the stovetop.

CALORIES: 210 · FAT: 15g · PROTEIN: 13g · TOTAL CARBS: 6.8g · DIETARY FIBER: 1.4g · NET CARBS: 5.4g

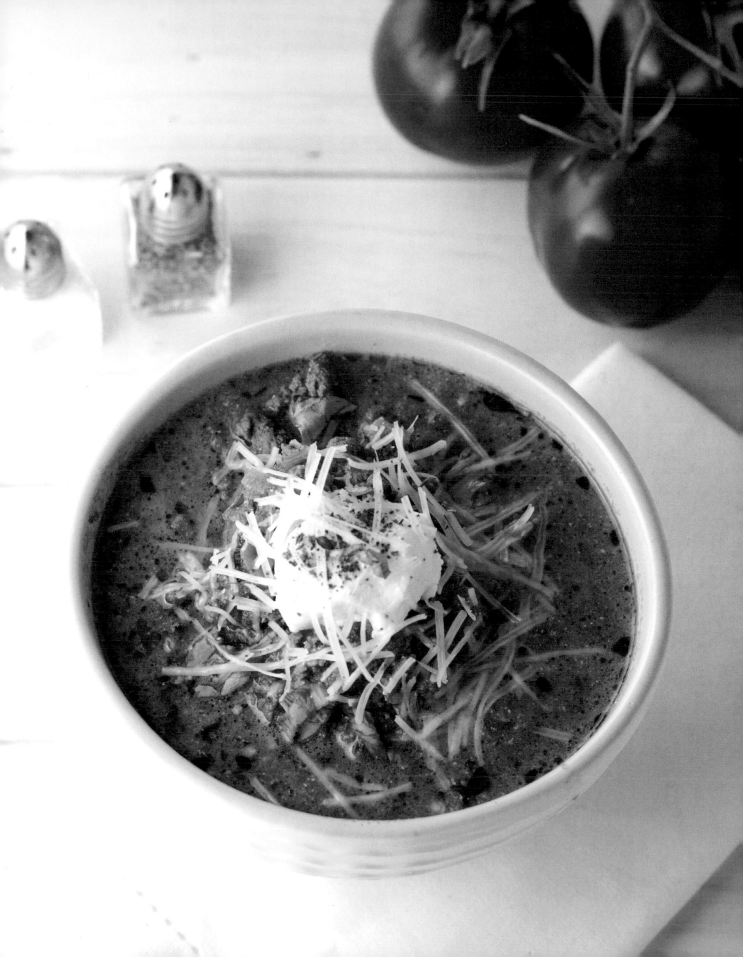

Mac Daddy Salad

makes 4 servings · prep time: 15 minutes · cook time: 15 minutes

I think we all remember the jingle—"Two all-beef patties, special sauce, lettuce, cheese, pickles, onions on a sesame seed bun"—and with that jingle, I'm sure you can instantly recall how it tastes. Well, I am here to tell you that this Mac Daddy Salad recaptures all of those delicious flavors in a healthy, non–fast food version. You will want to eat it time and time again.

ingredients

1 pound ground beef

1 small onion, diced (about ½ cup)

2 cloves garlic, minced

1 teaspoon sea salt

½ teaspoon ground black pepper

1 large head romaine lettuce, shredded

¾ cup shredded sharp cheddar cheese

⅓ cup sliced dill pickles

½ cup Thousand Island Dressing (page 330)

2 tablespoons toasted sesame seeds

directions

1. In a large skillet over medium-high heat, combine the ground beef, onion, garlic, salt, and pepper. Cook until the beef is browned and cooked all the way through. Set aside and let cool.

2. In a large mixing bowl, combine the lettuce, ground beef mixture, cheese, and pickles. Toss to combine.

3. Drizzle the dressing on top and sprinkle with the sesame seeds.

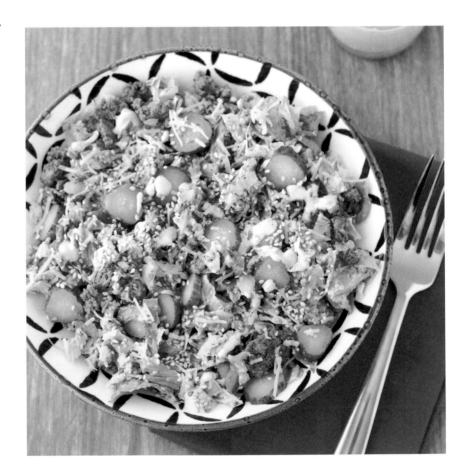

CALORIES: 400 · FAT: 28g · PROTEIN: 30g · TOTAL CARBS: 8.5g · DIETARY FIBER: 3.5g · NET CARBS: 5g

Shaved Brussels Sprouts Caesar Salad

makes 4 servings · prep time: 15 minutes

Brussels sprouts are miniature members of the cabbage family. They are a hearty, high-fiber vegetable. Unlike a salad made of lettuce, shaved Brussels sprouts hold up to the dressing, making leftovers a possibility. They keep their firm crunch even when they are dressed. Try adding some toasted almonds or pepitas and crispy bacon to this salad. I think you will be pleasantly surprised.

ingredients

1 pound Brussels sprouts

½ cup Garlic Parmesan Caesar Dressing (page 331), or more to taste

½ cup shaved Parmesan Romano cheese blend (or a blend of Parmesan, Romano, and Asiago), plus more for garnish

Cracked black pepper, for garnish (optional)

Lemon slices, for garnish (optional)

directions

1. Using a sharp knife or a mandoline, shave or thinly slice the Brussels sprouts into shreds.

2. In a large mixing bowl, combine the Brussels sprouts, dressing, and shaved cheese blend. Toss until the Brussels sprouts are well coated in the dressing. Garnish with additional cheese blend as well as cracked black pepper and lemon slices, if desired.

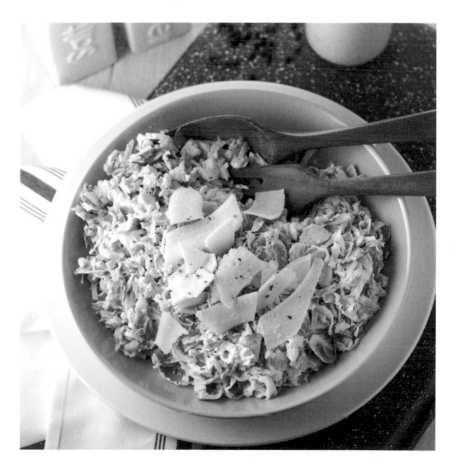

CALORIES: 259 · FAT: 21g · PROTEIN: 10g · TOTAL CARBS: 11g · DIETARY FIBER: 4g · NET CARBS: 7g

Roasted Cauliflower Mock Potato Salad

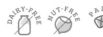

makes 6 servings · prep time: 20 minutes · cook time: 20 minutes

One of my favorite things about cauliflower is its ability to replicate so many other foods. While it isn't an exact texture replica, often I prefer the texture of cauliflower to the texture of the food it is supposed to be mimicking. I was never really a fan of potato salad because it always seemed so starchy, and I felt like each bite dried out my mouth instantly. But I did love the flavor combination in a classic potato salad, so using cauliflower for this recipe was a no-brainer. I dry-roast the cauliflower until it is perfectly crisp-tender. Cauliflower is like a sponge, so when you steam or boil it, it soaks up all the water, and that water usually ends up turning your dish into a soupy mess. When you dry-roast cauliflower, you don't get any of that excess moisture, and the end result is incredibly flavorful.

ingredients

1 large head cauliflower (about 2 pounds)

½ teaspoon sea salt

¼ teaspoon ground black pepper

4 hard-boiled eggs (see page 162), chopped

½ cup chopped dill pickles

2 ribs celery, chopped

2 tablespoons chopped fresh flat-leaf parsley

1 teaspoon chopped fresh dill weed

¾ cup mayonnaise, store-bought or homemade (page 336)

1 tablespoon apple cider vinegar

1 tablespoon Dijon mustard

directions

1. Preheat the oven to 425°F. Line a rimmed baking sheet with parchment paper.

2. Core the cauliflower and cut it into small florets. Spread the cauliflower in a single layer across the lined baking sheet. Sprinkle the salt and pepper over the cauliflower.

3. Roast the cauliflower for 15 to 20 minutes, until it is tender but not mushy.

4. Remove the cauliflower from the oven and allow to cool. Then chop it into bite-sized pieces and put them in a large mixing bowl.

5. To the bowl, add the eggs, pickles, celery, parsley, dill, mayonnaise, vinegar, and mustard. Mix until the ingredients are well incorporated. Taste and add more salt and pepper, if needed.

CALORIES: 270 · FAT: 24g · PROTEIN: 7g · TOTAL CARBS: 8.5g · DIETARY FIBER: 3.8g · NET CARBS: 4.7g

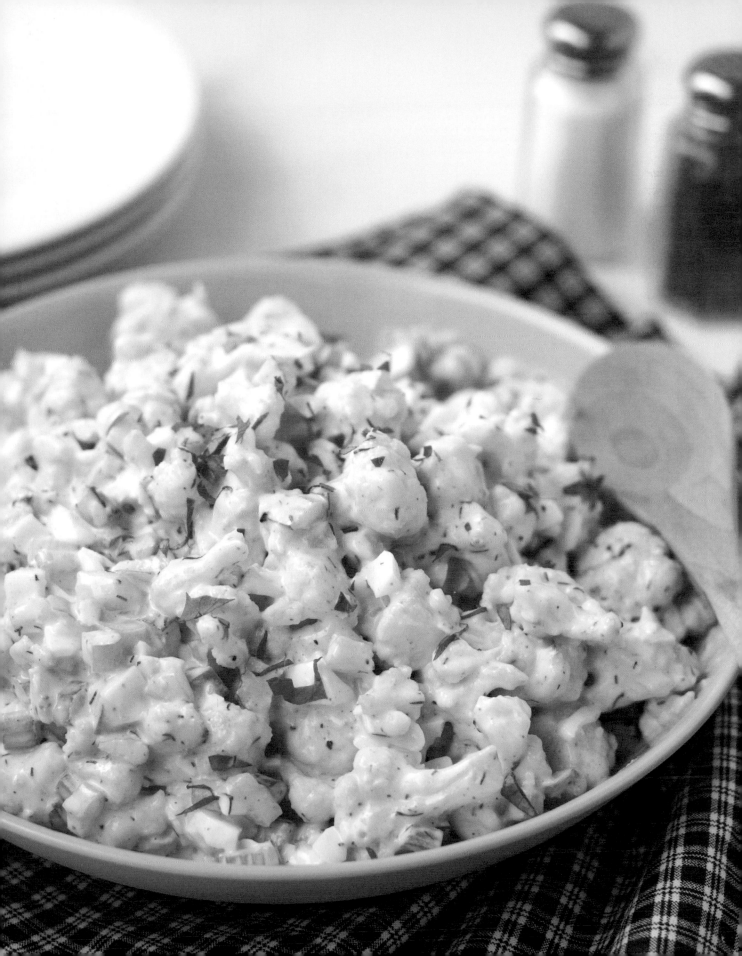

Dill Chicken Salad

makes 4 cups (½ cup per serving) · prep time: 10 minutes

When we bought our new home and were deep in the hustle and bustle of unpacking and settling in, I kept going to the grocery store and buying the dill chicken salad from the deli. I felt a little guilty each time I ordered it, because I knew that I could make a better-tasting, cleaner-ingredient version for way cheaper. Well, I finally did it, and this is the result. Just like my Favorite Buttery Herbed Eggs on page 126, this dish is in heavy rotation in my home.

ingredients

1 pound boneless, skinless chicken breast, cooked and cubed (see tips)

1 large rib celery, diced (about ½ cup)

⅓ cup finely chopped onions

3 tablespoons chopped fresh dill weed

¾ cup mayonnaise, store-bought or homemade (page 336), or more to taste

1 tablespoon plus 1 teaspoon Dijon mustard

Sea salt and ground black pepper, to taste

directions

In a large mixing bowl, mix all of the ingredients together until well combined. Store leftovers in the refrigerator for up to 1 week.

tips: My favorite way to cook the chicken for this recipe is to pan-sear it in butter. It gives the chicken excellent flavor and makes it incredibly juicy, but with a crispy, golden brown outside.

If you ask me, this salad tastes even better on days two and three.

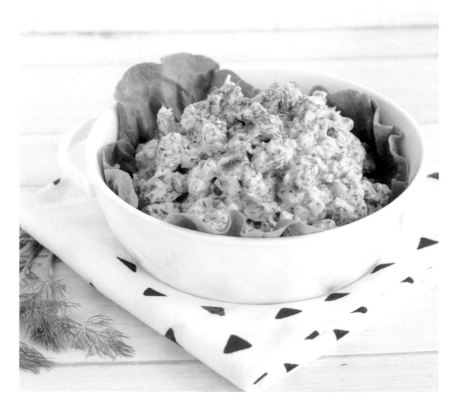

CALORIES: 236 · FAT: 16.5g · PROTEIN: 12g · TOTAL CARBS: 1.5g · DIETARY FIBER: 0.3g · NET CARBS: 1.3g

Creamy Cucumber Salad

 makes 8 servings · prep time: 15 minutes

If you aren't able to find mini seedless cucumbers, substitute Persian cucumbers. They both have the same great crunch and have a lower water content than regular cucumbers. I could seriously eat the dressing in this recipe with a spoon. Think tzatziki, but with a sour cream base instead of yogurt. I like to have a batch of it on hand at all times for dipping fresh veggies.

ingredients

1½ pounds mini seedless cucumbers, sliced

1 Roma tomato, diced

¼ cup thinly sliced red onions

¼ cup full-fat sour cream

2 tablespoons mayonnaise, store-bought or homemade (page 336)

1 tablespoon fresh lemon juice

1 tablespoon chopped fresh chives

1 teaspoon dried dill weed

1 clove garlic, minced

½ teaspoon sea salt

¼ teaspoon ground black pepper

¼ cup crumbled feta cheese

directions

1. In a large mixing bowl, combine the cucumbers, tomato, and onions.

2. In a separate mixing bowl, combine the sour cream, mayonnaise, lemon juice, chives, dill, garlic, salt, and pepper. Mix until the ingredients are well incorporated.

3. Fold the sauce mixture into the cucumbers, tomatoes, and onions a little at a time until they are sauced to your liking (see tips).

4. Top the dressed salad with the feta cheese before serving.

Tips: Because the cucumbers are so hearty, you can store this salad dressed in the refrigerator for up to 1 week.

Keep any extra sauce as a dip for crudités or as a salad dressing. It will keep in the refrigerator for up to 2 weeks.

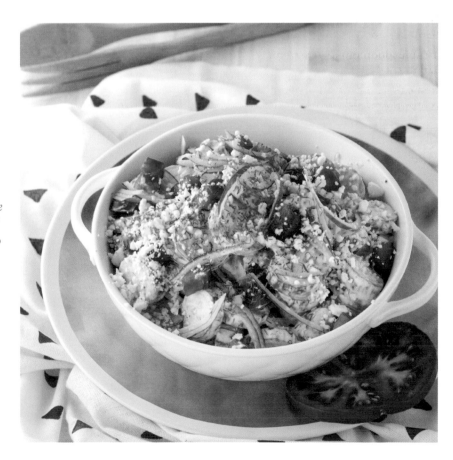

CALORIES: 70 · FAT: 5g · PROTEIN: 2g · TOTAL CARBS: 4.6g · DIETARY FIBER: 1.2g · NET CARBS: 3.4g

Asian Chicken Salad

NET CARBS
4g

 DAIRY-FREE · EGG-FREE · PALEO

makes 8 servings · prep time: 10 minutes

This quick-and-easy salad is great for weekly meal prep, as the cabbage in the coleslaw mix will hold up in the fridge for several days without wilting, even after being dressed. Using cabbage in place of lettuce gives this salad a nice crunchy heartiness.

ingredients

3 cups shredded cooked chicken

1 (14-ounce) bag coleslaw mix

1 small red bell pepper, seeded and cut into thin strips

4 green onions, thinly sliced on the bias

¼ cup torn fresh cilantro

¼ cup crushed roasted almonds

¼ cup toasted sesame seeds

½ cup Asian Vinaigrette (page 334)

directions

Place all of the ingredients in a large mixing bowl and toss until well combined. Store leftovers in the refrigerator for up to 4 days.

CALORIES: 201 · FAT: 9g · PROTEIN: 11g · TOTAL CARBS: 5.8g · DIETARY FIBER: 1.8g · NET CARBS: 4g

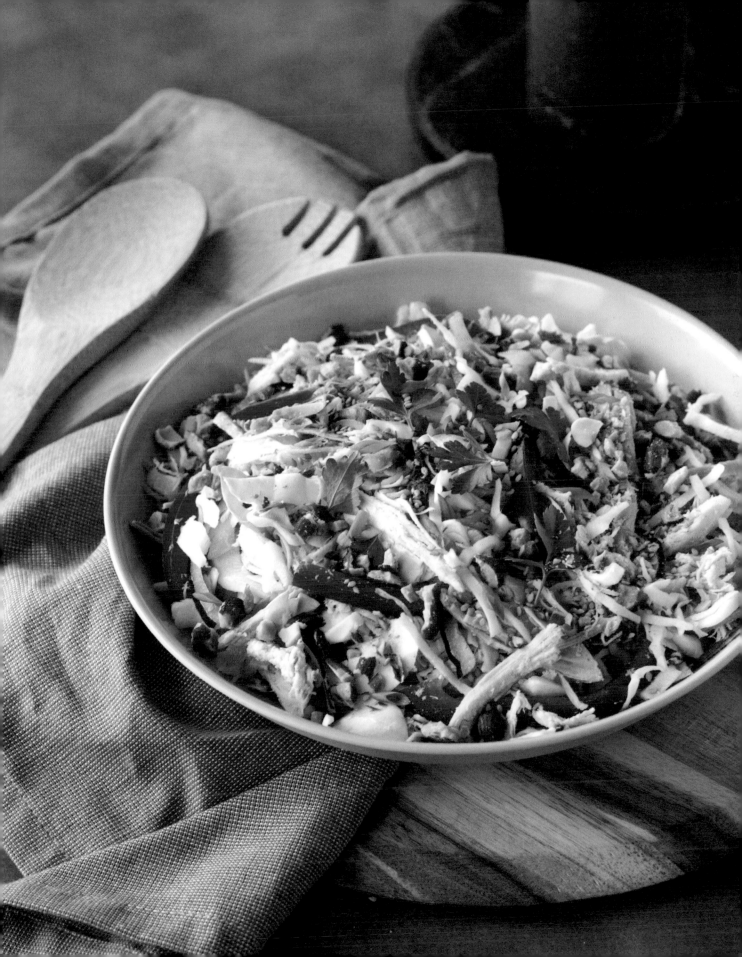

Creamy Caesar Salad with
Garlic Parmesan Cheese Crisps

g

 makes 4 servings · prep time: 10 minutes · cook time: 15 minutes

The cheese crisps in this recipe are so good that you will want to make batch after batch of them to eat as a snack. They also make the perfect "chip" to dip in a fresh batch of homemade guacamole. I just so happen to have a fabulous guacamole recipe, made by my handsome husband, on my website, peaceloveandlowcarb.com.

ingredients

1 cup shredded Parmesan cheese

2 teaspoons garlic powder

2 teaspoons Italian seasoning

1 large head romaine lettuce, chopped

¼ cup Garlic Parmesan Caesar Dressing (page 331), or more to taste

6 slices bacon, cooked crisp and crumbled

directions

1. Preheat the oven to 350°F. Line a rimmed baking sheet with parchment paper.

2. Spread the Parmesan cheese in a thin layer on the parchment paper. Sprinkle the garlic powder and Italian seasoning over the Parmesan cheese.

3. Bake the cheese until it is golden brown and crispy, about 10 minutes. Let it cool, then break it into bite-sized pieces.

4. In a large mixing bowl, combine the romaine lettuce, dressing, crumbled bacon, and cheese crisps. Toss and serve.

CALORIES: 261 · FAT: 19g · PROTEIN: 62g · TOTAL CARBS: 7.5g · DIETARY FIBER: 3.5g · NET CARBS: 4g

Soups & Salads

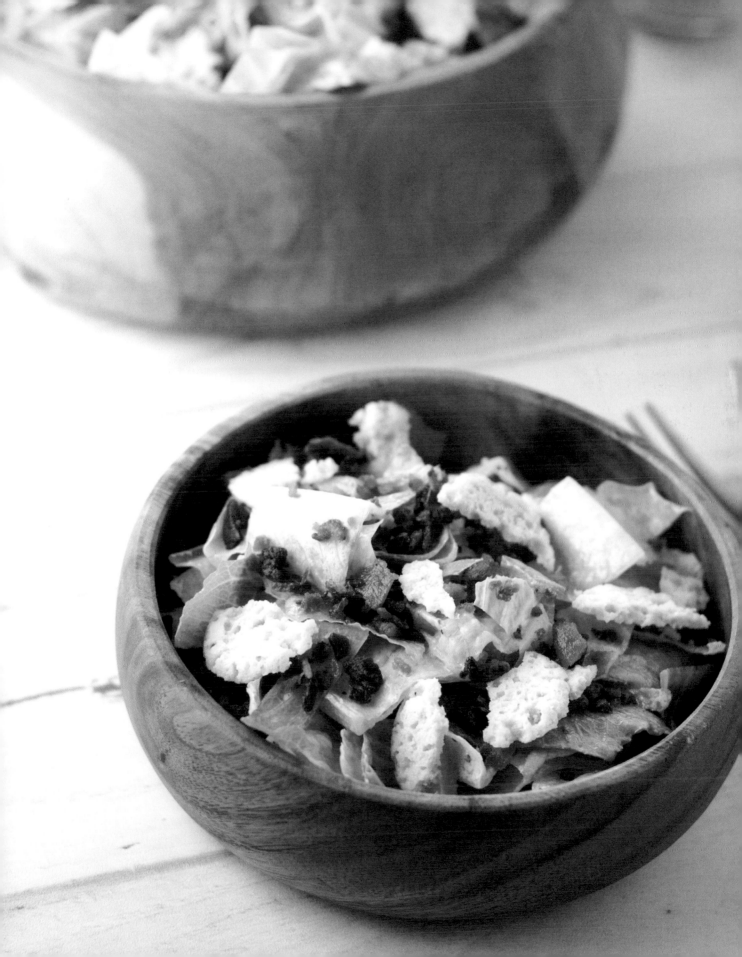

Cobb Salad

makes 4 servings · prep time: 20 minutes

This is one of my favorite dishes in the book simply because of all the beautiful colors. I truly believe that you eat with your eyes first. Pretty food just tastes better. My love of beautiful food, combined with all the years I spent in the restaurant industry, have me constantly styling my food and wiping the rims of plates, even when I am just plating a weeknight dinner for my family. There are few things I love more that an artfully plated dish of food. Cobb salads are traditionally served with blue cheese dressing, but I enjoy this salad with the Dill Pickle Vinaigrette on page 335.

ingredients

1 large head romaine lettuce, chopped

1 pound boneless, skinless chicken breasts or thighs, cooked and chopped

2 hard-boiled eggs (see page 162), chopped

1 small seedless cucumber, sliced

8 grape tomatoes, halved

½ small red onion, chopped

4 slices bacon, cooked and chopped

¼ cup raw cashews

¼ cup crumbled blue cheese

1 medium avocado, peeled, pitted, and cubed

Dressing of choice

directions

1. In a large serving bowl or on a large platter, spread the lettuce in an even layer.

2. Arrange the chicken, eggs, cucumber, tomatoes, onion, bacon, cashews, cheese, and avocado in even rows across the top of the romaine.

3. Drizzle with dressing before serving.

CALORIES: 442 · FAT: 26.5g · PROTEIN: 39g · TOTAL CARBS: 12.5g · DIETARY FIBER: 6.3g · NET CARBS: 6.3g

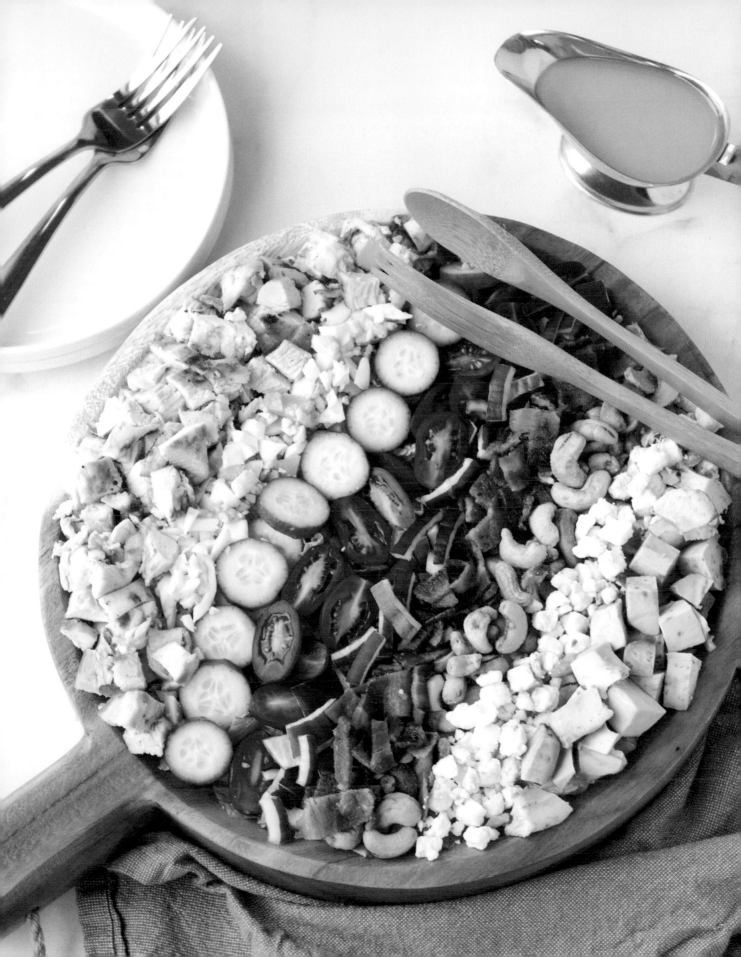

Chef Salad Skewers

NET CARBS
2.5g

 NUT-FREE makes 8 skewers (1 per serving) · prep time: 20 minutes · cook time: 20 minutes

I've decided that food is more fun when it is served on a stick. I think that's why fair food always draws such a huge crowd. My family loves these salad skewers so much so that they do not even use dressing with them. Personally, I really like to dip them in Avocado Green Goddess Dressing (page 333) or Ranch Dressing (page 332). These make for a beautiful presentation and are great to take to parties or get-togethers. It's always fun to bring something that looks fancy but takes little work to prepare. These are also a great way to sneak some extra veggies into your children's diet.

ingredients

4 slices thick-cut bacon

8 grape tomatoes, halved

8 romaine lettuce leaves

8 slices deli ham (about 8 ounces)

8 slices deli turkey (about 8 ounces)

4 hard-boiled eggs (see page 162), halved

3 ounces sharp cheddar cheese, cut into 8 thick slices or chunks

2 mini seedless cucumbers, thinly sliced lengthwise

Special equipment:

8 skewers, about 12 inches long

tip: Not all deli meats are created equal. Look for the cleanest brands possible. Sometimes they end up costing more, but in the end, they are worth it. Your health is worth it. YOU are worth it.

directions

1. Cook the bacon until it is beginning to get crispy but is still chewy. You want to be able to fold it. Cut each slice in half crosswise.

2. Divide all of the ingredients evenly among the 8 skewers, starting and finishing each skewer with a tomato half. Before threading the bacon, lettuce, deli meats, and cucumber ribbons onto the skewers, scrunch or fold each ingredient into a compact shape.

3. Store leftovers in the refrigerator for up to 1 week.

CALORIES: 173 · FAT: 9g · PROTEIN: 15g · TOTAL CARBS: 3.4g · DIETARY FIBER: 0.9g · NET CARBS: 2.5g

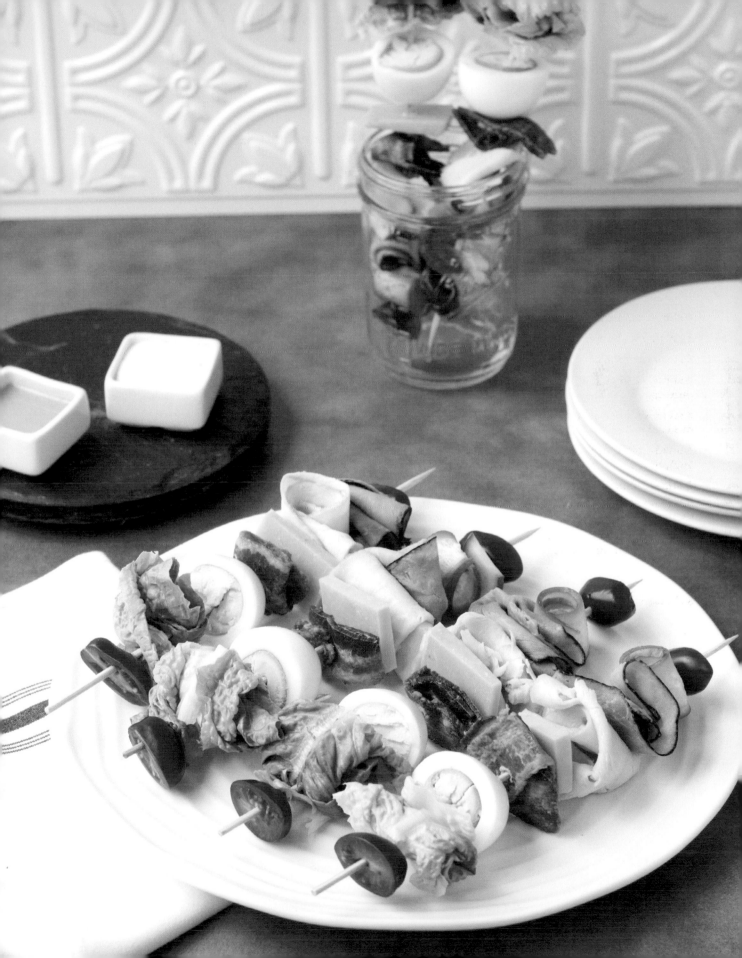

Deviled Ham and Egg Salad Wraps

makes 8 wraps (2 per serving) · prep time: 15 minutes

This is one of my favorite quick-and-easy weekday lunches. I like to make a double batch over the weekend so that Jon and I can eat it throughout the week. It is a lot easier to stay on track when you have healthy grab-and-go foods prepped in the fridge.

ingredients

4 hard-boiled eggs (see page 162), chopped

1 cup chopped ham steak

1 rib celery, finely chopped

2 tablespoons minced shallots

2 tablespoons dill pickle relish

1 tablespoon chopped fresh chives

¼ cup mayonnaise, store-bought or homemade (page 336)

1 tablespoon Dijon mustard

Sea salt and ground black pepper (optional)

8 large Bibb lettuce leaves, for the wraps

Chopped sun-dried tomatoes, for garnish (optional)

directions

1. In a large mixing bowl, combine the eggs, ham, celery, shallots, relish, chives, mayonnaise, and mustard. Mix until the ingredients are well combined. Taste and add salt and pepper, if desired.

2. Divide the mixture evenly among the lettuce leaves. Top with sun-dried tomatoes, if desired.

CALORIES: 243 · FAT: 17g · PROTEIN: 17g · TOTAL CARBS: 3.8g · DIETARY FIBER: 0.8g · NET CARBS: 3g

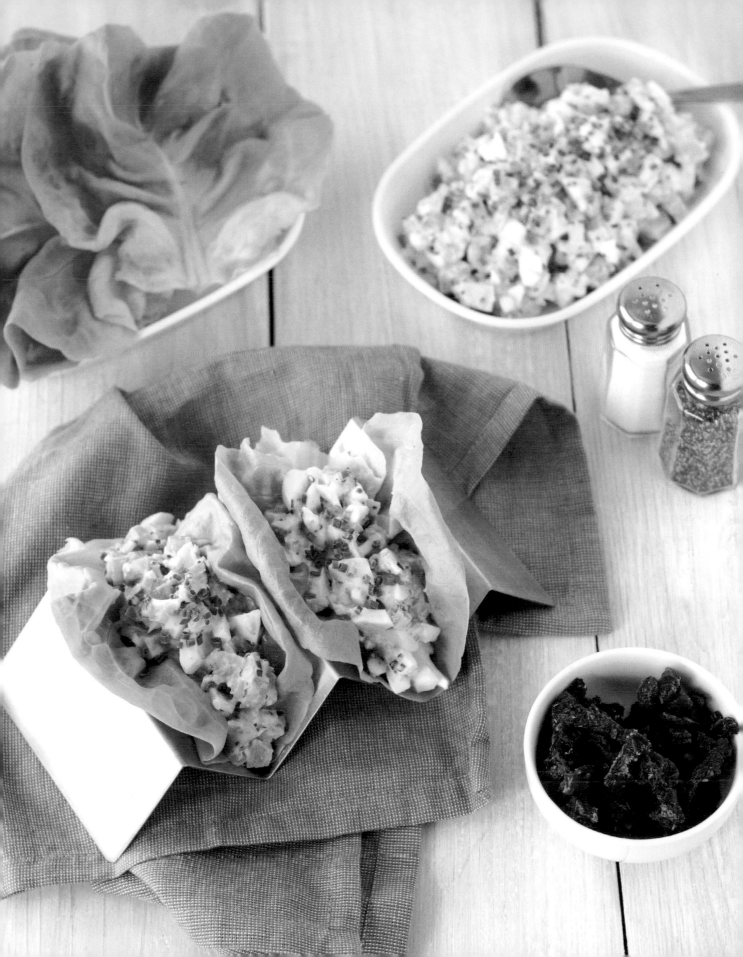

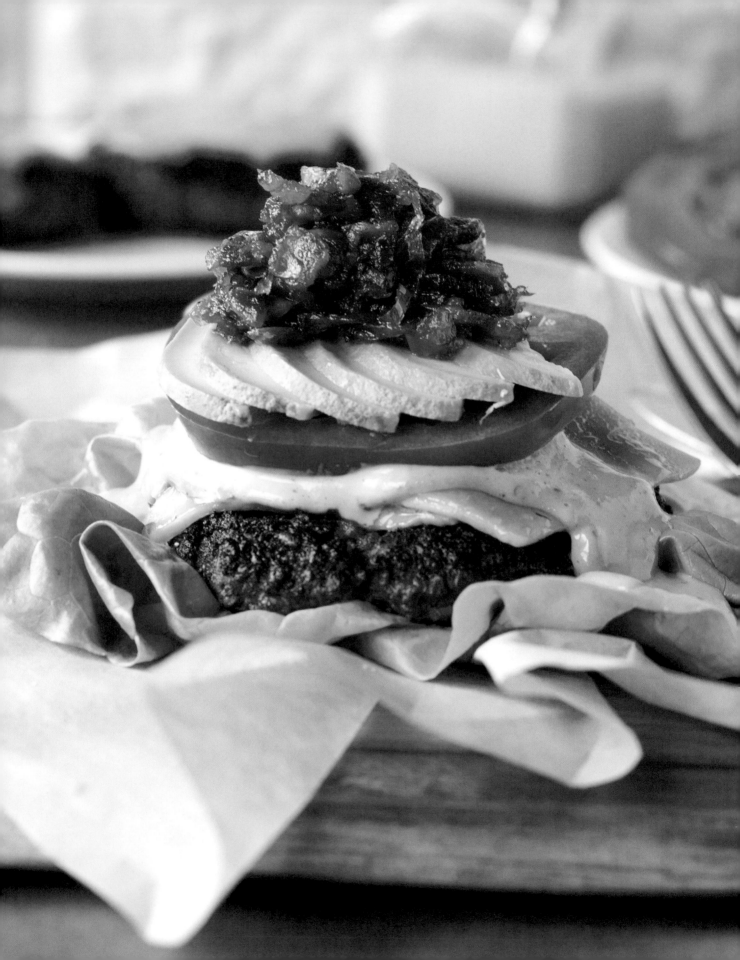

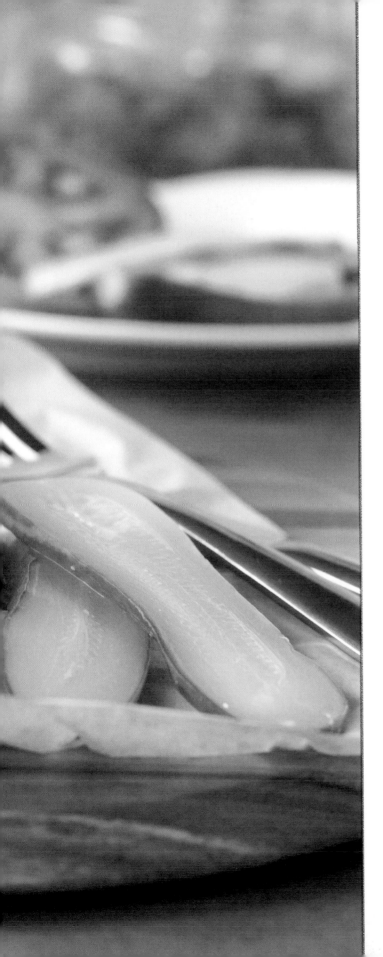

Main Dishes

Warm Taco Slaw

    makes 6 servings · prep time: 5 minutes · cook time: 15 minutes

I'm pretty sure that this book has established my vast love of all things taco and taco related. I think it's because my Mexican Seasoning Blend packs so much flavor. One simple seasoning blend can transform any dish from bland to grand.

ingredients

1 pound ground beef

4 tablespoons Mexican Seasoning Blend (page 350), divided

1 (10-ounce) can diced tomatoes and green chilies, with juices

1 (16-ounce) bag coleslaw mix

½ cup sliced black olives

Sea salt (optional)

½ cup full-fat sour cream, for garnish

1 large avocado, peeled, pitted, and sliced, for garnish

2 tablespoons torn fresh cilantro or flat-leaf parsley, for garnish (optional)

Pickled jalapeños, for garnish (optional)

directions

1. Heat a large skillet over medium heat. Put the ground beef and 2 tablespoons of the seasoning blend in the pan and cook until the meat is browned and cooked through, about 15 minutes.

2. To the skillet, add the diced tomatoes and green chilies, coleslaw mix, and remaining 2 tablespoons of the seasoning blend. Cook until the cabbage is tender, about 7 minutes.

3. Stir in the olives and cook until heated, about 2 minutes. Taste and add salt, if desired.

4. Top each serving with some sour cream and avocado slices as well as cilantro and/or pickled jalapeños, if desired.

5. Store leftovers in the refrigerator for up to 1 week.

tip: To make this dish dairy-free and Paleo compliant, omit the sour cream.

CALORIES: 278 · FAT: 19g · PROTEIN: 18g · TOTAL CARBS: 10g · DIETARY FIBER: 4.4g · NET CARBS: 5.6g

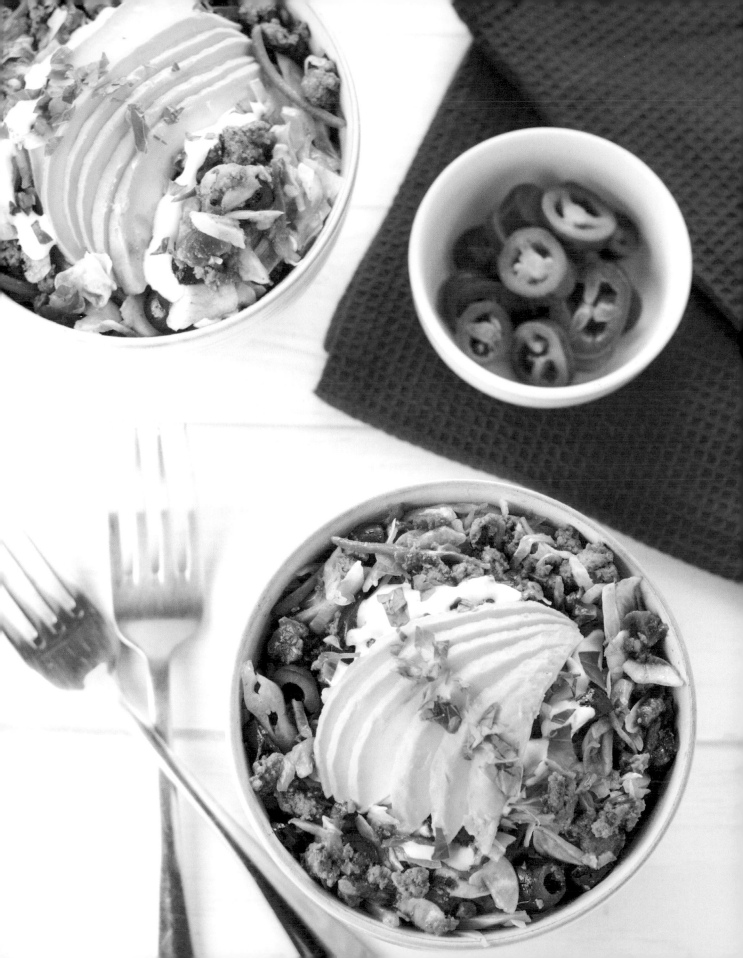

Steak Fajita Bowls

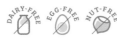

makes 6 servings · prep time: 25 minutes, plus up to 24 hours
to marinate · cook time: 15 minutes

In our house, we not only observe Taco Tuesday, but we also celebrate Fajita Friday. This is one of our favorite meals to prepare a double batch of for meals throughout the week. We use the leftovers for salads and for breakfast with eggs. These Steak Fajita Bowls are amazing served with Fiesta Cauliflower Rice (page 282).

ingredients

⅓ cup plus 2 tablespoons avocado oil or olive oil, divided

¼ cup coconut aminos or gluten-free soy sauce

4 tablespoons Mexican Seasoning Blend (page 350), divided

Grated zest and juice of 1 lime

3 cloves garlic, minced

2 pounds beef flank steak, sliced against the grain in ¼-inch-thick slices

1 medium onion, halved and thinly sliced (about 1 cup)

1 large green bell pepper, seeded and cut into ½-inch-wide strips

1 large yellow bell pepper, seeded and cut into ½-inch-wide strips

1 large red bell pepper, seeded and cut into ½-inch-wide strips

Full-fat sour cream, for topping (optional; omit for dairy-free and Paleo)

Fresh cilantro, for garnish (optional)

Sliced avocado, for garnish (optional)

directions

1. Make the marinade: In a small mixing bowl, whisk together ⅓ cup of the avocado oil, coconut aminos, 3 tablespoons of the seasoning blend, lime zest and juice, and garlic.

2. Place the steak in a gallon-sized resealable plastic bag. Pour the marinade into the bag and seal. Move the steak around to evenly coat the slices in the marinade. Refrigerate for 3 hours or up to 24 hours.

3. Heat the remaining 2 tablespoons of avocado oil in a large skillet over medium-high heat. Add the onion and bell peppers to the pan. Sprinkle the remaining tablespoon of seasoning blend over the peppers and onions and mix in. Cook the vegetables until they are crisp-tender and begin to char in spots. Remove the pan from the heat and set aside.

4. Heat a large grill pan over medium-high heat. Remove the strips of steak from the marinade and lay them across the hot grill pan in a single layer. You can do this step in batches, if necessary. Grill the steak for 2 to 3 minutes on each side for medium-done meat, or until it has reached your desired level of doneness.

5. Serve topped with sour cream, cilantro, and avocado slices, if desired. Store leftovers in the refrigerator for up to 1 week.

tips: You can change up this recipe in a lot of ways to make it work for you:

- *In place of the flank steak, you can use skirt steak or hanger steak.*

- *Try it as a sheet pan meal: Put the prepped veggies and marinated steak on a rimmed baking sheet and roast in a preheated 425°F oven until the meat is cooked to your desired level of doneness and the veggies are tender.*

- *You can cook the meat and veggies on a grill to add a little something special to an already amazing dish.*

CALORIES: 439 · FAT: 30g · PROTEIN: 32g · TOTAL CARBS: 10g · DIETARY FIBER: 2.5g · NET CARBS: 7.5g

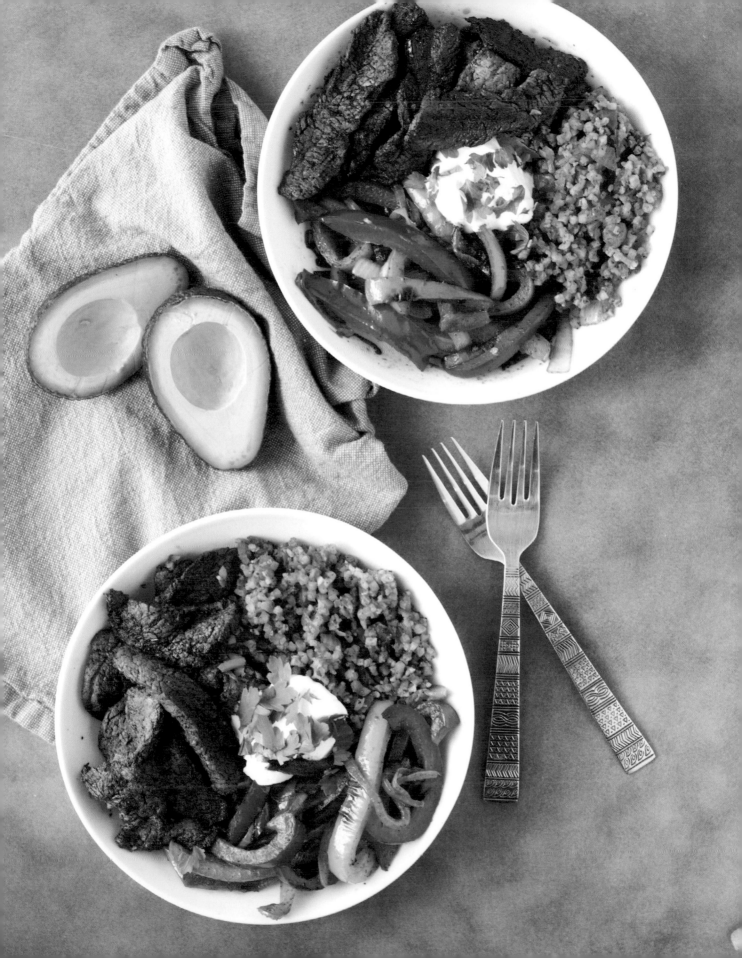

Everything Bagel Dogs

makes 6 servings · prep time: 15 minutes · cook time: 27 minutes

ingredients

For the dough:

¼ cup blanched almond flour

3 tablespoons coconut flour

1 teaspoon garlic powder

1 teaspoon onion powder

1 teaspoon Italian seasoning

1½ cups shredded low-moisture, part-skim mozzarella cheese

¼ cup (½ stick) butter or ghee

1 ounce full-fat cream cheese (2 tablespoons)

1 large egg

6 grass-fed beef hot dogs

For the topping:

2 tablespoons butter or ghee, melted

¼ cup Everything Bagel Seasoning (page 352)

Ketchup, mustard, relish, sauerkraut, and/or other condiments of choice, for serving

directions

1. Preheat the oven to 375°F. Line a rimmed baking sheet with parchment paper or a silicone baking mat.

2. To make the dough: In a small mixing bowl, whisk together the almond flour, coconut flour, garlic powder, onion powder, and Italian seasoning.

3. In a separate microwave-safe bowl, combine the mozzarella cheese, butter, and cream cheese. Microwave for 1 minute 30 seconds to soften. Mix together until everything is well combined. If it gets stringy or is not quite melted enough, put it back in the microwave for another 30 seconds.

4. To the cheese mixture, add the dry ingredients and the egg. Using your hands, mix until the ingredients are well incorporated. If you are having a hard time mixing the ingredients together, put the bowl back in the microwave for another 20 to 30 seconds. If the dough starts sticking to your hands, wet your hands slightly and continue working the dough.

5. Divide the dough into 6 equal portions.

6. Working on a silicone mat or sheet of parchment paper, use your hands to roll each portion of the dough into a thin cylinder about 10 inches long, resembling a breadstick. If the dough starts to get sticky, wet your hands with a little bit of water to prevent the dough from sticking to your hands.

7. Starting at one end of a hot dog, wrap the dough around the hot dog until you reach the other end. Repeat with the remaining dough portions and hot dogs.

8. Place the dough-wrapped hot dogs on the lined baking sheet. Brush each one generously with the melted butter, then top with the bagel seasoning.

9. Bake for 25 minutes or until golden brown. Serve with the condiments of your choice.

10. Store leftovers in the refrigerator for up to 1 week. Reheat in a preheated 250°F oven.

CALORIES: 377 · FAT: 31g · PROTEIN: 19g · TOTAL CARBS: 8g · DIETARY FIBER: 3.5g · NET CARBS: 4.5g

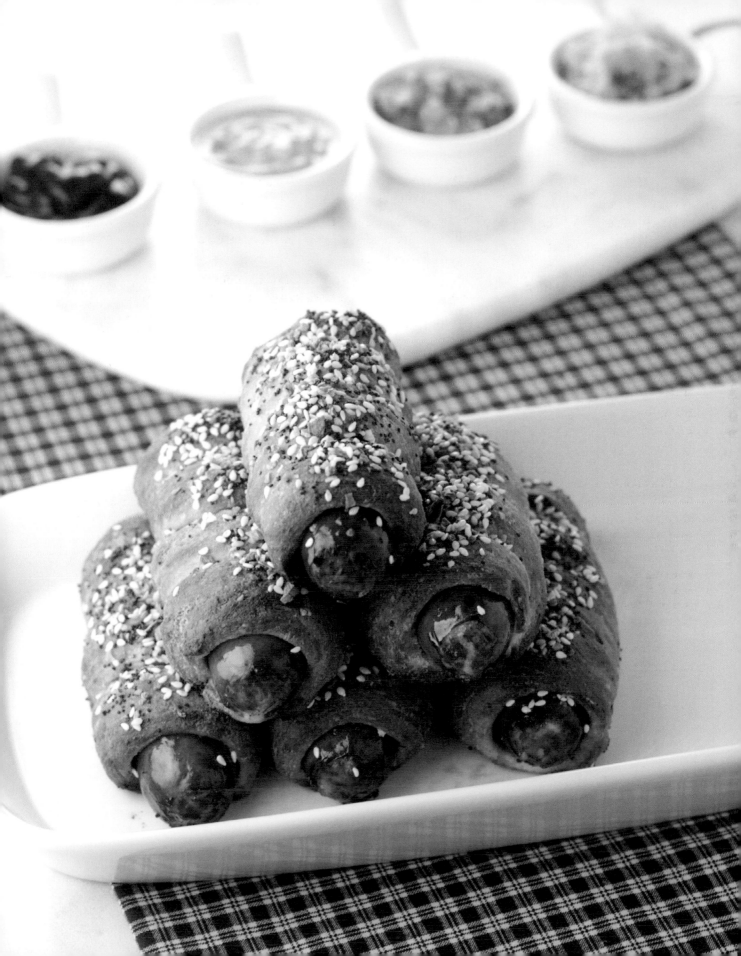

Spaghetti Squash Pork Lo Mein

   makes 8 servings · prep time: 20 minutes · cook time: 1 hour

Pork lo mein is traditionally made with Chinese egg noodles, but I lightened it up in this low-carb rendition by using spaghetti squash in place of the pasta. You could also make this with zucchini noodles, which will save you some time and lower the carb count. That's a win-win situation!

ingredients

1 small spaghetti squash (about 4 pounds)

1 tablespoon olive oil

Sea salt and ground black pepper

1 pound boneless pork tenderloin, cut into thin strips

3 tablespoons toasted sesame seeds, divided

5 tablespoons coconut aminos or gluten-free soy sauce, divided

4 cloves garlic, minced

1 tablespoon grated fresh ginger

½ cup chicken stock

2 tablespoons unseasoned rice wine vinegar

2 tablespoons toasted sesame oil, divided

1 red bell pepper, seeded and cut into thin strips

2 ribs celery, thinly sliced on the bias

1 (8-ounce) can bamboo shoots, drained

2 cups coleslaw mix

2 green onions, sliced on the bias, for garnish

directions

1. Preheat the oven to 400°F. Line a rimmed baking sheet with parchment paper or a silicone baking mat.

2. Cut the spaghetti squash in half lengthwise and, using a large spoon, scrape out the seeds. Place both halves of the squash cut side up on the lined baking sheet, drizzle with the olive oil, and sprinkle with a little salt and pepper. Roast for 45 minutes, or until the squash is easily pierced with a fork. Remove the squash from the oven and, once cool enough to handle, use a fork to scrape out the shreds of squash. Set aside.

3. When the spaghetti squash is nearly done roasting, combine the pork, 1 tablespoon of the sesame seeds, 2 tablespoons of the coconut aminos, garlic, and ginger in a mixing bowl and set aside.

4. In a small mixing bowl, combine the stock, remaining 3 tablespoons of coconut aminos, and vinegar.

5. Heat 1 tablespoon of the toasted sesame oil in a large deep-sided skillet or wok over medium-high heat. Add the bell peppers, celery, bamboo shoots, and coleslaw to the pan and stir-fry until the vegetables are tender, about 6 minutes.

6. Meanwhile, heat the remaining 1 tablespoon of sesame oil in a separate skillet over medium-high heat. Add the pork and its marinade to the pan. Stir-fry the pork until it is cooked through, 3 to 5 minutes.

7. Add the pork to the vegetables, along with the spaghetti squash and the sauce from Step 4, and stir-fry for an additional 5 minutes, until everything is well combined and heated through. Garnish with the green onions and remaining 2 tablespoons of sesame seeds before serving.

8. Store leftovers in the refrigerator for up to 1 week. Reheat in the microwave or on the stovetop.

CALORIES: 185 · FAT: 7.4g · PROTEIN: 12.5g · TOTAL CARBS: 7.6g · DIETARY FIBER: 1.9g · NET CARBS: 5.7g

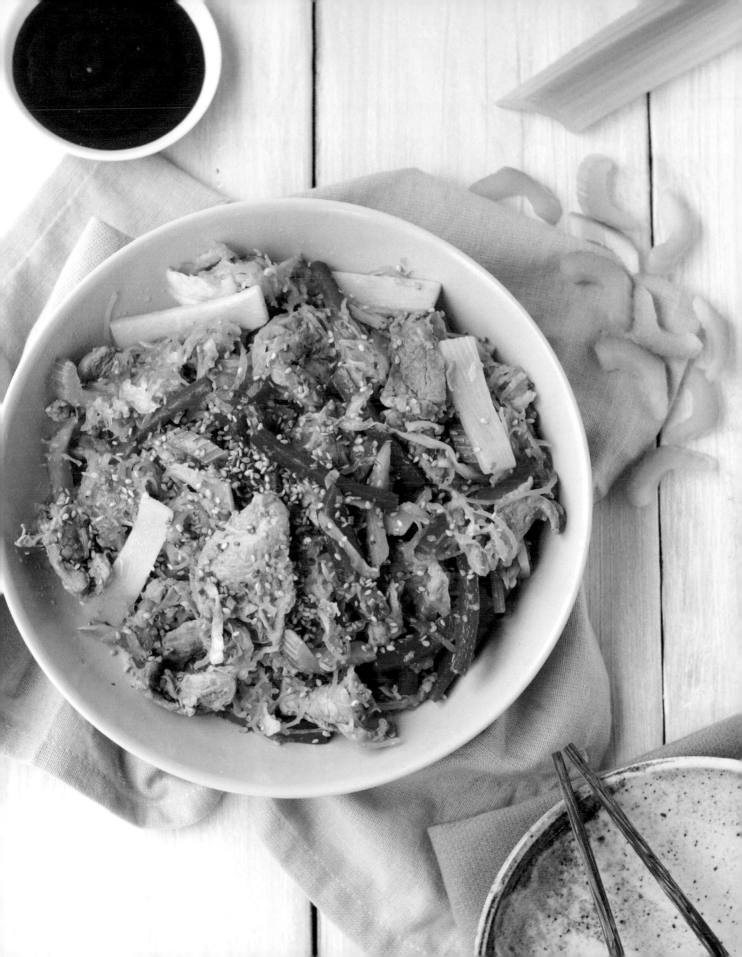

Slow Cooker Spiced Pork Tenderloin

   makes 10 servings · prep time: 15 minutes · cook time: 4 or 8 hours

I love how simply this recipe comes together. The slow cooker does all of the work for you. I like to serve this dish with Fiesta Cauliflower Rice (page 282). From time to time, I even use this in place of the beef in my Steak Fajita Bowls (page 210). This recipe makes a really large portion. It is great for meal prepping, as it freezes and reheats very well. I like to make a batch and then divide it into four portions and freeze them.

ingredients

2 tablespoons apple cider vinegar

6 cloves garlic, minced

1 tablespoon ground cumin

1 tablespoon smoked paprika

1 teaspoon dried oregano leaves

1 teaspoon onion powder

1 teaspoon sea salt

½ teaspoon ground black pepper

½ teaspoon ground coriander

¼ teaspoon ground cinnamon

2 tablespoons olive oil

4 pounds boneless pork tenderloin

1 (12-ounce) jar salsa verde

1 lime, cut into wedges, for garnish (optional)

A few sprigs fresh cilantro, for garnish (optional)

directions

1. Put the vinegar and garlic in a slow cooker and turn it on to the low setting.

2. Make the seasoning rub: In a small mixing bowl, mix together the cumin, paprika, oregano, onion powder, salt, pepper, coriander, and cinnamon.

3. Brush the olive oil over both sides of the pork tenderloin. Using half of the seasoning rub, generously coat one side of the pork, packing the seasoning down so that it sticks.

4. Place the pork tenderloin seasoned side down in the slow cooker. Coat the other side with the remaining seasoning rub. Cover and cook on low for 8 hours or on high for 4 hours.

5. Once the pork tenderloin has finished cooking, use two forks to shred the meat. Mix in half of the salsa verde.

6. Plate and top with the remaining salsa verde, lime wedges, and cilantro, if desired.

7. Store leftovers in the refrigerator for up to 1 week. Reheat in the microwave or on the stovetop.

tip: There are plenty of clean and Paleo-compliant brands of jarred salsa verde on the market. Just be sure to read the labels, as many salsas contain added sugar.

CALORIES: 384 · FAT: 25g · PROTEIN: 32g · TOTAL CARBS: 3.5g · DIETARY FIBER: 0.3g · NET CARBS: 3.2g

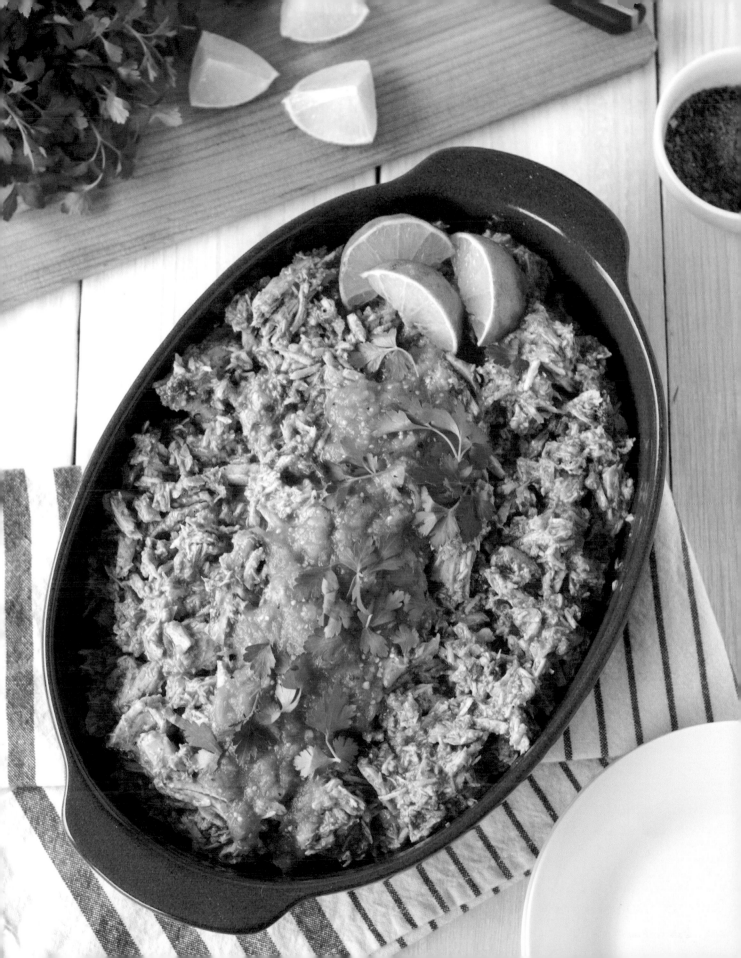

Slow Cooker Chinese Five-Spice Beef

DAIRY-FREE · EGG-FREE · NUT-FREE · PALEO

makes 8 servings · prep time: 20 minutes · cook time: 7 hours

My slow cooker is one of my absolute favorite things in my kitchen. It is perfect for a lazy weeknight dinner. It is amazing for comforting dishes in the cold of winter, and it is equally perfect for those hot summer days when you don't want to heat up your oven. You really can't go wrong when it comes to slow cooking. Perhaps one of my favorite things to slow cook is my Slow Cooker Kickin' Chili from my website; head to peacelove-andlowcarb.com to check it out! I love to serve this dish over cauliflower rice.

ingredients

2 pounds stew beef

Sea salt and ground black pepper

2 tablespoons olive oil

1 cup beef stock

½ cup cooking sherry

¼ cup coconut aminos or gluten-free soy sauce

2 tablespoons unseasoned rice wine vinegar

2 red bell peppers, seeded and sliced

8 ounces cremini mushrooms, quartered

2 large shallots, thinly sliced

3 cloves garlic, minced

1 (2-inch) piece fresh ginger, grated

1 tablespoon plus 1 teaspoon Chinese five-spice powder

1 teaspoon red pepper flakes

2 cups snow peas

1 batch Basic Cauliflower Rice (page 282), for serving (optional)

2 green onions, sliced on the bias, for garnish

2 tablespoons toasted sesame seeds, for garnish

directions

1. Preheat a slow cooker on the low setting. Season the stew beef generously with salt and pepper.

2. Heat the olive oil in a large skillet over medium-high heat. Add the beef and sear until browned on the outside, then transfer it, with juices, to the slow cooker.

3. To the slow cooker, add the stock, sherry, coconut aminos, vinegar, bell peppers, mushrooms, shallots, garlic, ginger, five-spice powder, and red pepper flakes. Stir to combine, cover, and cook for 6 hours.

4. Add the snow peas and cook for an additional hour.

5. Serve the beef and vegetable mixture over cauliflower rice, if desired, and top with green onions and sesame seeds.

6. Store leftovers in the refrigerator for up to 1 week. Reheat in the microwave or on the stovetop.

tip: To make this dish Paleo compliant, substitute extra beef stock for the cooking sherry.

CALORIES: 332 · FAT: 21.5g · PROTEIN: 23g · TOTAL CARBS: 8.5g · DIETARY FIBER: 1.5g · NET CARBS: 7g

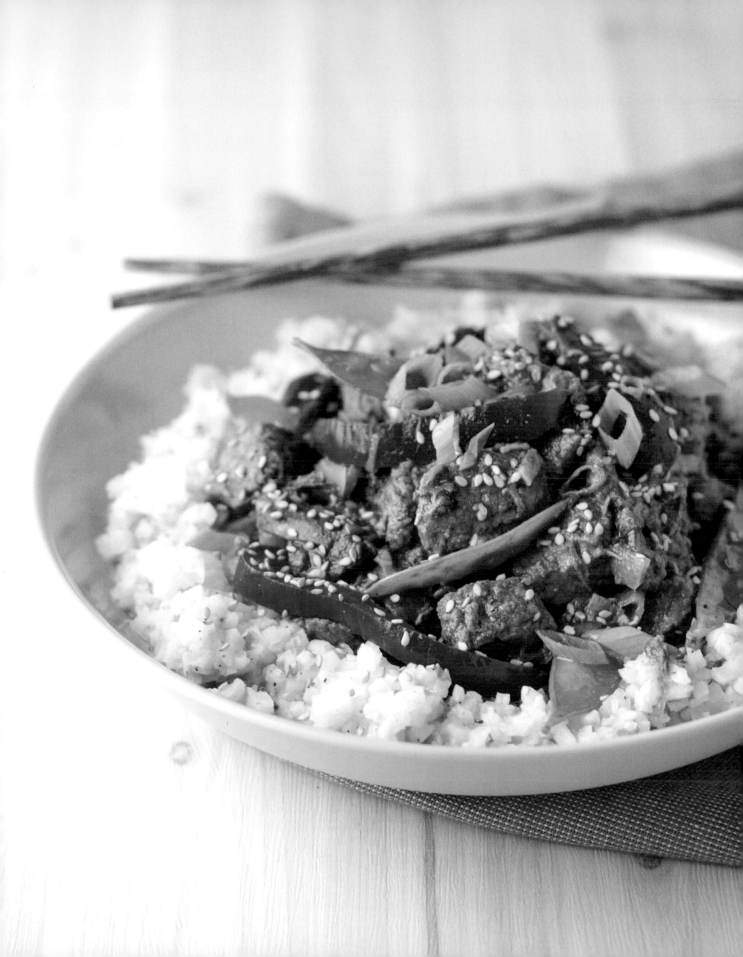

Shrimp and Cheesy Cauliflower Rice Stuffed Peppers

makes 4 servings · prep time: 15 minutes · cook time: 35 minutes

Psst...you wanna know a secret? The cauliflower rice mixture stuffed inside these peppers makes an awesome substitute for a traditional creamy risotto. When Jon and I were traveling in Monaco and France, nearly every menu we encountered had risotto, which I really, really love. I came home from that trip and started making as many different versions of cauliflower rice risotto as I could possibly think of. Using cauliflower in place of rice puts one of my favorite dishes back on the table while also bringing back memories of an amazing trip abroad.

ingredients

2 tablespoons butter or ghee

3 cloves garlic, minced

3 cups riced cauliflower (see page 76)

1 teaspoon Italian seasoning

1 teaspoon onion powder

1 teaspoon sea salt

½ teaspoon ground black pepper

¼ teaspoon red pepper flakes

4 red or yellow bell peppers, tops cut off and ribs and seeds removed

1 cup shredded mozzarella cheese

½ cup grated Parmesan cheese

⅓ cup heavy cream

2 tablespoons full-fat sour cream

1 pound medium-large shrimp (36/40), deveined and tails removed

¼ cup shredded Parmesan cheese, divided

Chopped fresh flat-leaf parsley, for garnish (optional)

directions

1. Preheat the oven to 400°F.

2. Heat the butter in a large skillet over medium-low heat. Add the garlic, riced cauliflower, Italian seasoning, onion powder, salt, black pepper, and red pepper flakes to the pan. Cook, stirring frequently, until the cauliflower rice is tender, about 15 minutes.

3. Meanwhile, bake the bell peppers: Place the peppers cut side up in an 8-inch square casserole dish. Bake for 20 minutes, until the peppers are crisp-tender.

4. When the rice is tender, add the mozzarella cheese, grated Parmesan cheese, heavy cream, and sour cream to the skillet. Stir in and cook until the cheeses are melted, about 5 minutes.

5. Add the shrimp to the cauliflower rice mixture and cook just until the shrimp are cooked through, 5 to 10 minutes. (When cooked through, they will no longer be translucent and will take on a pink color; do not overcook, or they will become tough.)

6. Divide the cauliflower rice and shrimp mixture evenly among the 4 peppers. Top each pepper with 1 tablespoon of the shredded Parmesan cheese.

7. Return the peppers to the oven and broil on high for 2 to 3 minutes, until the cheese on top is crispy and golden brown. Garnish with fresh parsley, if desired, before serving.

tips: To lower the overall carb count of this dish, make it as a casserole using 1 bell pepper, chopped up and added to the cauliflower rice.

You can use any size shrimp you have on hand, but if using extra-large or jumbo shrimp, chop them into smaller pieces.

This recipe calls for grated and shredded Parmesan cheese. If you have only one type on hand—shredded or grated—feel free to use all of one or the other.

CALORIES: 471 · FAT: 27g · PROTEIN: 37g · TOTAL CARBS: 14g · DIETARY FIBER: 4g · NET CARBS: 10g

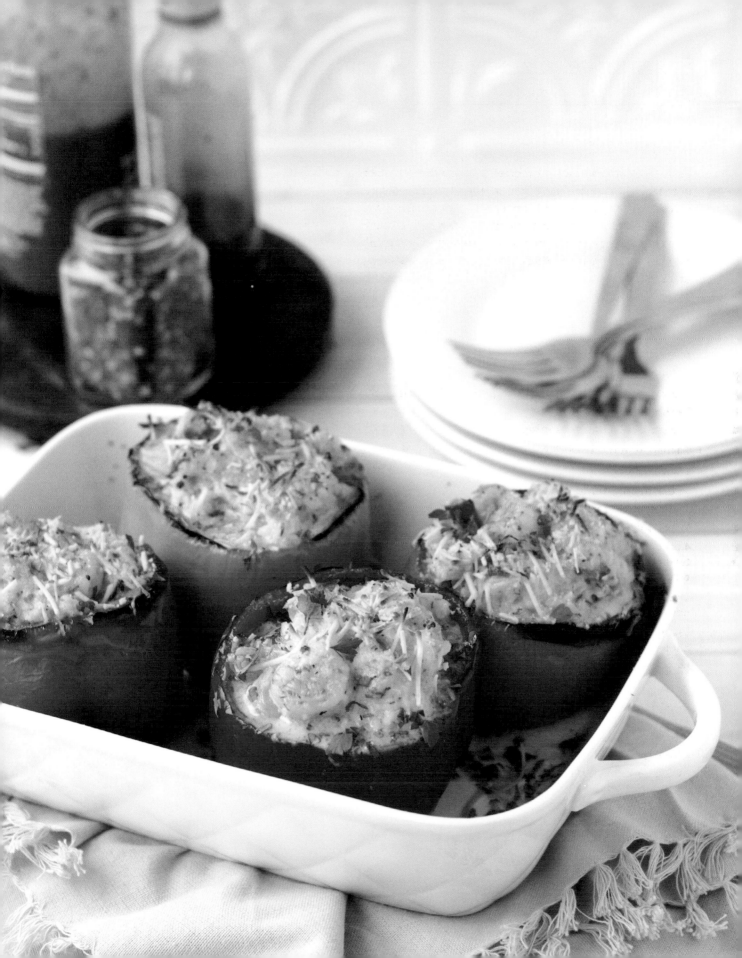

Seared Scallops with Sherry Beurre Blanc

   makes 4 servings · prep time: 10 minutes · cook time: 15 minutes

Scallops seem to be an intimidating food for many people. The main reason is that they have never actually tried them. I like to think of scallops as the gateway into seafood. They aren't fishy at all and actually have a deliciously meaty texture. They are mild and fairly neutral in flavor. Just be careful not to overcook them or they will become very chewy and almost rubbery. If you like the texture of crab and lobster, then I think you will love scallops. The sherry beurre blanc sauce is just the icing on the low-carb cake. It is rich and decadent and complements the scallops perfectly.

ingredients

1½ pounds sea scallops (16/20)

Sea salt and ground black pepper

2 tablespoons white wine vinegar

2 tablespoons cooking sherry

2 tablespoons minced shallots

1 bay leaf

¼ cup heavy cream

¾ cup (1½ sticks) cold butter, cut into chunks

2 tablespoons capers

4 slices bacon, cooked crisp and crumbled

2 tablespoons butter or ghee

2 tablespoons olive oil or avocado oil

Thinly sliced fresh chives, for garnish (optional)

directions

1. Season the scallops generously on both sides with salt and pepper; set aside.

2. Heat a large skillet over medium-high heat. Add the vinegar, sherry, shallots, and bay leaf. Bring to a low boil, then immediately reduce the heat to medium-low. Pour in the cream and whisk to combine. Simmer until the sauce has reduced by half.

3. Remove the bay leaf and reduce the heat to low. While whisking, add the cold butter, piece by piece, to the cream sauce. Continue whisking until the butter has melted into the sauce and the sauce has thickened, 3 to 4 minutes. Stir in the capers and bacon and slide the pan off the heat.

4. Heat the butter and olive oil in another large skillet over high heat. Add the scallops to the pan, making sure they are not touching, and sear for 1 to 1½ minutes on each side. They should have a nice golden-brown crust while still being translucent in the center.

5. Top the scallops with the sauce before serving. Garnish with fresh chives, if desired.

CALORIES: 644 · FAT: 55g · PROTEIN: 32g · TOTAL CARBS: 5.8g · DIETARY FIBER: 0.3g · NET CARBS: 5.5g

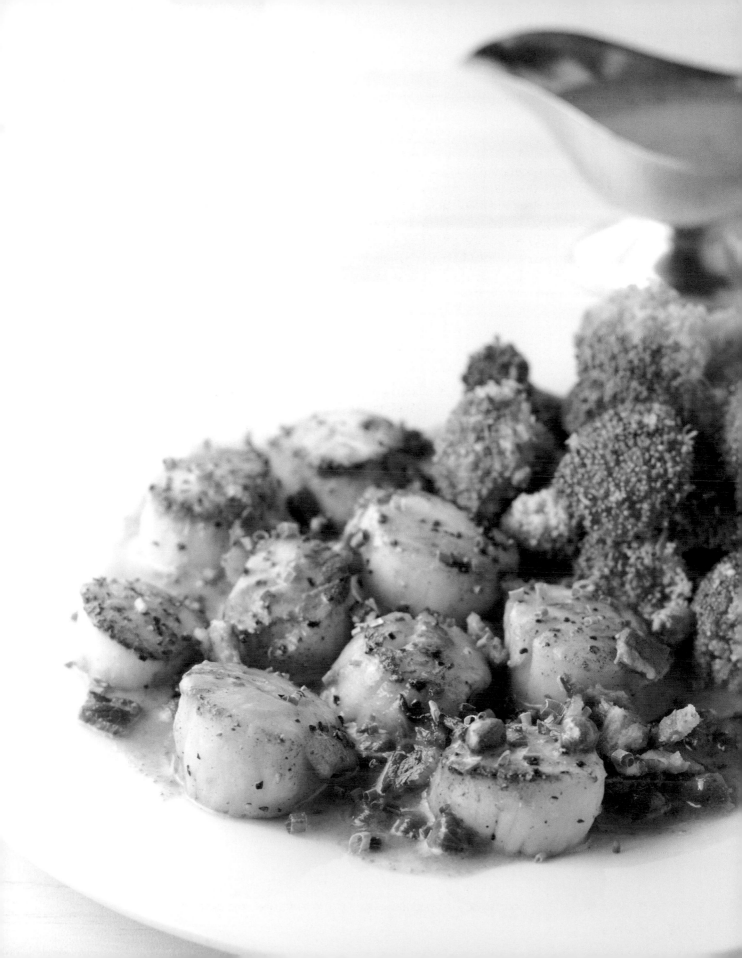

Sausage, Shrimp, and Chicken Jambalaya

makes 8 servings · prep time: 30 minutes · cook time: 40 minutes

Jambalaya makes me think of New Orleans, and New Orleans just plain makes my heart happy. I have a long history with that city; it truly feels like a second home to me. Some of my happiest life moments took place there—fun trips with friends, Jon proposing to me, and the first part of my honeymoon, to name just a few. The city is full of culture, history, and beautiful architecture. New Orleans comes alive with the sunrise and stays ablaze long after the sun sets. It's the kind of city that sets your soul on fire. Not to mention the incredible food at every turn. It's like the city is welcoming you and inviting you back with every bite. I can only hope that my low-carb rendition of a New Orleans staple does justice to the city I hold so dear.

ingredients

15 jumbo shrimp (20/25), peeled, deveined, and chopped

1 pound boneless, skinless chicken breasts or thighs, diced

2 tablespoons Cajun Seasoning (page 351)

2 tablespoons butter or ghee

1 medium onion, diced (about ½ cup)

1 small green bell pepper, seeded and diced

1 small orange bell pepper, seeded and diced

2 ribs celery, chopped

3 cloves garlic, minced

3 bay leaves

2 (10-ounce) cans diced tomatoes and green chilies

2 tablespoons Worcestershire sauce

4 cups riced cauliflower (see page 76)

2 smoked andouille sausage links (about 6 ounces), halved lengthwise and sliced into half-moons

½ cup chicken stock

Sea salt and ground black pepper

2 large green onions, sliced, for garnish

1 lemon, sliced, for serving (optional)

tip: To make this dish dairy-free and Paleo compliant, use ghee rather than butter.

directions

1. In a large mixing bowl, combine the shrimp and chicken. Toss with the Cajun seasoning until all of the pieces are well coated; set aside.

2. Heat the butter in a large skillet or Dutch oven over medium heat. Add the onion, bell peppers, celery, garlic, and bay leaves. Sauté until the vegetables are crisp-tender.

3. Remove the bay leaves. Add the diced tomatoes and green chilies, Worcestershire sauce, and riced cauliflower. Simmer over medium heat until the liquid is reduced by half, about 10 minutes.

4. Add the chicken, shrimp, andouille sausage, and stock and simmer until the meat is cooked all the way through and most of the liquid has evaporated, about 10 minutes. Taste and add salt and pepper, if needed.

5. Top with the green onions before serving. Serve with lemon slices, if desired.

6. Store leftovers in the refrigerator for up to 1 week, or freeze for later use. Reheat in the microwave or on the stovetop.

CALORIES: 223 · FAT: 10g · PROTEIN: 21g · TOTAL CARBS: 10g · DIETARY FIBER: 2.8g · NET CARBS: 7.3g

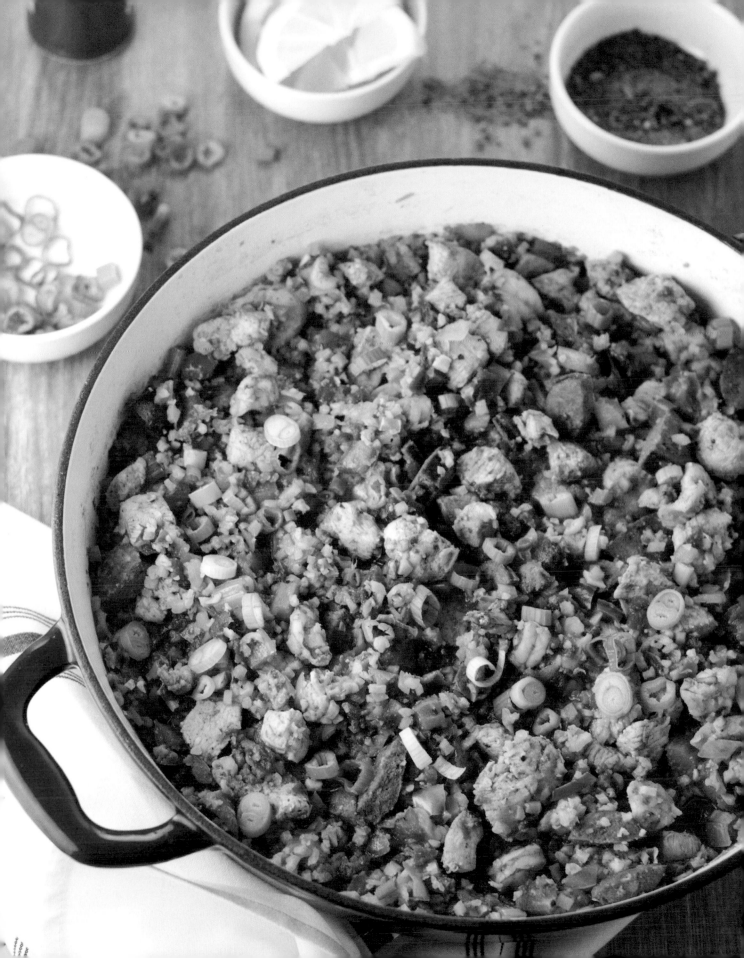

Reuben Biscuit Sandwiches

makes 5 sandwiches (1 per serving) · prep time: 15 minutes · cook time: 25 minutes

Remember how on page 104, in the introductory note to the Breakfast Pizza recipe, I refer to being a member of the "put an egg on it" society? Well, yes, that applies here, too! I love to turn this into a breakfast sandwich by adding a drippy, gooey, perfectly cooked poached egg. I'm pretty sure that means I should serve my sandwich with a bib. If you are anything like me and you add an egg, you might want to use a fork and knife for this sandwich.

ingredients

For the biscuits:

4 ounces full-fat cream cheese (½ cup), softened

1 large egg

1 teaspoon caraway seeds

½ teaspoon Italian seasoning

½ teaspoon onion powder

2 cloves garlic, minced

1½ cups blanched almond flour

1 cup shredded Swiss cheese

¼ cup heavy cream

¼ cup water

10 slices deli corned beef, warmed

5 slices Swiss cheese

1 cup sauerkraut

⅓ cup Thousand Island Dressing (page 330)

directions

1. Preheat the oven to 350°F. Line a rimmed baking sheet with parchment paper or a silicone baking mat.

2. In a mixing bowl, using a hand mixer, beat the cream cheese and egg until they are well combined and there are no visible clumps.

3. Add the caraway seeds, Italian seasoning, onion powder, garlic, almond flour, shredded Swiss cheese, cream, and water to the bowl. Mix with a rubber spatula until the ingredients are well incorporated.

4. Use a large spoon to drop the dough in 5 heaping mounds onto the prepared baking sheet. Bake for 25 minutes or until the biscuits are firm and golden brown on top.

5. Let the biscuits cool completely on the baking sheet before handling. Carefully slice each biscuit in half.

6. To assemble the sandwiches, top the bottom half of each biscuit with 2 slices of corned beef, 1 slice of Swiss cheese, a heaping spoonful of sauerkraut, and 1 tablespoon of dressing. Top with the other halves of the biscuits.

tip: I like to make these biscuits a day ahead of time and store them in the fridge. Once halved, they can be reheated in a toaster or toaster oven.

CALORIES: 656 · FAT: 53g · PROTEIN: 37g · TOTAL CARBS: 11g · DIETARY FIBER: 4g · NET CARBS: 7g

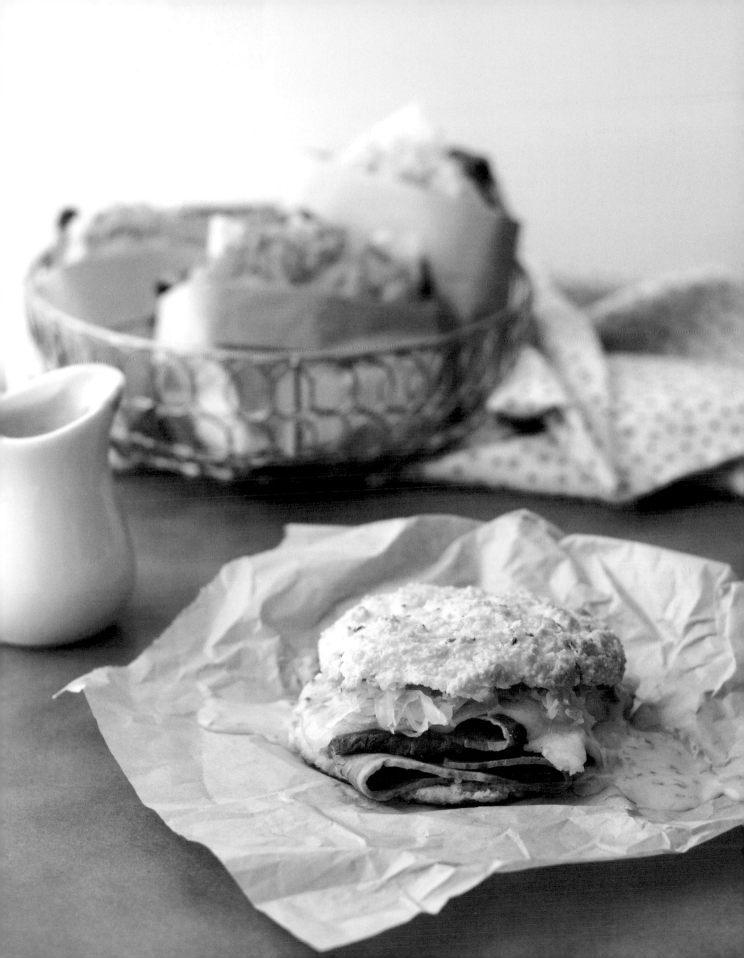

Pork Egg Roll in a Bowl

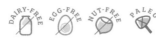

makes 6 servings · prep time: 10 minutes · cook time: 20 minutes

Pork Egg Roll in a Bowl, or "crack slaw," as it is affectionately called, is a staple in many low-carb, keto, and Paleo diets. It's packed with flavor and is quick and easy to prepare— on the table in under thirty minutes. You can't beat that! It also reheats well, making it the perfect dish for meal prep.

ingredients

2 tablespoons toasted sesame oil

1 medium onion, diced (about ½ cup)

3 cloves garlic, minced

5 green onions, sliced on the bias (white and green portions separated)

1 pound ground pork

½ teaspoon ginger powder

½ teaspoon sea salt

¼ teaspoon ground black pepper

1 tablespoon Sriracha sauce or garlic chili sauce, or more to taste

1 (14-ounce) bag coleslaw mix

3 tablespoons coconut aminos or gluten-free soy sauce

1 tablespoon unseasoned rice wine vinegar

2 tablespoons toasted sesame seeds, for garnish

directions

1. Heat the sesame oil in a large skillet over medium-high heat.

2. Add the onion, garlic, and white portions of the green onions to the skillet. Sauté until the green onions are translucent and the garlic is fragrant.

3. Add the ground pork, ginger, salt, pepper, and Sriracha sauce to the pan. Sauté until the pork is cooked through.

4. Add the coleslaw mix, coconut aminos, and vinegar and sauté until the coleslaw is tender.

5. Top with the green parts of the green onions and the sesame seeds before serving. Squirt some additional Sriracha over the top, if desired.

tip: This recipe is also great with ground chicken, beef, or turkey.

CALORIES: 297 · FAT: 20g · PROTEIN: 20g · TOTAL CARBS: 7g · DIETARY FIBER: 1.5g · NET CARBS: 5.5g

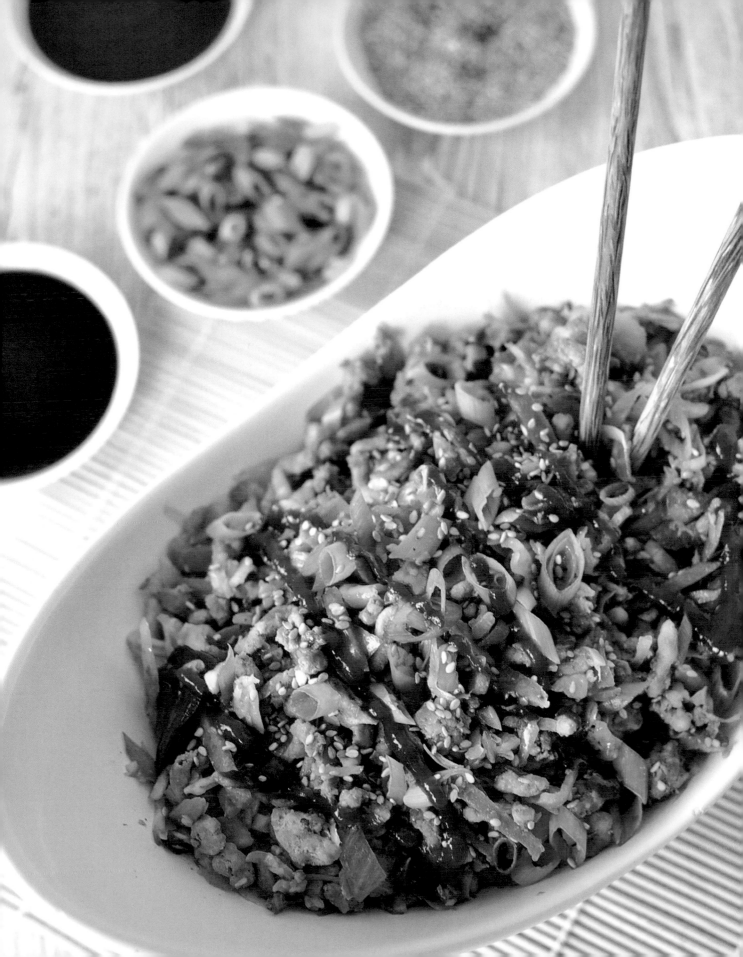

Philly Cheesesteak Casserole

makes 6 servings · prep time: 15 minutes · cook time: 30 minutes

This recipe is a quick-and-easy crowd pleaser. For a more traditional Philly cheesesteak, sauté some thinly sliced rib-eye steak with the peppers and onions before transferring the skillet to the oven. Or, better yet, go one step further and add a package of cream cheese and make a hot Philly cheesesteak dip.

ingredients

1 large green bell pepper

1 large yellow bell pepper

1 large red bell pepper

2 tablespoons butter or ghee

1 small onion, thinly sliced (about ½ cup)

3 cloves garlic, minced

8 ounces cremini mushrooms, thinly sliced

1½ pounds precooked deli-style roast beef, thinly sliced

6 slices provolone cheese (about 6 ounces)

1 cup shredded low-moisture, part-skim mozzarella cheese

directions

1. Cut the tops off the peppers, remove the ribs and seeds, and thinly slice the peppers. Set aside.

2. Heat the butter in a large deep-sided ovenproof skillet or Dutch oven over medium-low heat. Add the onion and garlic and cook until the onion is translucent and the garlic is fragrant, about 7 minutes.

3. Add the mushrooms and peppers to the skillet. Cook until the mushrooms release their liquid and the peppers are crisp-tender, about 10 minutes.

4. Preheat the oven to 350°F.

5. Add the roast beef to the skillet and mix with the vegetables. Top with the provolone cheese, then sprinkle the mozzarella cheese over the top.

6. Bake for 15 minutes, then finish under the broiler for 2 to 3 minutes, until the cheese is browned and bubbling.

CALORIES: 272 · FAT: 16g · PROTEIN: 27g · TOTAL CARBS: 7g · DIETARY FIBER: 1.7g · NET CARBS: 5.3g

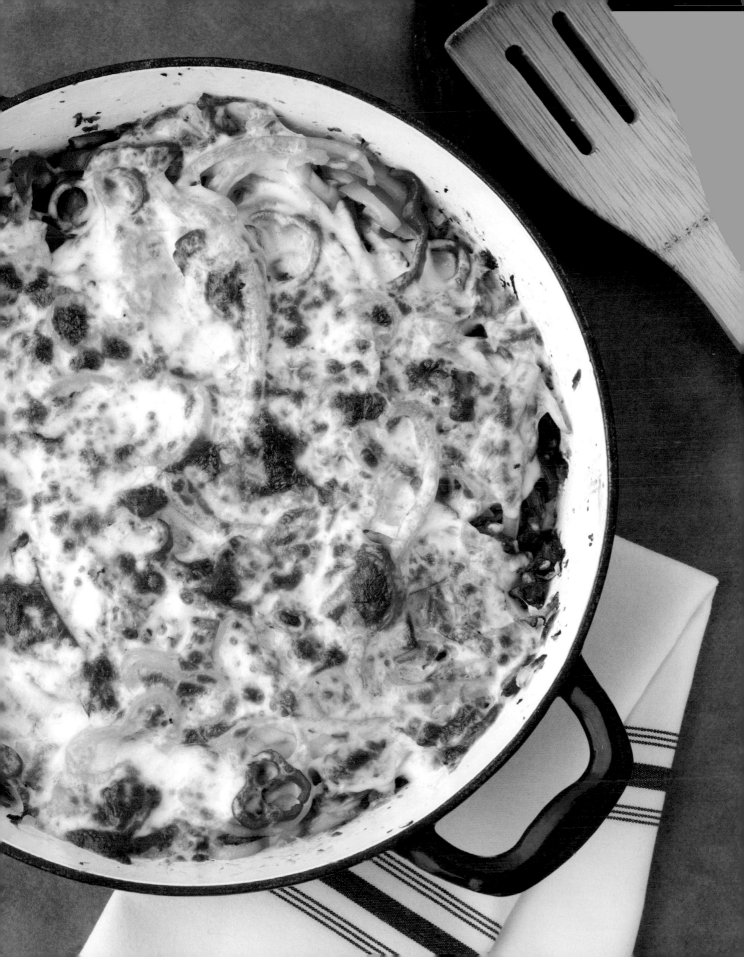

Peanut Chicken Skillet

makes 4 servings · prep time: 10 minutes · cook time: 20 minutes

When you think of peanut butter, chicken isn't usually the next thing that comes to mind. If we were playing a word association game, you would likely answer jelly. But trust me when I tell you that peanut butter is equally good paired with chicken.

ingredients

1½ pounds chicken tenderloins (see tip)

Sea salt and ground black pepper

2 tablespoons butter or ghee

2 tablespoons olive oil

1 red bell pepper, seeded and cut into thin strips

3 cloves garlic, minced

¾ cup chicken stock

⅓ cup reduced-sugar creamy peanut butter

3 tablespoons coconut aminos or gluten-free soy sauce

½ teaspoon red pepper flakes

3 green onions, sliced, for garnish

directions

1. Season the chicken on both sides with a little salt and pepper.

2. Heat the butter and olive oil in a large skillet over medium-high heat. Add the chicken to the skillet and sear for 5 to 10 minutes, until browned on both sides.

3. Reduce the heat to medium-low and add the pepper strips and garlic to the skillet. Cook, stirring often, for 5 minutes, being careful not to scorch the garlic.

4. In a mixing bowl, combine the stock, peanut butter, coconut aminos, and red pepper flakes. Whisk until the ingredients are well incorporated.

5. Pour the sauce into the skillet. Bring to a boil over medium-high heat, then reduce the heat to low and simmer, stirring frequently, for 5 minutes, until the sauce has thickened.

6. Sprinkle the green onions over the top before serving.

tip: You can also use 1½ pounds of boneless, skinless breasts. Simply cut them lengthwise into tenderloin-sized strips, about 1½ inches wide.

CALORIES: 502 · FAT: 33g · PROTEIN: 44g · TOTAL CARBS: 12g · DIETARY FIBER: 3.8g · NET CARBS: 8.3g

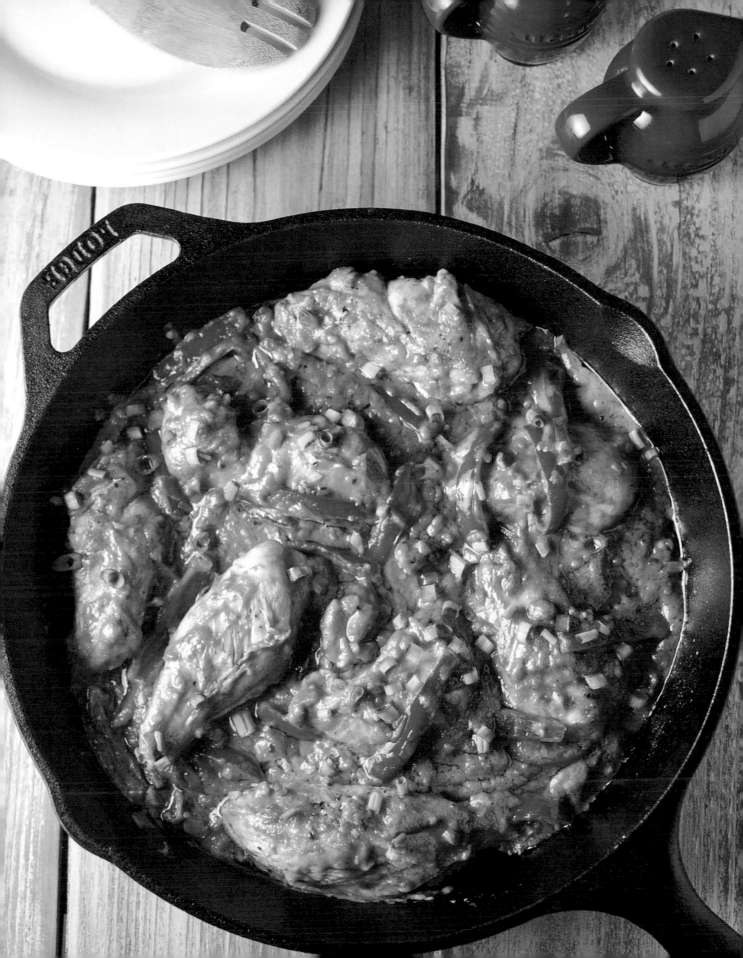

Pan-Seared Chicken with Balsamic Cream Sauce, Mushrooms, and Onions

NET CARBS
6.5g

makes 4 servings · prep time: 20 minutes · cook time: 40 minutes

This recipe will have your friends and family feeling like they are eating at a fine-dining restaurant. The acidity of the balsamic vinegar and the richness of the heavy cream come together to create an amazingly flavorful sauce. You will want to make it time and time again.

ingredients

1½ pounds boneless, skinless chicken breasts

Sea salt and ground black pepper

5 tablespoons butter or ghee, divided

1 medium onion, thinly sliced

½ cup chicken stock

1 cup heavy cream

2 tablespoons balsamic vinegar

8 ounces cremini mushrooms, halved (quartered if large)

½ cup grated Parmesan cheese

2 tablespoons chopped fresh flat-leaf parsley, for garnish (optional)

directions

1. Lightly season the chicken on both sides with salt and pepper and set aside.

2. Melt 2 tablespoons of the butter in a large skillet over medium-low heat. Add the onion and cook until it is nice and caramelized, about 20 minutes. Remove the pan from the heat and set aside.

3. Preheat another large skillet over medium-high heat. Melt the remaining 3 tablespoons of butter in the pan, then add the chicken. Pan-sear until browned on both sides, then remove from the pan and set aside. (The chicken will not be fully cooked at this time.)

4. Deglaze the pan with the stock; use a rubber spatula to scrape the bottom and mix in any remaining bits of chicken. Simmer for 5 minutes.

5. Reduce the heat to low, then add the cream, vinegar, mushrooms, and a little salt and pepper. Simmer for 10 minutes, until the mushrooms are tender and the sauce has reduced by a third.

6. Add the chicken back to the pan and simmer until it is cooked all the way through, 10 to 15 minutes. (When done, the chicken will no longer be pink in the center.)

7. Remove the chicken from the pan and plate. Add the Parmesan cheese and caramelized onions to the sauce and stir until the cheese is melted into the sauce. Pour the sauce over the top of the chicken. Garnish with fresh parsley, if desired, before serving.

CALORIES: 670 · FAT: 46g · PROTEIN: 48g · TOTAL CARBS: 7.5g · DIETARY FIBER: 1g · NET CARBS: 6.5g

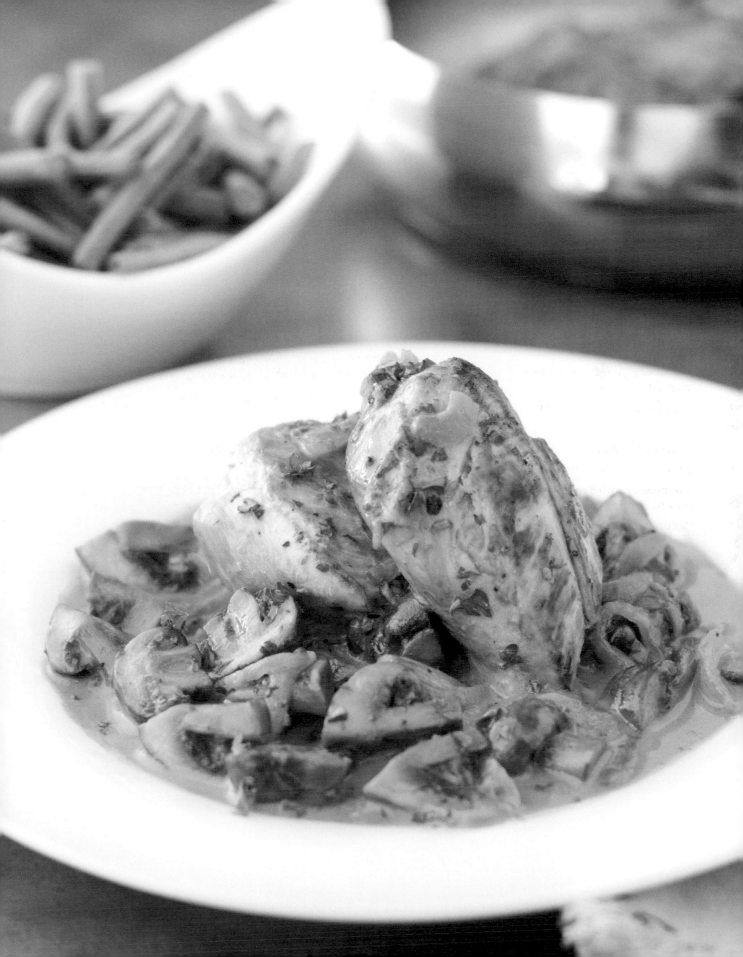

Lemon Sherry Chicken

NET CARBS 3.8g

EGG-FREE   NUT-FREE   makes 4 servings · prep time: 10 minutes · cook time: 20 minutes

With only five main ingredients, this recipe couldn't be easier to prepare. Any meal that dirties only one pan and can be on the table in less than thirty minutes is a keeper—perfect for those busy weeknight dinners.

ingredients

¼ cup cooking sherry

1½ pounds chicken tenderloins (see tip)

⅔ cup heavy cream

2 tablespoons fresh lemon juice

1 tablespoon lemon pepper seasoning

1 cup shredded low-moisture, part-skim mozzarella cheese

2 tablespoons chopped fresh flat-leaf parsley, divided

directions

1. Pour the sherry into a large skillet over medium heat.

2. When the skillet is hot, add the chicken and cook until nearly all of the sherry has evaporated, about 10 minutes.

3. Whisk in the cream, lemon juice, and lemon pepper seasoning. Reduce the heat to low and simmer until the chicken is cooked all the way through, about 15 minutes.

4. Add the mozzarella cheese and 1 tablespoon of the parsley to the sauce. Stir and simmer until the sauce has thickened.

5. Garnish the chicken with the remaining tablespoon of parsley before serving.

tip: You can also use 1½ pounds boneless, skinless chicken breasts. Simply cut them lengthwise into tenderloin-sized strips, about 1½ inches wide.

CALORIES: 329 · FAT: 16g · PROTEIN: 43g · TOTAL CARBS: 3.8g · DIETARY FIBER: 0 · NET CARBS: 3.8g

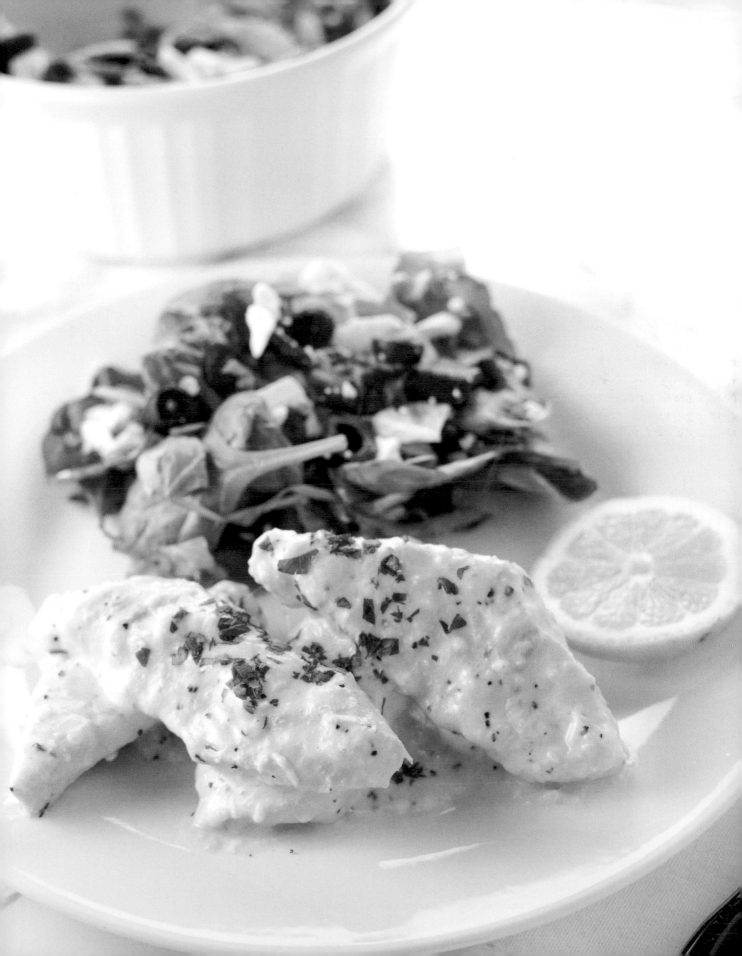

Lasagna Zucchini Roll-Ups

makes 20 roll-ups (4 per serving)
prep time: 10 minutes, plus time to rest zucchini slices · cook time: 30 minutes

These roll-ups make for an impressive table presentation. They are also a great way to sneak some extra vegetables into your children's diet. Lasagna is one of my favorite dishes to re-create in healthier low-carb versions. Check out my website, peaceloveandlowcarb. com, for more low-carb lasagna variations, including Lasagna Stuffed Peppers and Eggplant Lasagna with Meat Sauce.

ingredients

3 large zucchini (about 10 inches), sliced lengthwise in ⅛- to ¼-inch-thick planks (about 20 total)

3 teaspoons sea salt, divided

1 pound ground beef

2 cups Garlic and Herb Marinara Sauce (page 344), divided

1 cup full-fat ricotta cheese

½ cup shredded mozzarella cheese, divided

½ cup shredded Parmesan cheese, divided

1 tablespoon chopped fresh chives

1 tablespoon chopped fresh flat-leaf parsley, plus more for garnish (optional)

½ teaspoon ground black pepper

directions

1. Lay the zucchini slices in a single layer on a bed of paper towels. Sprinkle them with 2 teaspoons of the salt and let rest for about 20 minutes. The salt will help draw out the excess moisture, which will keep your lasagna from being soupy. When the noodles have released liquid, use a fresh paper towel to dry them, then set the noodles aside.

2. Heat a large skillet over medium heat. Add the ground beef and cook, crumbling the meat with a spatula, until it is browned and cooked through. Drain the excess grease from the pan. Stir 1½ cups of the marinara sauce into the meat, then set the pan aside.

3. Pour the remaining ½ cup of marinara sauce into a 10-inch square baking dish. Use a spoon to spread it into a thin, even layer.

4. In a mixing bowl, combine the ricotta cheese, ¼ cup of the mozzarella cheese, ¼ cup of the Parmesan cheese, chives, parsley, remaining teaspoon of salt, and pepper. Mix until well combined.

5. Preheat the oven to 400°F.

6. Spread a thin layer of the cheese mixture on each zucchini noodle. Spread a layer of the meat sauce on top of the cheese.

7. Gently roll up each zucchini noodle and place spiral side up in the baking dish. Push each new roll up against the one before it to help keep them all rolled up.

8. Top the roll-ups with any remaining meat sauce and the remaining ¼ cup of mozzarella cheese and ¼ cup of Parmesan cheese.

9. Bake for 30 minutes, until the zucchini is tender and the cheese on top is golden brown and bubbling. Garnish with chopped parsley, if desired, before serving.

CALORIES: 371 · FAT: 22g · PROTEIN: 33g · TOTAL CARBS: 10g · DIETARY FIBER: 2g · NET CARBS: 8g

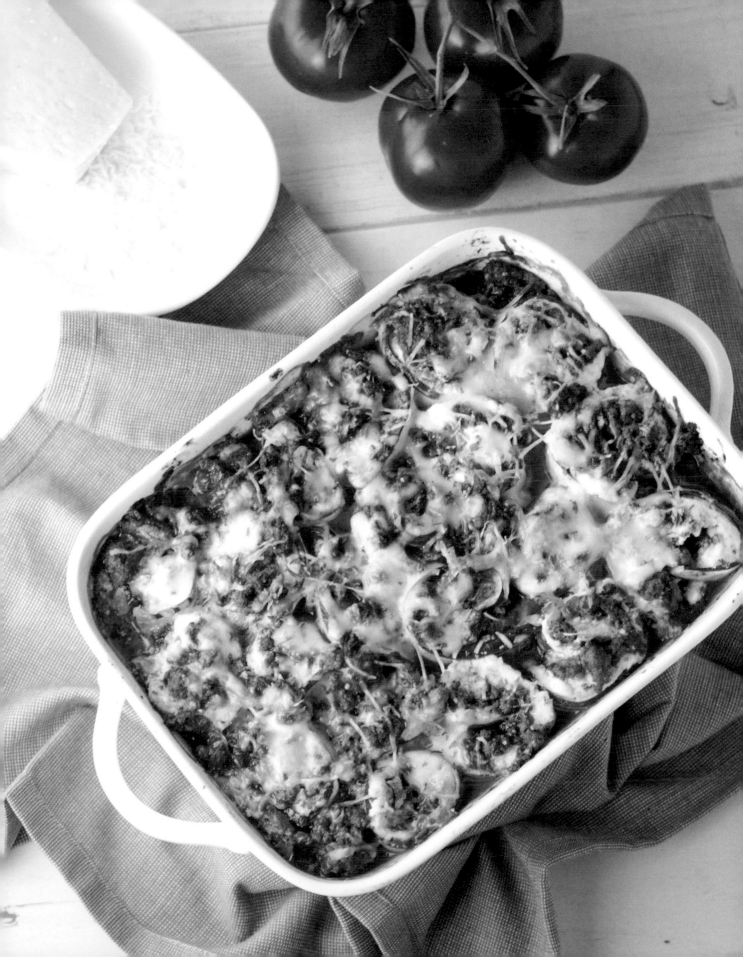

"Just Like the Real Thing" Lasagna

 makes 6 servings · prep time: 30 minutes · cook time: 1 hour

This one is a little more labor-intensive than most of the recipes in the book, but if you are thinking of skipping it, don't. You will be seriously missing out. And for every person who buys this book but doesn't make this recipe, a shelter pup doesn't get adopted. You don't want to be responsible for homeless dogs, do you? But seriously, run, don't walk, to your kitchen and make this lasagna, and I'll adopt all the lonely pups.

ingredients

For the "noodles":

4 ounces full-fat cream cheese (½ cup), softened

2 large eggs

¼ cup grated Parmesan cheese

¼ teaspoon Italian seasoning

¼ teaspoon garlic powder

¼ teaspoon onion powder

1¼ cups shredded low-moisture, part-skim mozzarella cheese

For the filling:

1 pound ground beef

1 tablespoon dried minced onions

1 teaspoon dried basil

1 teaspoon dried oregano leaves

1 teaspoon garlic powder

1½ cups Garlic and Herb Marinara Sauce (page 344), divided

¾ cup shredded low-moisture, part-skim mozzarella cheese

6 tablespoons full-fat ricotta cheese

1 teaspoon Italian seasoning

Fresh basil leaves, for garnish (optional)

directions

To make the "noodles":

1. Place an oven rack in the middle position. Preheat the oven to 375°F. Line a 13 by 9-inch baking dish with parchment paper.

2. In a large mixing bowl, using a hand mixer, cream the cream cheese and eggs.

3. Add the Parmesan cheese, Italian seasoning, garlic powder, and onion powder to the bowl. Stir until the ingredients are well combined.

4. Using a rubber spatula, fold in the mozzarella cheese until well incorporated. Spread the mixture in the baking dish, forming a nice even layer.

5. Bake for 20 to 25 minutes, until golden brown and firm.

6. When the "noodles" are done baking, place in the fridge to cool for about 20 minutes, then cut the noodles crosswise into thirds. This makes three perfectly sized layers for an 8½ by 4½-inch loaf pan.

To make the filling:

1. In a large skillet over medium-high heat, combine the ground beef, dried minced onions, basil, oregano, and garlic powder. Cook until the meat is browned, about 15 minutes.

2. Drain the excess grease from the skillet and add 1 cup of the marinara sauce to the meat. Reduce the heat to low and simmer for 10 minutes.

CALORIES: 399 · FAT: 27g · PROTEIN: 33.5g · TOTAL CARBS: 6.3g · DIETARY FIBER: 0.7g · NET CARBS: 5.6g

To assemble:

1. Pour ¼ cup of the marinara sauce into an 8½ by 4½-inch loaf pan. Place the first noodle layer on top of the sauce.

2. On top of the noodles, layer a third of the meat sauce. Top the sauce with ¼ cup of the mozzarella cheese and 3 tablespoons of the ricotta cheese. Cover with another noodle layer. Repeat this step once more.

3. Cover the top noodle layer with the remaining meat sauce, remaining ¼ cup of marinara sauce, and remaining ¼ cup of mozzarella cheese. Sprinkle the Italian seasoning over the top.

4. Bake for 20 minutes, until the cheese on top is bubbling. Let the lasagna rest for 10 minutes before serving. Garnish with fresh basil leaves before serving, if desired.

5. Store leftovers in the refrigerator for up to 1 week.

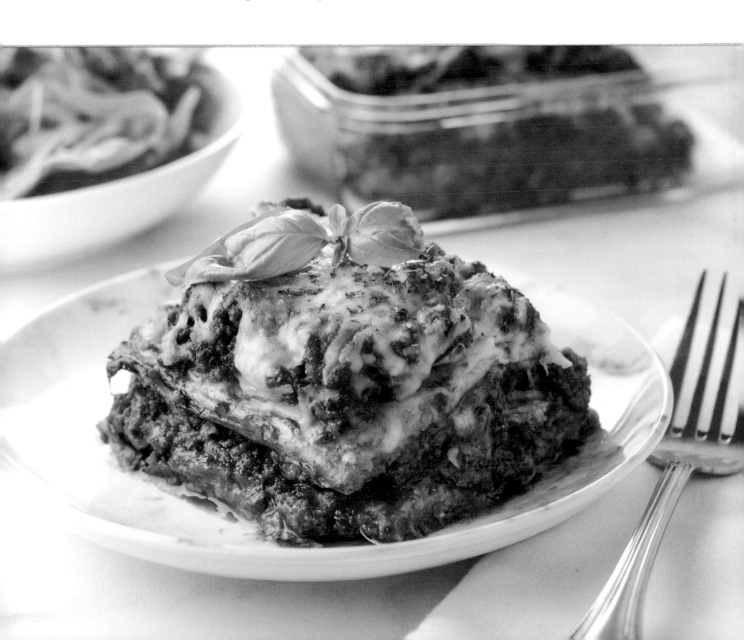

Fried Cabbage with Kielbasa

   makes 8 servings · prep time: 10 minutes · cook time: 20 minutes

You've got to love any recipe that uses inexpensive ingredients, is quick to make, and tastes like you spent hours on it. That's pretty much the food trifecta. This recipe meets all three criteria. Add the fact that it's low-carb and gluten-free, and it's like winning the food lottery. Cabbage has become an increasingly popular low-carb staple. Did you know that it is the second-most consumed vegetable, next to potatoes?

ingredients

6 tablespoons (¾ stick) butter or ghee, divided

1 large onion, diced (about 1 cup)

4 cloves garlic, minced

2 tablespoons red wine vinegar

1 (14-ounce) kielbasa, thinly sliced on the bias

1 large head green cabbage, cored and roughly chopped

1 teaspoon smoked paprika

Sea salt and ground black pepper (optional)

¼ cup roughly chopped fresh flat-leaf parsley, for garnish (optional)

1 teaspoon red pepper flakes, for garnish (optional)

directions

1. In a large skillet over medium heat, melt 3 tablespoons of the butter. Add the onion and garlic and sauté until the onion is translucent and the garlic is fragrant.

2. Add the vinegar and kielbasa to the skillet and cook until the kielbasa is slightly browned.

3. Add the remaining 3 tablespoons of butter, cabbage, and paprika to the skillet. Toss to mix the ingredients together and coat the cabbage. Taste and add salt and pepper, if needed.

4. Continue cooking until the cabbage is wilted and slightly browned, about 15 minutes.

5. Top with fresh parsley and red pepper flakes, if desired, before serving. Store leftovers in the refrigerator for up to 1 week.

Tips: To make this dish dairy-free and Paleo compliant, use ghee rather than butter.

Finding a clean brand of kielbasa can be tricky. Pederson's Natural Farms is a brand I know and love.

CALORIES: 370 · FAT: 29g · PROTEIN: 6g · TOTAL CARBS: 16.5g · DIETARY FIBER: 7g · NET CARBS: 9.5g

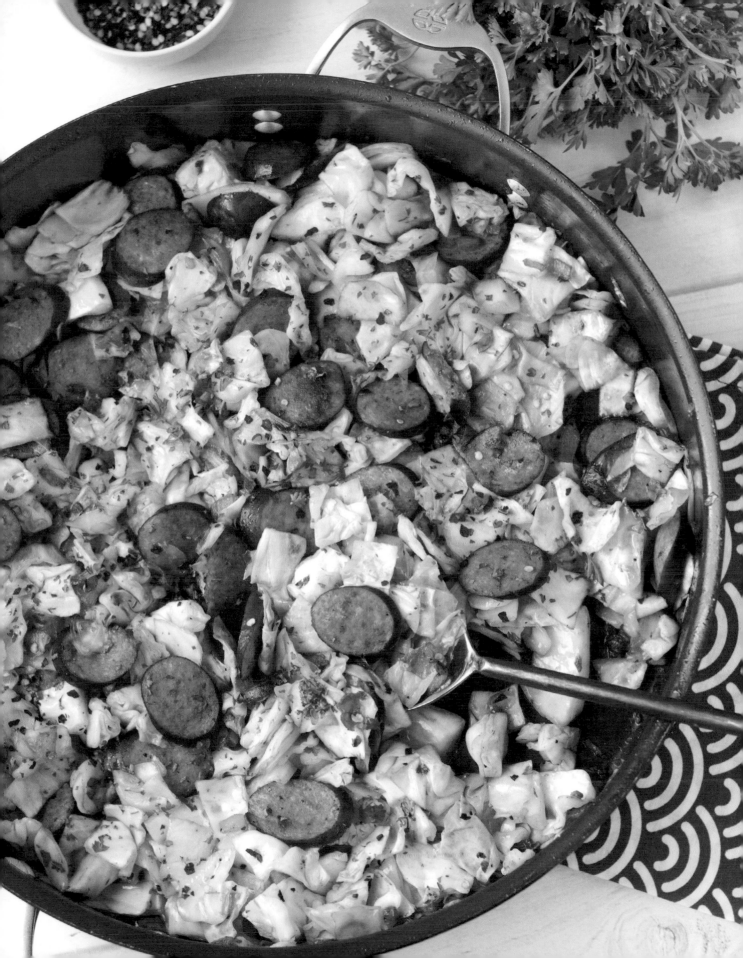

Barbecue Dry Rub Ribs

makes 6 servings · prep time: 20 minutes · cook time: 2½ hours

I'm always surprised by how many people have never made their own ribs at home. It is one of the easiest meals to cook: just a few minutes to prep the meat and the oven does the rest. I love to serve these ribs with Dill Pickle Coleslaw (page 280).

ingredients

2 pounds pork baby back ribs

2 tablespoons olive oil

1 batch Barbecue Dry Rub (page 353)

directions

1. Preheat the oven to 300°F. Line a rimmed baking sheet with aluminum foil.

2. Remove the thin membrane from the back, or concave side, of the ribs. Start by slicing into the membrane with a sharp knife, then pull the skin away from the ribs. Place the ribs on the lined baking sheet.

3. Brush the olive oil evenly over the ribs. Pour the dry rub over the ribs and work it evenly onto both sides.

4. Bake until the ribs are tender and juicy on the inside and nice and crispy on the outside, about 2½ hours. Store leftovers in the refrigerator for up to 1 week.

CALORIES: 400 · FAT: 43g · PROTEIN: 43g · TOTAL CARBS: 3.8g · DIETARY FIBER: 1g · NET CARBS: 2.8g

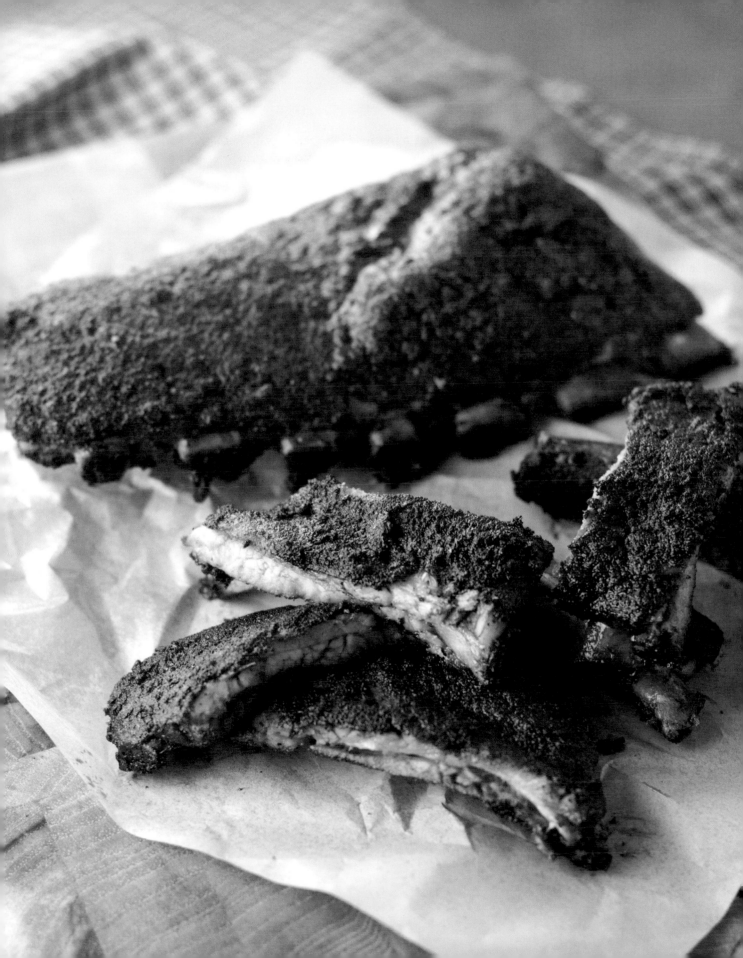

Dill Pickle Juice Brined Fish and Chips

makes 4 servings · prep time: 20 minutes, plus 24 hours to marinate
cook time: 30 minutes

When you first started living a low-carb, ketogenic lifestyle, did you ever dream that you would still be able to eat fried fish dipped in a fantastic tartar sauce? Anything is possible with a little time and creativity. How about I take care of the creativity part for you so that you only have to worry about the time? Deal? Deal!

ingredients

1½ pounds fresh wild-caught cod fillets

1 cup dill pickle juice

2 large eggs

1 batch Nut-Free Keto Breading Mix (page 355)

Cooking oil, such as avocado oil or tallow, for deep-frying

½ cup Garlic Dill Tartar Sauce (page 339), for serving (optional)

Lemon wedges, for serving (optional)

directions

1. Place the cod fillets and pickle juice in a gallon-sized resealable plastic bag. Marinate the fish in the fridge for 24 hours.

2. Crack the eggs into a shallow bowl and whisk with a fork.

3. Pour the breading mix onto a plate and spread into a thin layer.

4. Dip a cod fillet in the egg wash, then dredge it in the breading mix, making sure that both sides are evenly coated. Lay the breaded fillet on another plate and repeat with the remaining fish.

5. Heat 2 inches of oil in 4-inch-deep (or deeper) skillet or Dutch oven over medium heat. When the oil is hot and begins to bubble slightly, drop 2 or 3 of the breaded cod fillets one at a time into the hot oil and fry until they are golden brown and crispy, about 3 minutes per side.

6. Remove the fish from the oil and place on paper towels to absorb the excess grease before serving. Repeat with the remaining fish. Serve with the tartar sauce and lemon wedges, if desired.

CALORIES: 312 · FAT: 17g · PROTEIN: 39g · TOTAL CARBS: 1.3g · DIETARY FIBER: 0 · NET CARBS: 1.3g

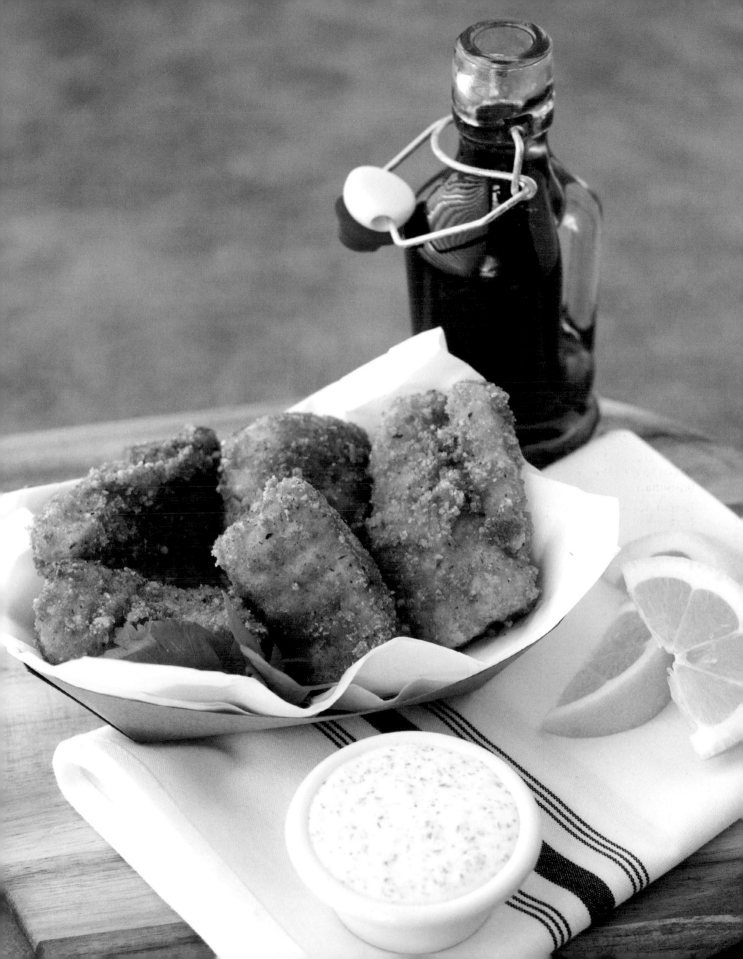

Crispy Chicken Thigh and Vegetable Sheet Pan Dinner

  makes 4 servings · prep time: 20 minutes · cook time: 20 minutes

We are really big on meat and vegetables in our house. More often than not, our dinner consists of a protein and a huge mound of vegetables. I often get asked questions like, "Doesn't eating that many vegetables put you over your carb limit for the day?" To which I always respond, "I don't think any of us got overweight in the first place from eating too many vegetables." It is always one of those light-bulb moments for people.

ingredients

20 cremini mushrooms, halved

1 large head broccolini, trimmed, and divided into individual stalks

1 red bell pepper, seeded and sliced

1 yellow bell pepper, seeded and sliced

1 small red onion, sliced

2 tablespoons olive oil

2 tablespoons butter or ghee

8 bone-in, skin-on chicken thighs

Sea salt and ground black pepper

1 whole head garlic, cloves separated and peeled

2 sprigs fresh rosemary

directions

1. Preheat the oven to 400°F.

2. Arrange the mushrooms, broccolini, bell peppers, and onion on a rimmed baking sheet and drizzle with the olive oil.

3. Heat the butter in a large skillet over medium-high heat. Season the chicken thighs on both sides with a little salt and pepper. Add the chicken, garlic cloves, and rosemary sprigs to the pan. Sear the chicken on both sides until the skin is crispy and golden brown. (The chicken will not be fully cooked at this stage.) As the garlic starts to brown, remove it from the pan and place it on the baking sheet with the vegetables. Do the same with the rosemary sprigs.

4. Place the chicken thighs on top of the vegetables and pour any pan drippings over the top of everything.

5. Transfer the baking sheet to the oven and bake the chicken and vegetables for 20 minutes, until the chicken is cooked through and the vegetables are tender but not mushy.

tip: *To make this dish dairy-free and Paleo compliant, use ghee rather than butter.*

CALORIES: 616 · FAT: 44g · PROTEIN: 53g · TOTAL CARBS: 10.3g · DIETARY FIBER: 2.3g · NET CARBS: 8g

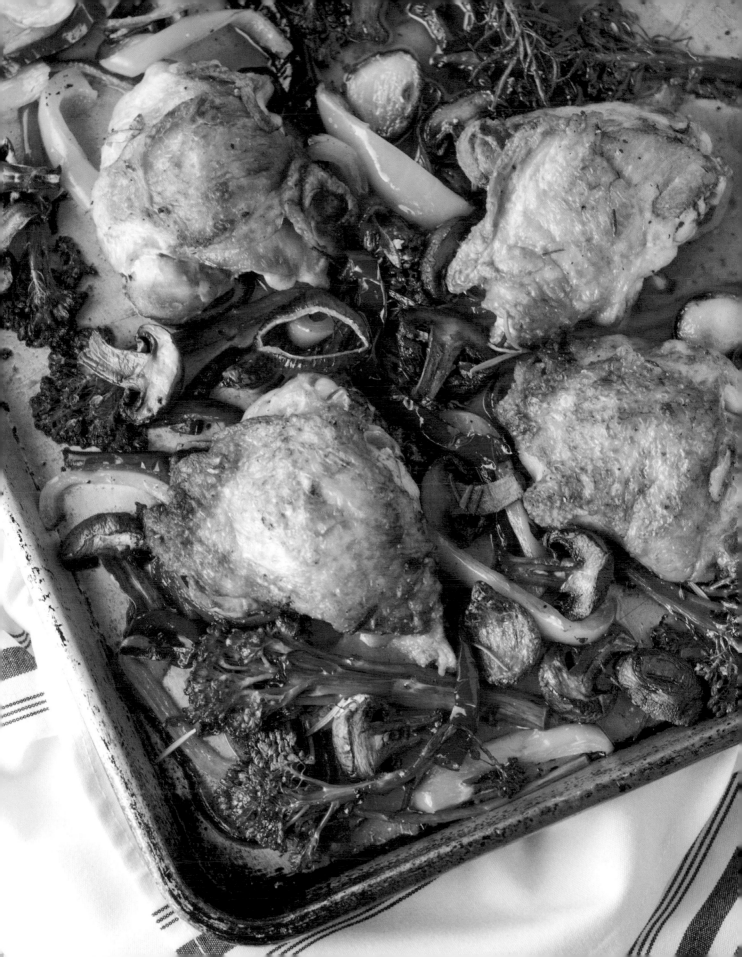

Creamy Pesto Chicken Zucchini Pasta

NET CARBS
5.5g

makes 6 servings · prep time: 20 minutes, plus time to rest zucchini noodles
cook time: 30 minutes

With so much flavor packed into one dish, you will forget that you are not eating regular pasta. For years I worked in various Italian restaurants, and I really grew to love the strong, sharp flavors of pesto and goat cheese, especially when combined. I'm pretty confident that there won't be any leftovers when you make this recipe, but on the off chance that there are, try mixing them with some whisked eggs and then baking it to make a delicious leftover-surprise frittata.

ingredients

4 medium zucchini (about 8 inches), spiral-sliced into noodles (see page 78)

1½ pounds boneless, skinless chicken breasts or thighs, cut into chunks

Sea salt and ground black pepper

2 tablespoons butter or ghee

2 cloves garlic, minced

½ cup chicken stock

½ cup heavy cream

¼ cup pesto, store-bought or homemade (page 340)

½ cup grated Parmesan cheese, divided

½ cup pine nuts, divided

½ cup pitted Kalamata olives, halved

½ cup sun-dried tomatoes

¼ cup crumbled fresh (soft) goat cheese

A few fresh basil leaves, for garnish

directions

1. Lay the zucchini noodles in a single layer on a bed of paper towels. Sprinkle them 2½ teaspoons of salt and let rest for 10 to 15 minutes. The salt will help draw out the excess moisture so that the pasta isn't soupy. When the noodles have released liquid, place a layer of fresh paper towels on top and dab away the excess moisture, then set the noodles aside.

2. Meanwhile, prepare the rest of the ingredients: Season the chicken with a little salt and pepper.

3. Heat the butter in a large skillet over medium heat. Add the chicken and sauté until the chunks are cooked through and browned on all sides. Add the garlic to the pan and sauté for 2 minutes. Remove the chicken from the pan and set aside.

4. Deglaze the skillet with the stock, using a rubber spatula to scrape up and mix in any bits of chicken and garlic stuck to the bottom of the pan. Reduce the heat to medium-low.

5. Add the cream, pesto, and ¼ cup of the Parmesan cheese to the skillet. Simmer, stirring continuously, until the sauce begins to thicken, 3 to 5 minutes.

6. Return the chicken to the skillet. Add the zucchini noodles and toss to coat the chicken and noodles in the sauce. Taste and add salt and pepper, if needed. Cook the noodles in the sauce for 5 to 7 minutes. Don't cook them too long or they will get mushy.

7. Toss in ¼ cup of the pine nuts, the olives, and the sun-dried tomatoes.

8. Transfer to a serving bowl and top with the remaining ¼ cup of Parmesan, remaining ¼ cup of pine nuts, goat cheese, and basil leaves before serving. Store leftovers in the refrigerator for up to 1 week.

CALORIES: 436 · FAT: 33g · PROTEIN: 31g · TOTAL CARBS: 7.5g · DIETARY FIBER: 2g · NET CARBS: 5.5g

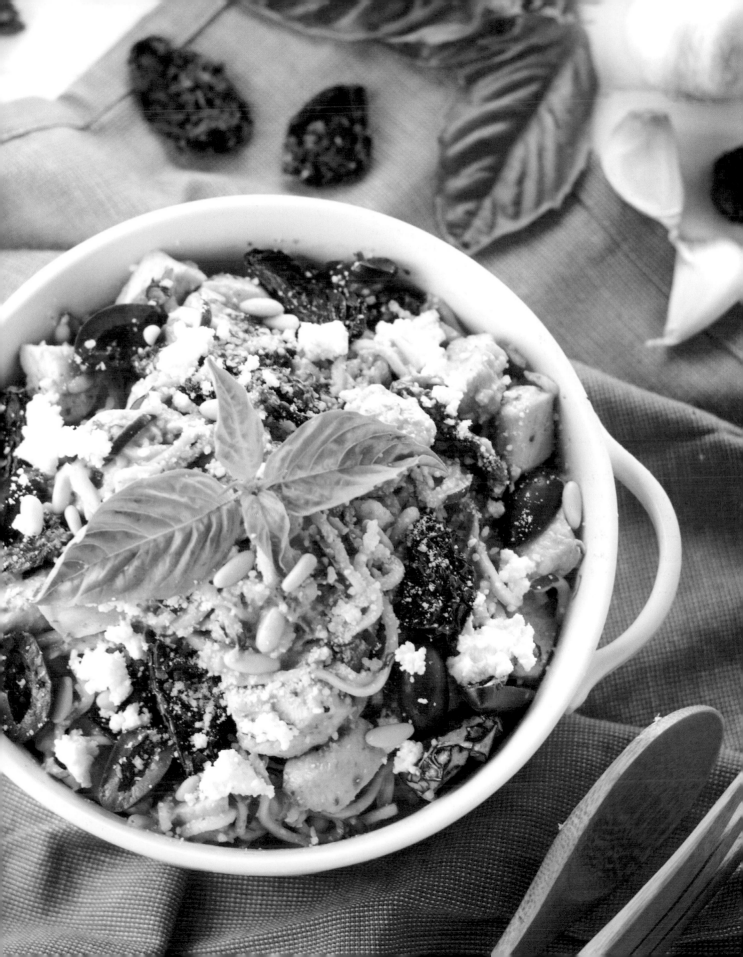

Chicken Zoodle Alfredo

makes 4 servings · prep time: 20 minutes, plus time to rest zucchini noodles
cook time: 20 minutes

I always hear people talking about how much they wish they could still eat Alfredo sauce on their low-carb meal plan. Well, guess what? You can! A traditional Alfredo sauce has a base of butter, cream, and Parmesan cheese. Unfortunately, many restaurants add flour to the sauce to thicken it and make it go farther, which makes it far from low-carb or gluten-free. Then there is the matter of the pasta, which is definitely not low-carb or keto-friendly. Well, with this recipe, chicken Alfredo is back on the table with the use of zucchini noodles and a more traditional sauce recipe. This one comes kid and husband approved!

ingredients

4 medium zucchini (about 8 inches), spiral-sliced into noodles (see page 78)

1 pound boneless, skinless chicken thighs, cut into bite-sized pieces

Sea salt and ground black pepper

1 tablespoon butter or ghee

1 batch Garlic Parmesan Cream Sauce (page 342)

¼ cup shredded Parmesan cheese

2 teaspoons chopped fresh flat-leaf parsley

directions

1. Lay the zucchini noodles in a single layer on a bed of paper towels. Sprinkle them with 2½ teaspoons of salt and let rest for 10 to 15 minutes. The salt will help draw out the excess moisture so that the pasta isn't soupy. When the noodles have released liquid, place a layer of fresh paper towels on top and dab away the excess moisture, then set the noodles aside.

2. Season the chicken with a little salt and pepper.

3. Heat the butter in a large skillet over medium-high heat. Add the chicken and sauté until the pieces are cooked through and golden brown.

4. Add the zucchini noodles to the skillet and sauté until they are tender, 2 to 3 minutes.

5. Toss with the cream sauce until heated through. Top with the Parmesan cheese and parsley before serving.

CALORIES: 433 · FAT: 28g · PROTEIN: 37g · TOTAL CARBS: 9.5g · DIETARY FIBER: 2g · NET CARBS: 7.5g

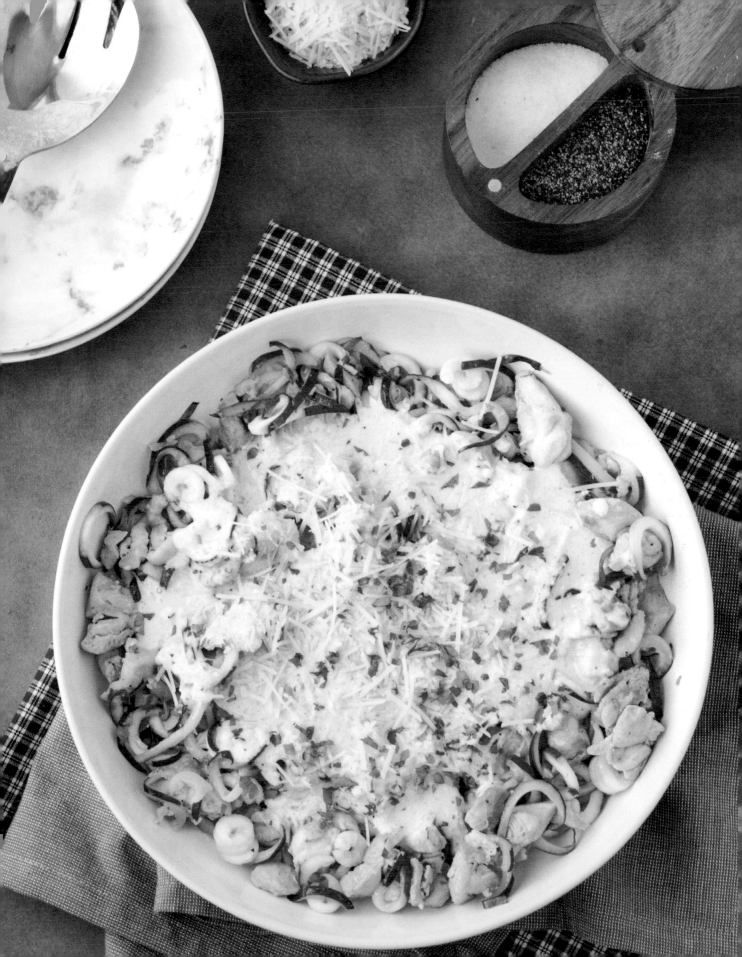

Chicken Parmesan Zucchini Boats

makes 8 servings · prep time: 15 minutes · cook time: 45 minutes

One of my favorite things to do with food is to stuff it inside another food. On my website, peaceloveandlowcarb.com, I have several recipes for stuffed peppers, stuffed zucchini, stuffed mushrooms, and even stuffed avocado boats. If you are also a fan of food inside of food, be sure to check out my recipes for Beef Enchilada Stuffed Spaghetti Squash (page 266) and Beef Stuffed Poblanos with Lime Crema (page 264).

ingredients

2 tablespoons olive oil

1 pound boneless, skinless chicken breasts, cubed

½ teaspoon sea salt

¼ teaspoon ground black pepper

4 large zucchini (about 10 inches long)

1 cup marinara sauce, store-bought (see tips) or homemade (page 344)

1 cup shredded mozzarella cheese

½ cup shredded Parmesan cheese

1 teaspoon Italian seasoning

Fresh basil crowns and basil chiffonade, for garnish

directions

1. Heat the olive oil in a large skillet over medium-high heat. Add the chicken, salt, and pepper and cook for 8 to 10 minutes, until the chicken is cooked through.

2. While the chicken cooks, prepare the zucchini. Cut each zucchini in half lengthwise and, using a spoon, scoop out the center, leaving about ¼ inch of flesh in each one.

3. Line the zucchini halves cut side up in a 13 by 9-inch baking dish.

4. Preheat the oven to 400°F.

5. Pour the marinara sauce over the chicken and stir to coat. Divide the sauced chicken evenly among all 8 zucchini halves.

6. Divide the mozzarella cheese evenly over the tops of the zucchini boats. Repeat with the Parmesan cheese. Sprinkle the Italian seasoning over the top.

7. Bake for 30 minutes. Top each zucchini boat with fresh basil before serving.

8. Store leftovers in the refrigerator for up to 1 week. Reheat in a preheated 300°F oven until warmed through.

tips: To cut down on prep time, you can use a store-bought sauce, but be sure to read the labels and look for a sauce that contains only vegetables, healthy fats, and seasonings.

To increase the fat content of this dish, you can substitute boneless chicken thighs for the chicken breasts.

If you want to add a little bit of crunch to this dish, try sprinkling some crushed pork rinds or almond flour over the top before baking.

CALORIES: 196 · FAT: 8.5g · PROTEIN: 24.5g · TOTAL CARBS: 4.8g · DIETARY FIBER: 1.3g · NET CARBS: 3.5g

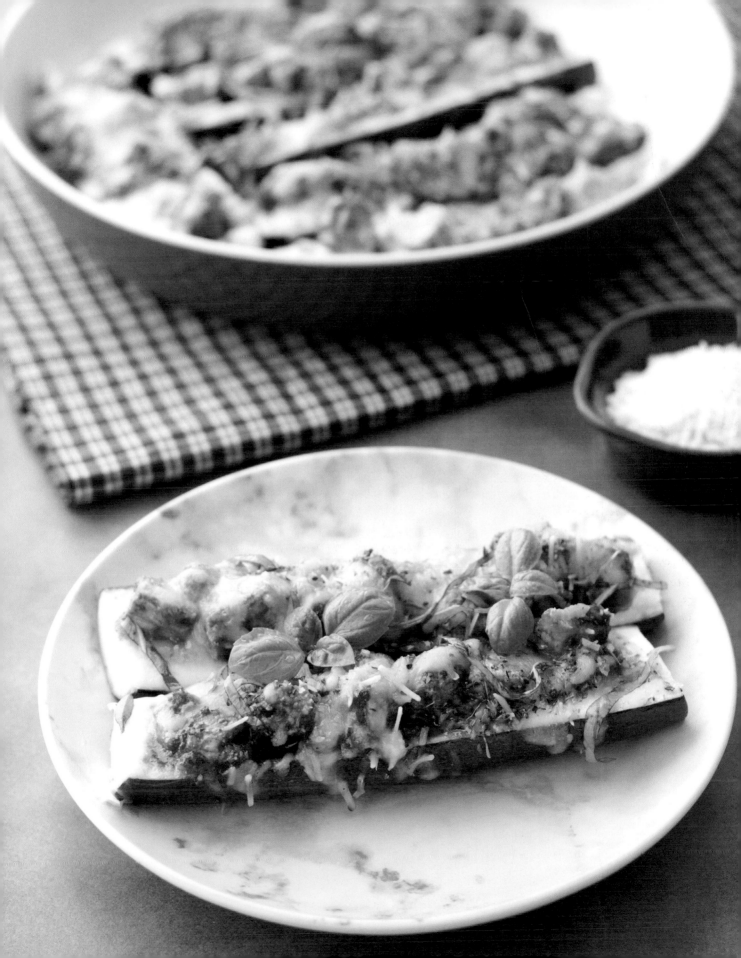

Chicken Cordon Bleu Pizza

makes 8 servings · prep time: 15 minutes · cook time: 15 minutes

I've always loved a good white sauce pizza. To be honest, I just love pizza. In my world, even mediocre pizza is good pizza. But not everyone feels that way, so it's a good thing that *this* pizza is far better than mediocre. It is rich and creamy, and usually just one or two slices will do the trick.

ingredients

1 baked Pizza Crust (page 356)

½ cup Garlic Parmesan Cream Sauce (page 342)

4 slices Swiss cheese (about 4 ounces)

6 ounces ham or Canadian bacon, thinly sliced

8 ounces boneless, skinless chicken breasts, cooked and cubed

½ cup shredded mozzarella cheese

2 tablespoons chopped fresh chives

directions

1. Preheat the oven to 425°F. Lightly grease a pizza pan or rimmed baking sheet.

2. Place the pizza crust on the greased pan. Spread the cream sauce over the top of the baked crust, covering it evenly.

3. Place the slices of Swiss cheese on top of the sauce. Next, layer on the ham and chicken. Sprinkle the mozzarella cheese evenly over the top of the pizza.

4. Bake for 10 to 15 minutes, until the cheese is melted and bubbly.

5. Sprinkle the chives over the top of the pizza, then cut it into 8 slices and serve. Store leftovers in the refrigerator for up to 1 week. Reheat in the oven.

tip: For a nut-free version, use a Nut-Free Pizza Crust (page 358). And if you are not a fan of white sauce on pizza, try it with Garlic and Herb Marinara Sauce (page 344) instead.

CALORIES: 336 · FAT: 22.5g · PROTEIN: 29g · TOTAL CARBS: 4.8g · DIETARY FIBER: 1.2g · NET CARBS: 3.6g

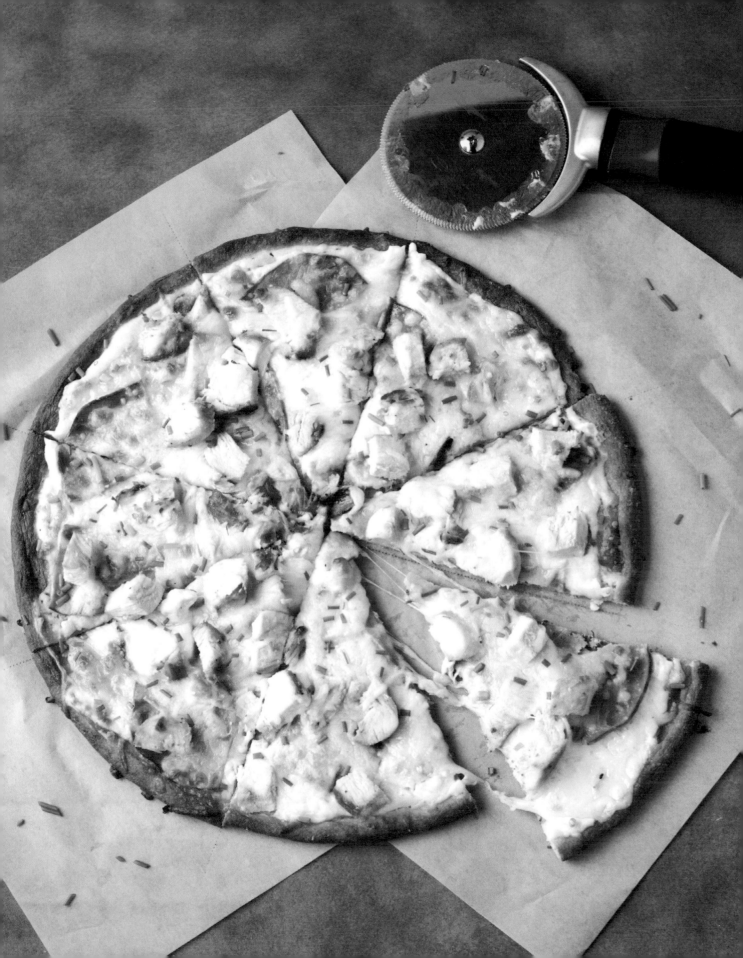

Cheesy Smoked Sausage and Cabbage Casserole

makes 8 servings · prep time: 15 minutes · cook time: 35 minutes

When I make this casserole, I usually take half, vacuum-seal it, and freeze it for a future dinner; it reheats perfectly. This is a great budget-friendly recipe that will please the whole family.

ingredients

2 tablespoons olive oil

2 tablespoons butter or ghee

1 medium head green cabbage, cored and sliced

1 yellow bell pepper, seeded and chopped

1 large onion, diced (about 1 cup)

4 cloves garlic, minced

1 teaspoon sea salt

½ teaspoon ground black pepper

1 (14½-ounce) can diced tomatoes

1½ cups crushed tomatoes

1 (14-ounce) smoked beef sausage, halved lengthwise and sliced into half-moons

1½ cups shredded mozzarella cheese

¼ cup roughly chopped fresh flat-leaf parsley

directions

1. Preheat the oven to 400°F.

2. Heat the olive oil and butter in a large skillet over medium heat. Once the butter has melted and the pan is hot, add the cabbage, bell pepper, onion, garlic, salt, and pepper. Sauté until the bell pepper is crisp-tender and the cabbage is wilted, about 10 minutes.

3. Mix in the diced tomatoes, crushed tomatoes, and smoked sausage. Cook for an additional 10 minutes. Taste and add more salt and pepper, if needed.

4. Transfer the mixture to a large casserole dish, top with the mozzarella cheese, and bake for 15 minutes, until the cheese is melted and bubbling.

5. Top with fresh parsley before serving. Store leftovers in the refrigerator for up to 1 week.

CALORIES: 322 · FAT: 23.5g · PROTEIN: 14.8g · TOTAL CARBS: 11.8g · DIETARY FIBER: 4.2g · NET CARBS: 7.6g

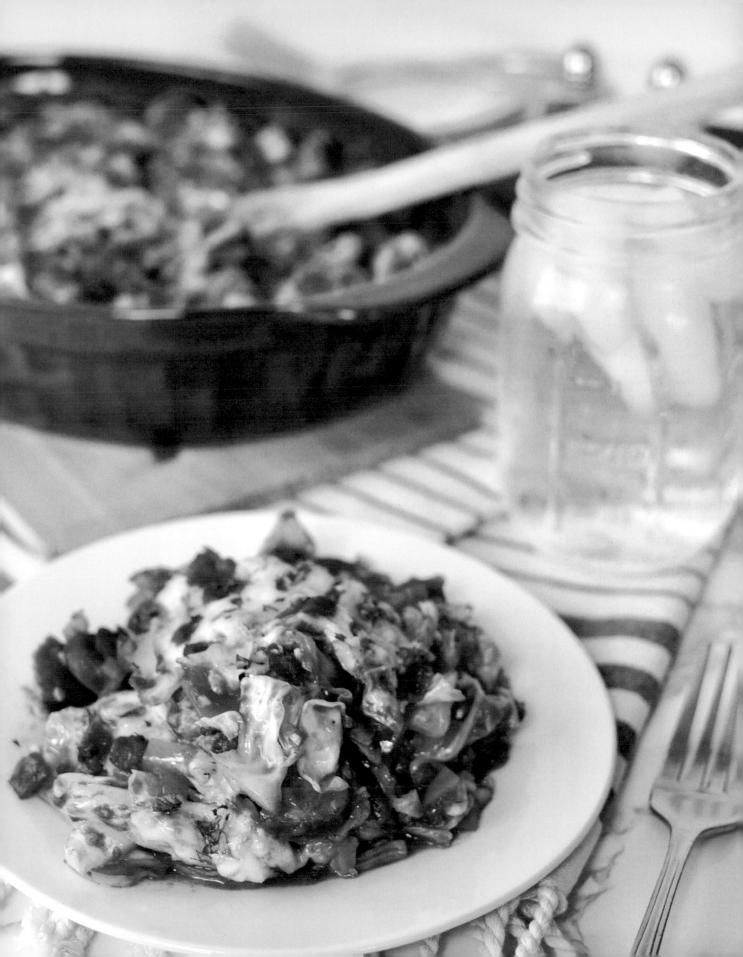

Best-Ever Fork and Knife Pub Burger

NET CARBS
5.1g

 makes 6 burgers (1 per serving) · **prep time: 20 minutes** · **cook time: 30 minutes**

This is one of my favorite meals to serve when we are entertaining. I make a complete burger bar on my kitchen counter and everyone builds their own custom burger. It is always a big hit. If you aren't a fan of burger sauce, be sure to make the 2-Minute Mayo on page 336.

ingredients

2 pounds ground beef

2 cloves garlic, minced

2 tablespoons dried minced onions

Sea salt and ground black pepper

2 tablespoons butter or ghee

6 slices sharp cheddar cheese

6 large Bibb lettuce leaves

½ cup Not-So-Secret Burger Sauce (page 347)

1 large tomato, sliced

1 medium avocado, pitted and sliced

1 batch Bacon Jam (page 341)

2 large dill pickles, thinly sliced

directions

1. In a large mixing bowl, combine the ground beef, garlic, and dried minced onions. Mix until the ingredients are well incorporated.

2. Divide the mixture into 6 equal portions and form into patties about ¾ inch thick. Season both sides of the patties generously with salt and pepper.

3. Using your thumb, make a depression in the center of each patty. The burgers will plump as you cook them, and making this depression will help them stay flat and even.

4. Heat the butter in a large skillet over medium-high heat. Place the first 3 patties in the pan. For medium-done burgers, sear until browned and slightly charred on the first side, 3 to 5 minutes. Flip the patties over and do the same on the second side.

5. Top each patty with a slice of cheese and let the cheese melt before removing the patties from the pan. Repeat this process with the remaining 3 patties.

6. Put each burger patty on top of a lettuce leaf and top with a spoonful of the burger sauce, a tomato slice, a few avocado slices, and a spoonful of bacon jam. Serve the burgers with pickle slices.

7. Store leftovers in the refrigerator for up to 1 week.

CALORIES: 650 · FAT: 49g · PROTEIN: 44g · TOTAL CARBS: 7.8g · DIETARY FIBER: 2.7g · NET CARBS: 5.1g

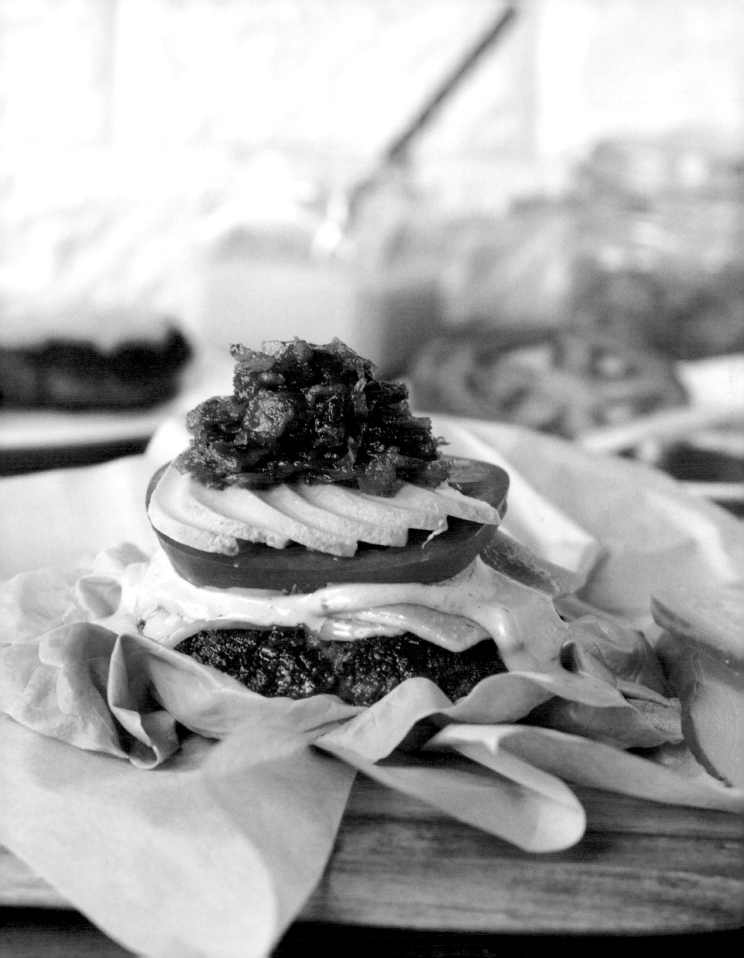

Beef Tips in Mushroom Brown Gravy

makes 6 servings · prep time: 15 minutes · cook time: 20 minutes

All during my childhood, if anyone asked me what my favorite food was, I would loudly and emphatically exclaim that it was mashed potatoes and gravy. That unwavering love lasted well into adulthood. In fact, it would still be alive and well today if I could get away with eating that many potatoes. I came up with a lot of creative cauliflower recipes that helped curb the potato craving, but coming up with a tasty low-carb and gluten-free gravy was definitely necessary, too. I love to serve this dish over Basic Cauliflower Rice (page 282) or Creamy Herbed Slow Cooker Cauliflower Mash (page 284). It just screams comfort food! To make it a complete meal, serve it with your favorite vegetable. Mine is broccoli.

ingredients

2 pounds stir-fry beef

Sea salt and ground black pepper

2 tablespoons olive oil

2 tablespoons butter or ghee

1 small shallot, finely chopped

2 cloves garlic, minced

2 tablespoons Worcestershire sauce

8 ounces cremini mushrooms, sliced

1 cup beef stock

¼ cup heavy cream

directions

1. Generously season the pieces of beef with salt and pepper.

2. Heat the olive oil in a large skillet over medium-high heat. Once the pan is hot, add the beef and sear on both sides until nice and browned.

3. Remove the beef from the skillet and set aside. Reduce the heat to medium-low.

4. Add the butter, shallot, and garlic to the skillet and cook for 2 to 3 minutes, until the shallot is translucent and the garlic is fragrant.

5. Add the Worcestershire sauce and mushrooms to the skillet. Sauté until the mushrooms have released their liquid and the liquid has evaporated.

6. Deglaze the pan with the stock, using a rubber spatula to scrape up and mix in any bits stuck to the bottom of the pan.

7. Whisk in the cream and bring to a boil over medium heat. Reduce the heat to low and simmer, stirring occasionally, until the sauce has started to thicken, about 10 minutes.

8. Return the beef to the pan and toss to coat in the sauce. Continue to cook for an additional 5 to 10 minutes, until the meat is tender and the sauce has finished thickening.

9. Store leftovers in the refrigerator for up to 1 week.

CALORIES: 298 · FAT: 16.3g · PROTEIN: 35g · TOTAL CARBS: 3.5g · DIETARY FIBER: 0.5g · NET CARBS: 3g

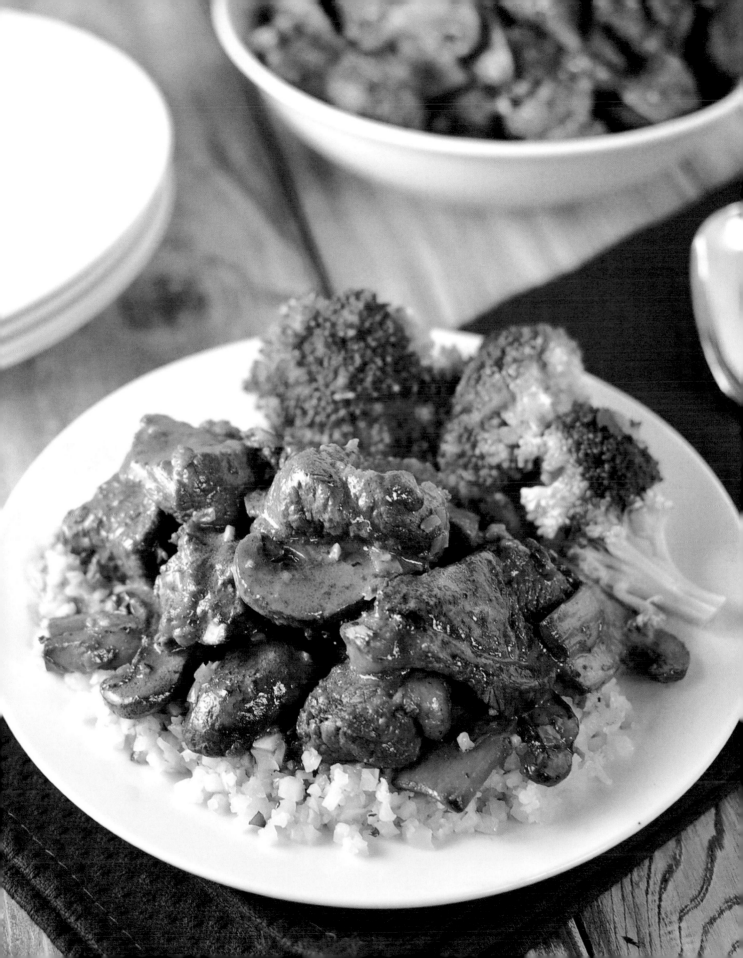

NET CARBS

11g

Beef Stuffed Poblanos with Lime Crema

EGG-FREE

makes 4 servings · prep time: 15 minutes · cook time: 40 minutes

This recipe was inspired by a delicious meal I had at a restaurant called Barrio in Seattle. It was the kind of meal that I thought about over and over afterward. Even before we got home, I already wanted to go back and order another one. That is the mark of an inspired dish. I knew right then that I needed to work my low-carb magic and create my own version. This is easily one of my favorite recipes in this book.

ingredients

4 poblano peppers (see tips)

2 tablespoons olive oil

Sea salt and ground black pepper

1 tablespoon butter or ghee

1 small red onion, thinly sliced (about ½ cup)

3 cloves garlic, minced

1 pound ground beef

2 cups riced cauliflower (see page 76)

¼ cup tomato paste

1 tablespoon ground cumin

¼ cup roasted and salted pepitas

¼ cup no-sugar-added dried cranberries (optional; see tips)

¼ cup Mexican crema or full-fat sour cream

Juice of ½ lime

2 tablespoons torn fresh cilantro, for garnish (optional)

Lime wedges, for serving (optional)

directions

1. Preheat the oven to 500°F. Place the poblanos on a rimmed baking sheet, drizzle with the olive oil, and sprinkle with salt and pepper. Roast for 5 to 7 minutes, until the skins are browned and blistered. Remove from the oven and set aside to cool.

2. While the peppers are cooling, heat the butter in a large skillet over medium-low heat. Add the onion and garlic and cook until the onion is translucent and the garlic is fragrant.

3. Increase the heat to medium and add the ground beef and riced cauliflower to the skillet. Sauté until the beef is browned and cooked through, 10 to 15 minutes.

4. Stir in the tomato paste, cumin, 1 teaspoon of salt, and ½ teaspoon of pepper. Cook for an additional 2 to 3 minutes. Add the pepitas and dried cranberries, if using, and mix in.

5. Cut a lengthwise slit in each of the roasted poblanos and remove the ribs and seeds. Stuff each pepper with the meat mixture.

6. Combine the crema and lime juice and drizzle some over each poblano. Top each pepper with fresh cilantro and serve with lime wedges, if desired.

tips: The heat of a pepper lives in the ribs and seeds. For a spicier dish, you can leave some of the ribs and seeds in. If spicy isn't your thing, you can skip the poblanos altogether and use bell peppers instead.

If you can't find no-sugar-added dried cranberries, you can either omit them or make your own by dehydrating fresh cranberries in a low-temperature oven.

CALORIES: 460 · FAT: 30g · PROTEIN: 31g · TOTAL CARBS: 17.5g · DIETARY FIBER: 6.5g · NET CARBS: 11g

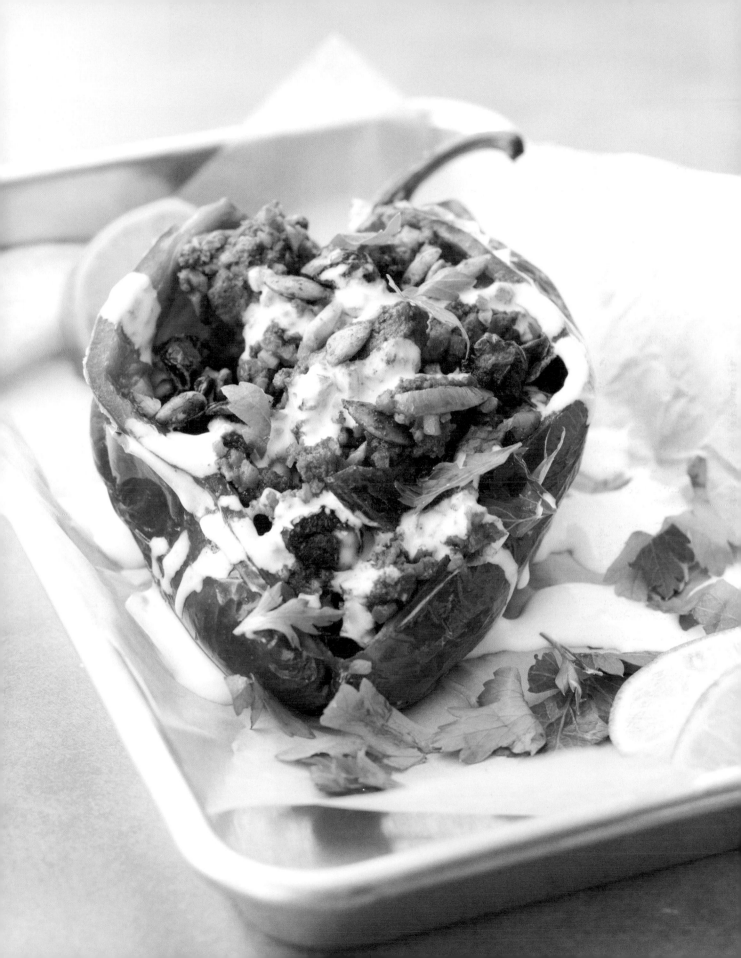

Beef Enchilada Stuffed Spaghetti Squash

NET CARBS

12 g

 EGG-FREE · NUT-FREE   makes 6 servings · prep time: 20 minutes · cook time: 1 hour

If there is a Taco Tuesday and a Fajita Friday, can we all agree that there should be an Enchilada Every Day? If you aren't yet convinced, I'm sure you will be once you taste this dish. To make it even lower in carbs, try stuffing the meat mixture into zucchini instead of spaghetti squash. I love to serve this with Fiesta Cauliflower Rice (page 282).

ingredients

1 large spaghetti squash

2 tablespoons olive oil

Sea salt and ground black pepper

2 tablespoons butter or ghee

1 small onion, diced (about ½ cup)

2 cloves garlic, minced

1 pound ground beef

2 cups Enchilada Sauce, divided (page 346)

1½ cups shredded sharp cheddar cheese, divided

¼ cup sliced black olives

1 (4-ounce) can diced green chilies

¼ cup full-fat sour cream

2 green onions, sliced

2 tablespoons torn fresh cilantro

directions

1. Preheat the oven to 400°F. Line a rimmed baking sheet with parchment paper or a silicone baking mat.

2. Cut the spaghetti squash in half lengthwise and, using a large spoon, scrape out the seeds. Place the squash halves cut side up on the lined baking sheet. Drizzle the squash with the olive oil and sprinkle with a little salt and pepper. Roast for 45 minutes, until the squash is tender and shreds easily. When the squash is done, rake a fork over the shreds to loosen them.

3. While the spaghetti squash is roasting, prepare the filling: Heat the butter in a large skillet over medium heat. Add the onion and garlic and sauté until the onion is translucent and the garlic is fragrant.

4. Add the ground beef to the skillet and cook until it is browned all the way through. Drain the excess grease from the pan. Pour 1 cup of the enchilada sauce into the skillet and stir to combine with the meat mixture.

5. Pour ½ cup of the remaining enchilada sauce over each of the spaghetti squash halves. Using two forks, mix it in with the shreds. Top each squash half with ¼ cup of the cheese.

6. Divide the meat mixture evenly between the spaghetti squash halves. Divide the remaining 1 cup of cheese between the squash halves.

7. Lower the oven temperature to 350°F and return the stuffed squash to the oven for an additional 15 minutes.

8. Remove the squash halves from the oven and top with the olives, chilies, sour cream, green onions, and cilantro.

9. Cut each squash half into thirds before serving. Store leftovers in the refrigerator for up to 1 week.

CALORIES: 466 · FAT: 33g · PROTEIN: 25g · TOTAL CARBS: 17g · DIETARY FIBER: 5g · NET CARBS: 12g

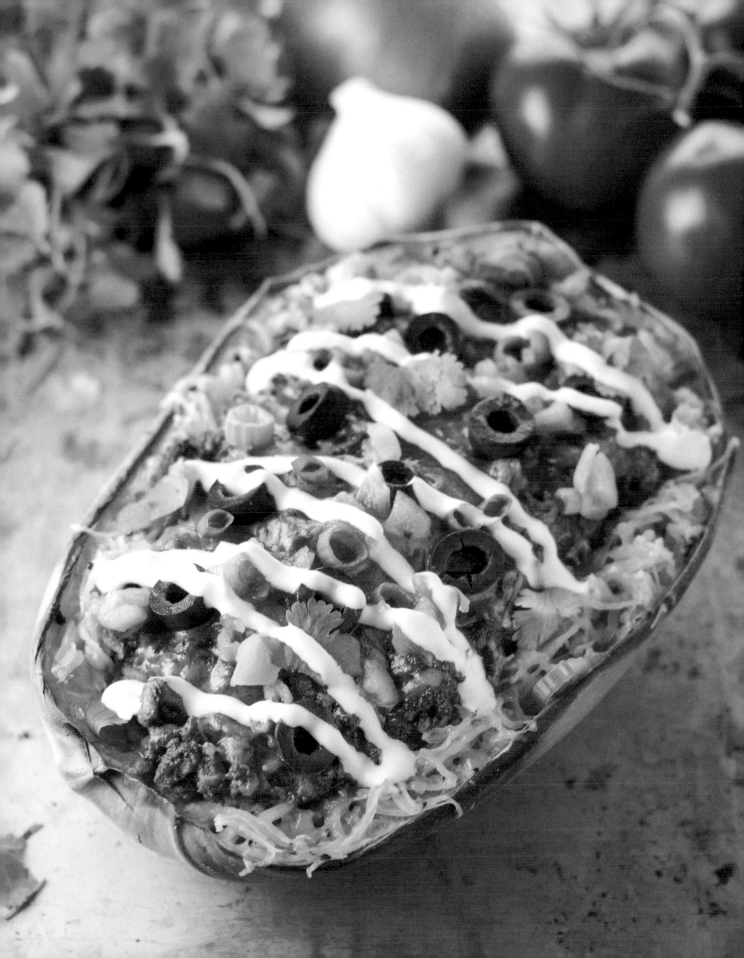

Asian Beef Skewers

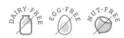

makes 6 skewers · prep time: 10 minutes, plus up to 24 hours to marinate
cook time: 7 minutes

These skewers are amazing paired with Ginger Lime Slaw (page 278). The spiciness of the Sriracha paired with the saltiness of the coconut aminos and the sweetness of the brown sugar sweetener are a match made in heaven. This recipe is also terrific when made with chicken.

ingredients

1½ pounds beef tenderloin, cut into large chunks

2 cloves garlic, minced

½ cup coconut aminos or gluten-free soy sauce

2 tablespoons brown sugar erythritol

2 teaspoons Sriracha sauce

1 tablespoon olive oil

1 teaspoon toasted sesame seeds, for garnish (optional)

Lime wedges, for serving (optional)

Special equipment:

6 skewers, about 12 inches long

directions

1. In a medium mixing bowl, combine the beef chunks, garlic, coconut aminos, brown sugar erythritol, and Sriracha. Place in the refrigerator to marinate for several hours; 24 hours is best.

2. Thread the beef onto the skewers, leaving a small space between pieces to allow the meat to cook evenly.

3. Brush a grill pan with the olive oil and preheat the pan over medium-high heat. Place the skewers in a single layer across the pan. Cook for about 7 minutes, turning halfway through, until the meat has reached the desired level of doneness.

4. Sprinkle the sesame seeds over the top of the beef before serving with the lime wedges, if desired. Store leftovers in the refrigerator for up to 1 week.

CALORIES: 416 · FAT: 30g · PROTEIN: 27g · TOTAL CARBS: 5.2g · DIETARY FIBER: 1g · NET CARBS: 4.2g · ERYTHRITOL: 3.5g

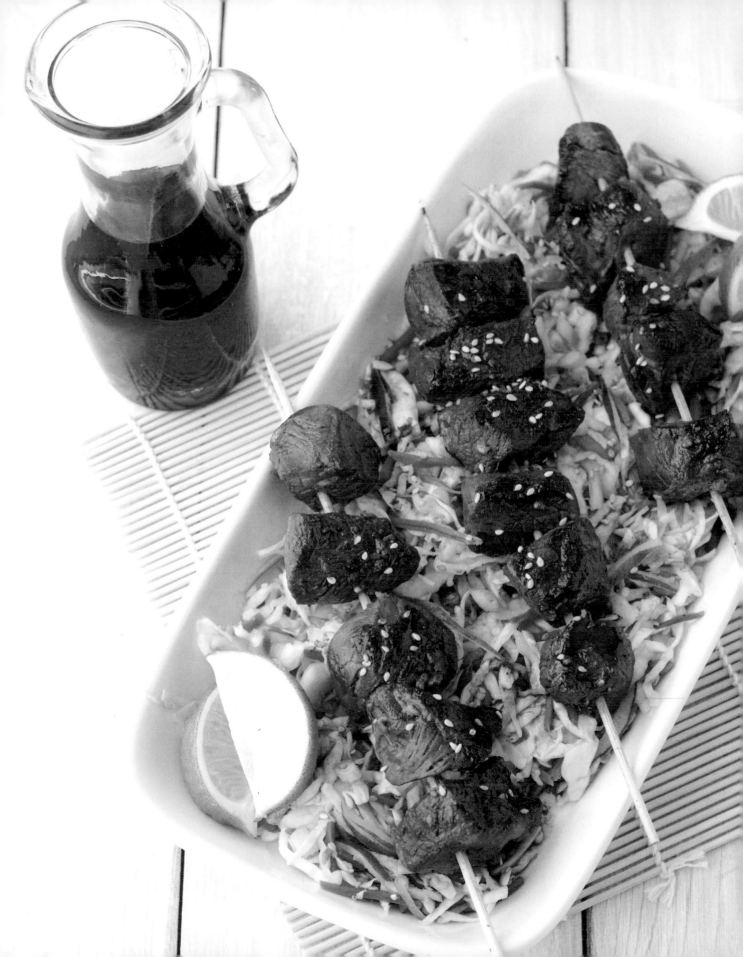

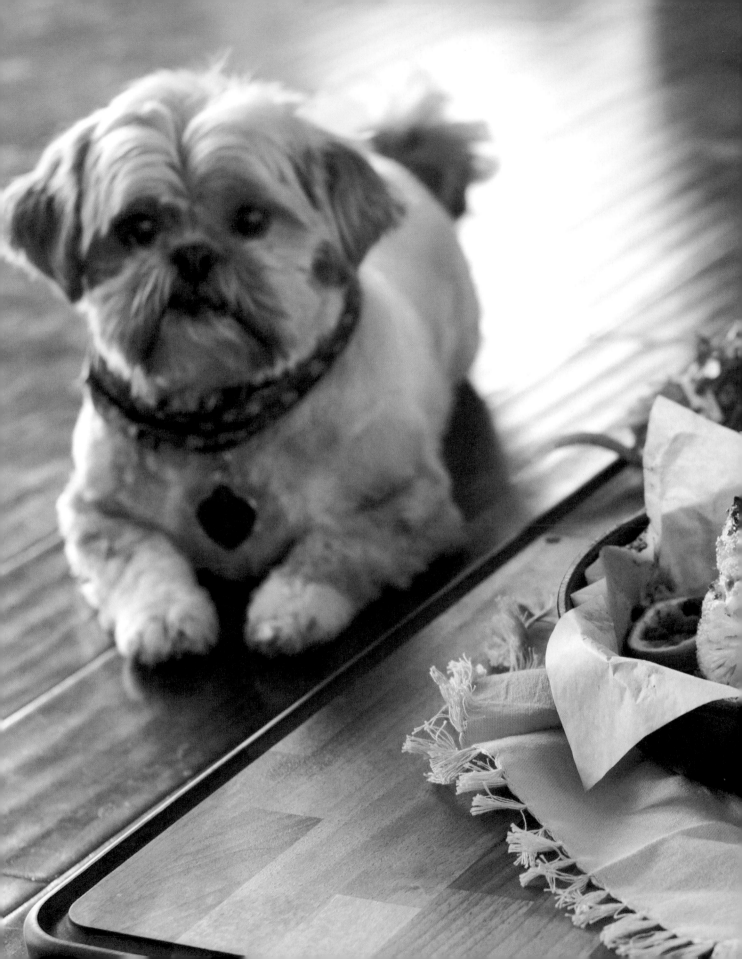

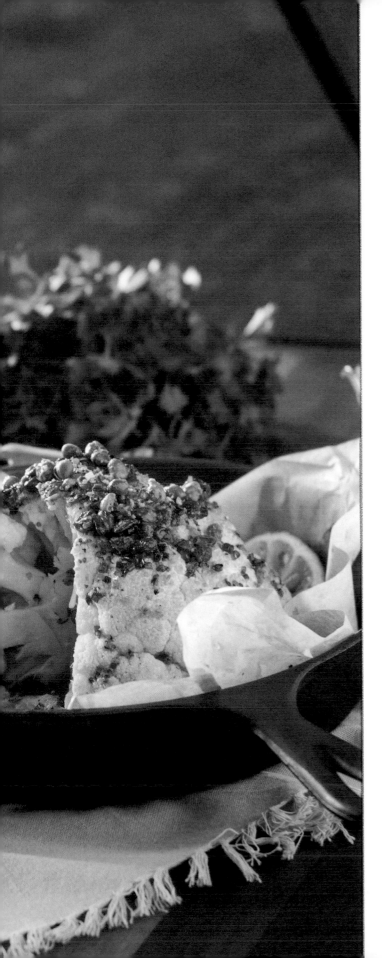

Sides

Oven-Roasted Cabbage Wedges with Dijon Bacon Vinaigrette

   makes 8 servings · prep time: 10 minutes · cook time: 24 minutes

The Dijon bacon vinaigrette in this recipe also makes a delicious salad dressing. It can be stored in the fridge for up to two weeks. If you are having trouble getting your cabbage wedges to stay together, you can chop up all the cabbage, roast it for fifteen to twenty minutes, and then toss it in the vinaigrette before serving. It may look different, but it will still have the same amazing taste.

ingredients

1 medium head green cabbage, halved and then quartered (leave the core intact)

2 tablespoons butter or ghee, melted

Sea salt and ground black pepper

For the vinaigrette:

½ cup avocado oil

2 tablespoons chopped shallots

2 cloves garlic, minced

2 tablespoons Dijon mustard

4 slices thick-cut bacon, diced and cooked until crispy

1 tablespoon chopped fresh chives

Pinch of ground black pepper

Juice of ½ lemon

directions

1. Preheat the oven to 400°F. Line a rimmed baking sheet with a silicone baking mat or parchment paper.

2. Lay the cabbage wedges in a single layer across the prepared baking sheet. Drizzle each wedge with a little melted butter and then sprinkle with salt and pepper. Roast for 10 to 12 minutes on each side, until the outer leaves are just starting to char.

3. In a small mixing bowl, combine the ingredients for the vinaigrette. Whisk vigorously until the ingredients are well combined.

4. Drizzle the vinaigrette over the roasted cabbage wedges before serving. Store leftovers in the refrigerator for up to 1 week. For best results, reheat the cabbage in the oven.

tip: To make this dish dairy-free and Paleo compliant, use ghee rather than butter.

CALORIES: 192 · FAT: 18.5g · PROTEIN: 2.5g · TOTAL CARBS: 4.4g · DIETARY FIBER: 1.6g · NET CARBS: 2.8g

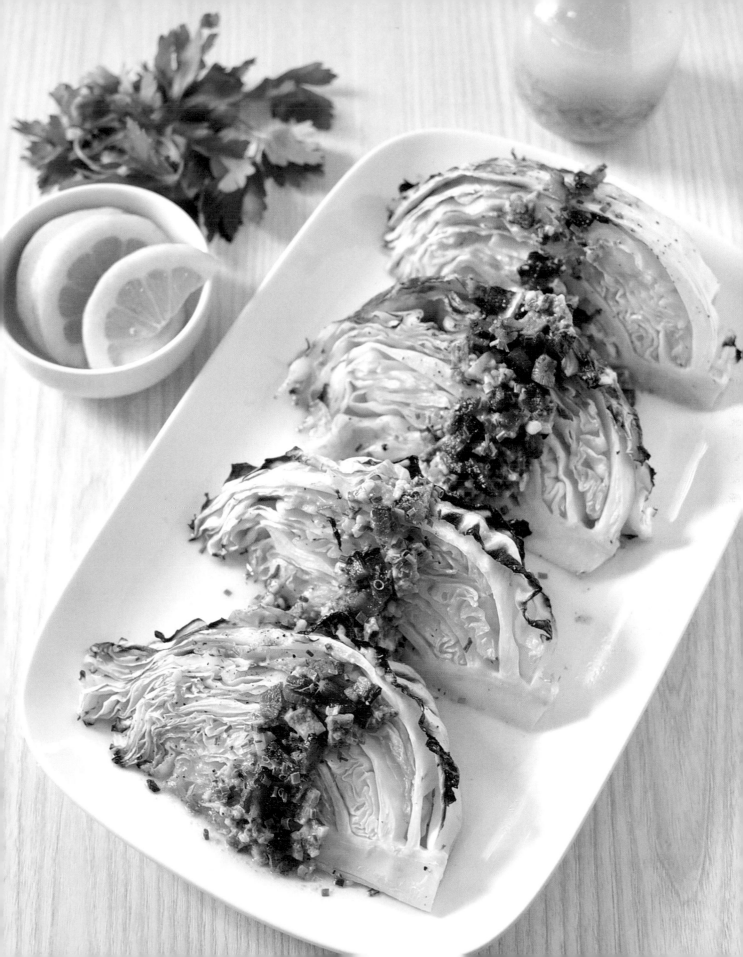

Mascarpone Creamed Greens

makes 8 servings · prep time: 15 minutes · cook time: 20 minutes

Have you ever seen the photo floating around social media that shows a pile of raw spinach a mile high in a pan, and then, after it's cooked, it's in a tablespoon? Although it's a joke, it's surprisingly accurate. This may seem like way too many greens as you start preparing the recipe, but trust me when I tell you that they will cook down considerably and maybe even leave you scratching your head, wondering where all the food went.

ingredients

3 tablespoons butter or ghee

1 large onion, chopped (about 1 cup)

3 cloves garlic, minced

1½ teaspoons sea salt

½ teaspoon ground black pepper

1 large bunch rainbow chard, stemmed and chopped

1 large bunch Lacinato kale, stemmed and chopped

1 pound fresh spinach, stemmed

¼ teaspoon ground nutmeg

¾ cup heavy cream

½ cup shredded Parmesan cheese

4 ounces mascarpone cheese

directions

1. In an extra-large skillet or a large Dutch oven, melt the butter over medium heat. Add the onion, garlic, salt, and pepper to the pan. Sauté until the onion is translucent and the garlic is fragrant.

2. Add the chard, kale, and spinach to the skillet and cook until they are wilted. Remove the greens from the pan and drain them. You may need to press the greens in a colander to help remove the excess moisture. Once the greens are thoroughly drained, set them aside.

3. To the skillet, add the nutmeg, cream, and Parmesan and mascarpone cheeses. Stir to combine. Reduce the heat to low and simmer until the sauce has thickened, 5 to 10 minutes.

4. Add the wilted greens back to the skillet and toss until they are rewarmed and evenly coated in the cheese sauce.

5. Store leftovers in the refrigerator for up to 4 days. Reheat on the stovetop.

tip: If you don't have any mascarpone on hand, feel free to substitute cream cheese. Additionally, you can use any cheeses you have on hand for the sauce. If chard and kale aren't your thing, you can make this dish with all spinach or any greens you prefer.

CALORIES: 151 · FAT: 13g · PROTEIN: 4g · TOTAL CARBS: 5g · DIETARY FIBER: 1.4g · NET CARBS: 3.6g

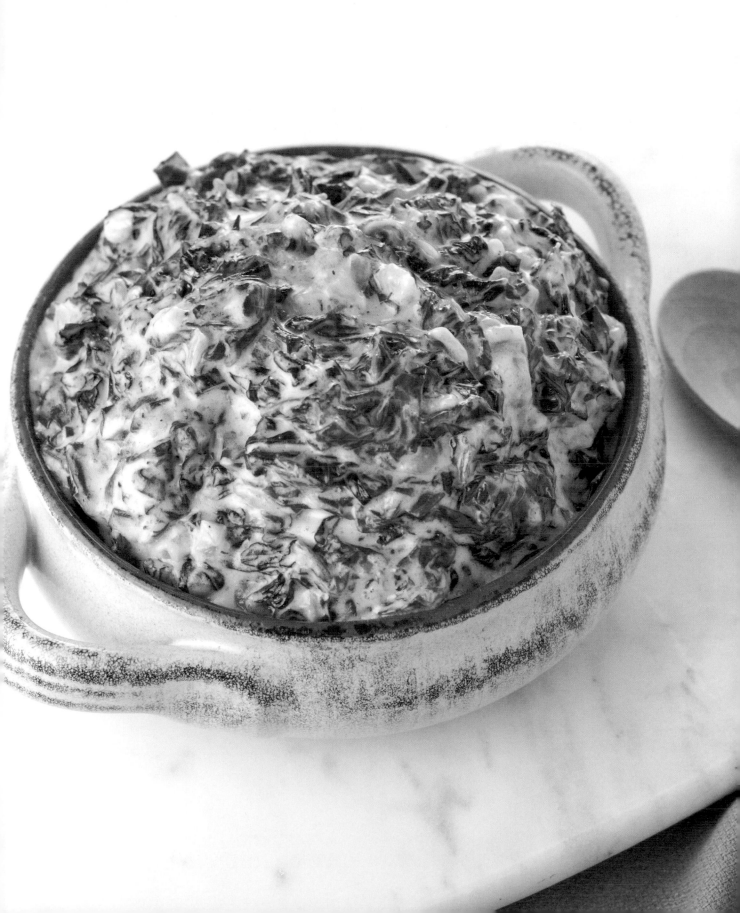

Green Beans with Shallots and Pancetta

NET CARBS
7g

   makes 6 servings · prep time: 10 minutes · cook time: 20 minutes

This side dish is super simple but doesn't skimp on flavor. Feel free to use regular bacon in place of the pancetta. The shallot is a perfect complement to the other flavors in this dish. I love cooking with shallots. They are milder and sweeter than onions, and they have a far less pungent odor. They are also a great natural immune booster, and whenever possible, I prefer food to be my medicine.

ingredients

1½ pounds fresh green beans, ends trimmed

4 ounces pancetta, chopped

1 tablespoon butter or ghee

1 shallot, thinly sliced

Sea salt and ground black pepper (optional)

tip: To make this dish dairy-free and Paleo compliant, use ghee rather than butter. Alternatively, you can use olive oil, coconut oil, or avocado oil.

directions

1. Bring a large pot of salted water to a boil over high heat. Add the green beans and blanch for 4 minutes. Remove the beans and transfer them to an ice bath to shock them and stop the cooking process. Drain and set aside.

2. Heat a large skillet over medium heat. Put the pancetta in the pan and cook, stirring occasionally, until crisped, 3 to 4 minutes. Using a slotted spoon, remove the pancetta from the skillet. Transfer to a plate and set aside.

3. In the same skillet, melt the butter over medium heat. Add the shallot and sauté until it is soft and slightly caramelized.

4. Put the pancetta back in the pan and add the green beans. Toss until the beans are coated and heated through. Taste and add salt and pepper, if desired. Store leftovers in the refrigerator for up to 1 week.

CALORIES: 107 · FAT: 6.7g · PROTEIN: 5g · TOTAL CARBS: 9g · DIETARY FIBER: 2g · NET CARBS: 7g

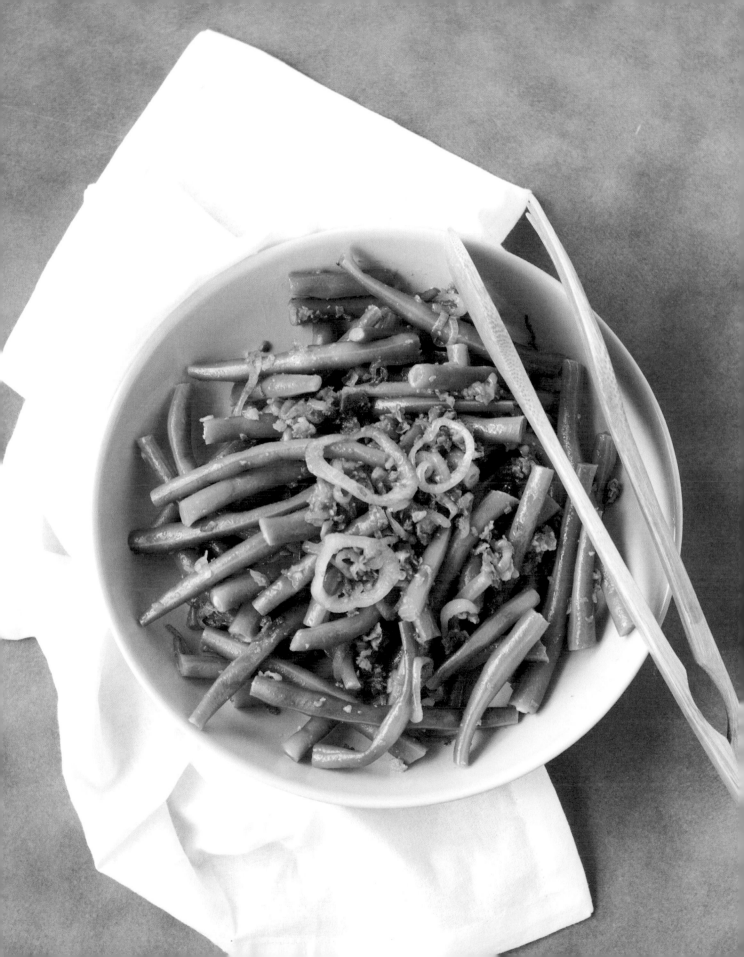

Ginger Lime Slaw

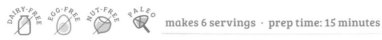

makes 6 servings · prep time: 15 minutes

This dish is so fresh and light and comes together in a matter of minutes—perfect for a quick-and-easy weeknight side dish. The cabbage in the coleslaw mix holds up well against the sauce without getting mushy like lettuce, making it a great make-ahead option. I love to serve this slaw with the Asian Beef Skewers on page 268. From time to time, I like to grill prawns, mix them into the slaw, and make a meal out of it.

ingredients

1 (16-ounce) bag coleslaw mix

A few thin slices red onion

3 green onions, sliced on the bias

2 tablespoons toasted sesame oil

2 tablespoons unseasoned rice wine vinegar

2 teaspoons grated fresh ginger

Juice of ½ lime

¼ cup coconut aminos or gluten-free soy sauce

2 tablespoons toasted sesame seeds

Lime wedges, for serving (optional)

directions

1. In a large mixing bowl, combine the coleslaw mix, red onion, and green onions.

2. In a separate small mixing bowl, combine the sesame oil, vinegar, ginger, lime juice, and coconut aminos. Whisk until the ingredients are well incorporated.

3. Pour the sauce over the top of the coleslaw mixture and toss to combine.

4. Sprinkle the sesame seeds over the top of the slaw or mix them in. Serve with lime wedges, if desired.

CALORIES: 72 · FAT: 5.5g · PROTEIN: 0.7g · TOTAL CARBS: 5.3g · DIETARY FIBER: 0.8g · NET CARBS: 4.5g

NET CARBS
4.5g

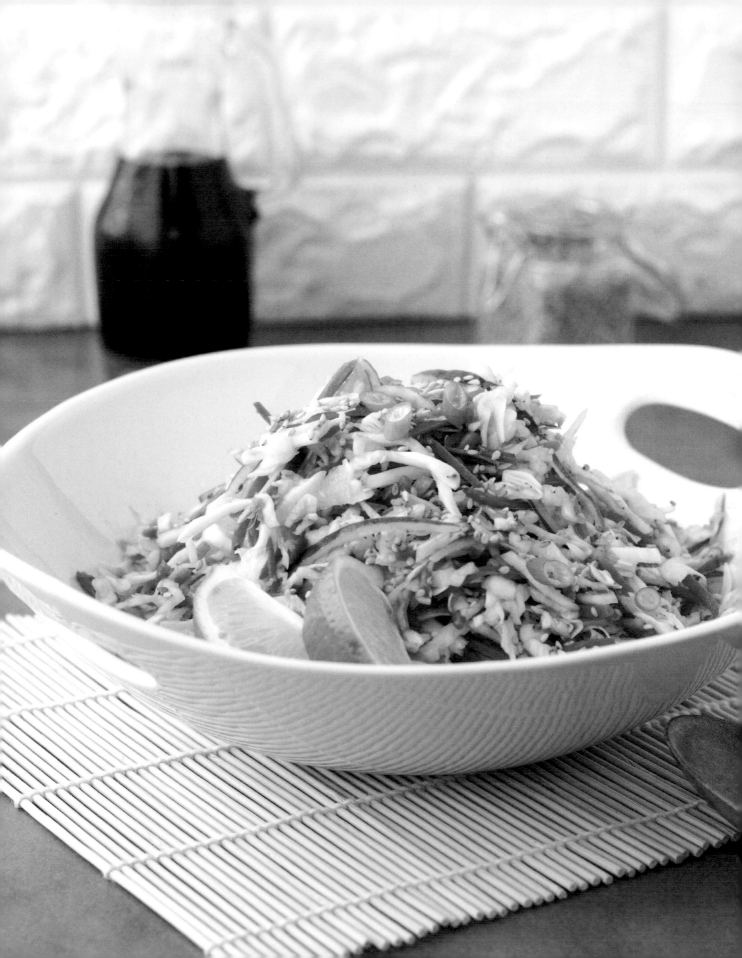

Dill Pickle Coleslaw

makes 6 servings · prep time: 10 minutes, plus 1 to 2 hours to refrigerate

If you have followed my blog or social media over the years, then you already know that I am only slightly obsessed with all things dill pickle flavored. This recipe hits the dill trifecta for me—pickles, pickle juice, and fresh dill. I think I've died and gone to pickle heaven! I love to serve this slaw with the Everything Bagel Dogs on page 212. It is the perfect summertime cookout food, year-round.

ingredients

1 (14-ounce) bag coleslaw mix

1 cup chopped dill pickles

⅓ cup mayonnaise, store-bought or homemade (page 336), or more to taste

2 tablespoons dill pickle juice (from the jar of pickles)

1 tablespoon apple cider vinegar

1 tablespoon Dijon mustard

1 tablespoon chopped fresh chives

1 teaspoon chopped fresh dill weed

Sea salt and black pepper

directions

1. In a large mixing bowl, combine all of the ingredients and mix until well incorporated. Taste and add salt and pepper, if desired.

2. Refrigerate for 1 to 2 hours before serving. Store leftovers in the refrigerator for up to 1 week.

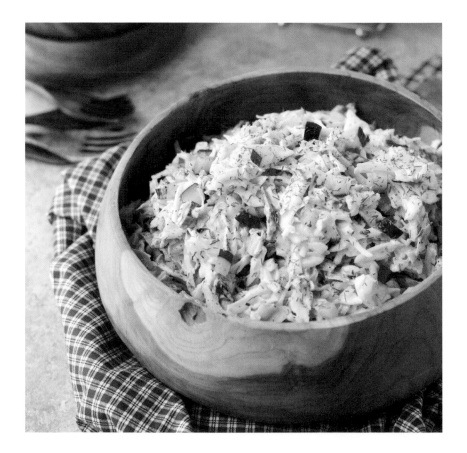

CALORIES: 94 · FAT: 9g · PROTEIN: 0.5g · TOTAL CARBS: 2.5g · DIETARY FIBER: 1g · NET CARBS: 1.5g

Parmesan Roasted Broccoli

NET CARBS
5.8g

  makes 4 servings · prep time: 10 minutes · cook time: 20 minutes

Even when I was a child, broccoli was my favorite vegetable. I have always preferred vegetables over fruit, which made switching to a low-carb way of life a little easier. Did you know that 1 cup of chopped broccoli has the same amount of vitamin C as an orange? They can keep their oranges; I'll take a plate full of broccoli any day!

ingredients

1 large head broccoli, trimmed and cut into florets

2 tablespoons olive oil

½ teaspoon garlic powder

½ teaspoon onion powder

½ teaspoon sea salt

½ teaspoon ground black pepper

½ cup shredded Parmesan cheese

directions

1. Preheat the oven to 450°F. Line a rimmed baking sheet with parchment paper.

2. Arrange the broccoli in a single layer on the prepared baking sheet and drizzle with the olive oil.

3. In a small bowl, combine the garlic powder, onion powder, salt, and pepper. Sprinkle the seasoning mixture over the broccoli.

4. Roast, without stirring, until the edges of the broccoli are crispy and the stalks are crisp-tender, 10 to 15 minutes.

5. Top the broccoli with the Parmesan cheese and roast for an additional 5 minutes. Taste and season with more salt, if needed.

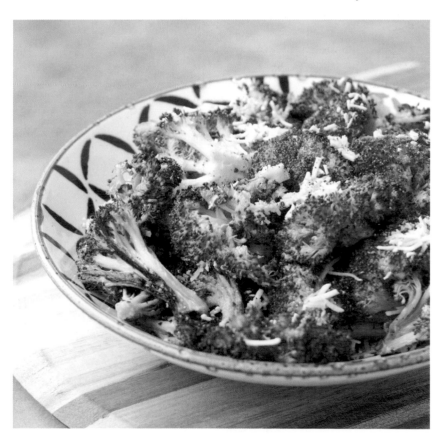

CALORIES: 144 · FAT: 10g · PROTEIN: 7.3g · TOTAL CARBS: 9g · DIETARY FIBER: 3.3g · NET CARBS: 5.8g

Fiesta Cauliflower Rice

   makes 6 servings · prep time: 10 minutes · cook time: 20 minutes

Most grocery stores now carry frozen riced cauliflower, making recipes like this one a breeze. If you aren't able to find it at your local store, you can always use a box grater or food processor to grate or chop a head of cauliflower into "rice" (see page 76). Making your own riced cauliflower is far more cost-effective than buying it and adds just a little more prep time to recipes.

This rice has a nice kick to it. If spicy isn't your thing, you can use diced tomatoes in place of the tomatoes and green chilies. Also, a squeeze of fresh lime juice helps counter-act the spiciness. I love to serve this rice alongside the Steak Fajita Bowls on page 210. If you're looking for a simple cauliflower rice that will go with every recipe in this book, no matter the seasonings, see the variation below for Basic Cauliflower Rice.

ingredients

2 tablespoons butter or ghee

1 medium onion, diced (about 1 cup)

½ teaspoon sea salt

¼ teaspoon ground black pepper

3 cups riced cauliflower (see page 76)

1 (10-ounce) can diced tomatoes and green chilies

1 tablespoon Mexican Seasoning Blend (page 350)

Chopped fresh flat-leaf parsley, for garnish

Lime wedges, for serving (optional)

directions

1. Heat the butter in a large skillet over medium heat. Add the onion, salt, and pepper and sauté until the onion is translucent and soft.

2. Add the riced cauliflower, tomatoes and green chilies, and seasoning blend to the skillet and mix until the ingredients are well combined. Cook for an additional 15 minutes, until the rice is tender.

tips: To make this dish dairy-free and Paleo compliant, use ghee rather than butter.

From my experience, the key to getting cauliflower to have more of a true ricelike texture is to cook it longer. The great thing about cauliflower is that it won't dry out from an extended cook time.

Variation: Basic Cauliflower Rice. Complete Step 1 above, adding 2 cloves of minced garlic, then add the riced cauliflower and ½ cup of chicken stock to the skillet and stir to combine. Continue to cook until all of the liquid has evaporated and the rice is tender. Garnish with freshly grated Parmesan cheese and chopped fresh flat-leaf parsley.

CALORIES: 70 · FAT: 4g · PROTEIN: 1.8g · TOTAL CARBS: 7g · DIETARY FIBER: 2.3g · NET CARBS: 4.8g

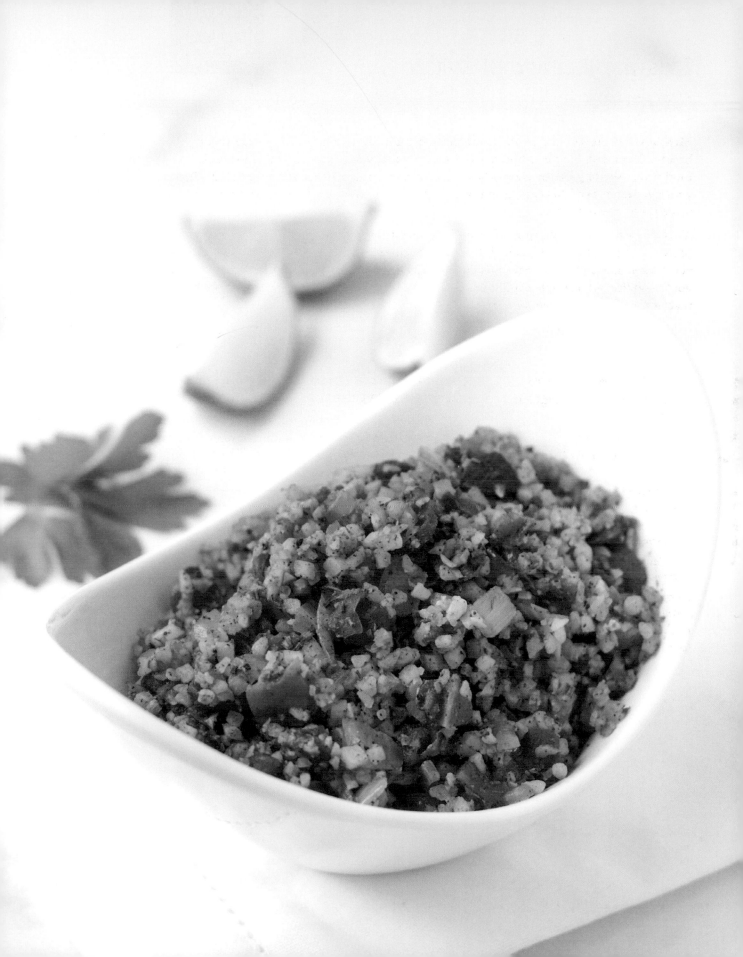

Creamy Herbed Slow Cooker Cauliflower Mash

makes 8 servings · prep time: 15 minutes, plus 30 minutes to rest cook time: 6 hours

There is something so magical about cooking with fresh herbs. They are so fragrant and have such vivid colors. The great thing about this recipe is how versatile it is. You can mix and match any herbs you like; the same goes with the cheeses.

ingredients

1 large head or 2 small heads cauliflower (about 3 pounds)

4 large cloves garlic, peeled

1 bay leaf

1½ teaspoons sea salt

½ teaspoon ground black pepper

4 cups chicken stock

1 tablespoon chopped fresh chives, plus more for garnish

1 tablespoon chopped fresh flat-leaf parsley, plus more for garnish

1 tablespoon chopped fresh rosemary, plus more for garnish

1 teaspoon chopped fresh thyme, plus more for garnish

4 ounces full-fat cream cheese (½ cup)

½ cup grated Parmesan cheese

½ cup heavy cream

¼ cup (½ stick) butter or ghee, plus more for garnish

directions

1. Preheat a slow cooker on the low setting.

2. Clean and core the cauliflower, then cut it into florets.

3. Put the cauliflower, garlic cloves, bay leaf, salt, pepper, and stock in the slow cooker. Cover and cook on low for 6 hours.

4. Remove the bay leaf from the slow cooker and drain all of the stock from the cauliflower.

5. Add the herbs, cream cheese, Parmesan cheese, cream, and butter. Using a hand mixer or an immersion blender, mix until smooth and creamy. Taste and add more salt and pepper, if desired. Cover and let sit off the heat for 30 minutes.

6. Garnish with extra herbs and butter before serving.

tips: If using dried herbs, a good general rule is 1 teaspoon of dried herbs for every 1 tablespoon of fresh herbs.

You can cut the time in half by cooking on high for 3 hours.

CALORIES: 188 · FAT: 15.5g · PROTEIN: 6.8g · TOTAL CARBS: 7.4g · DIETARY FIBER: 2.8g · NET CARBS: 4.7g

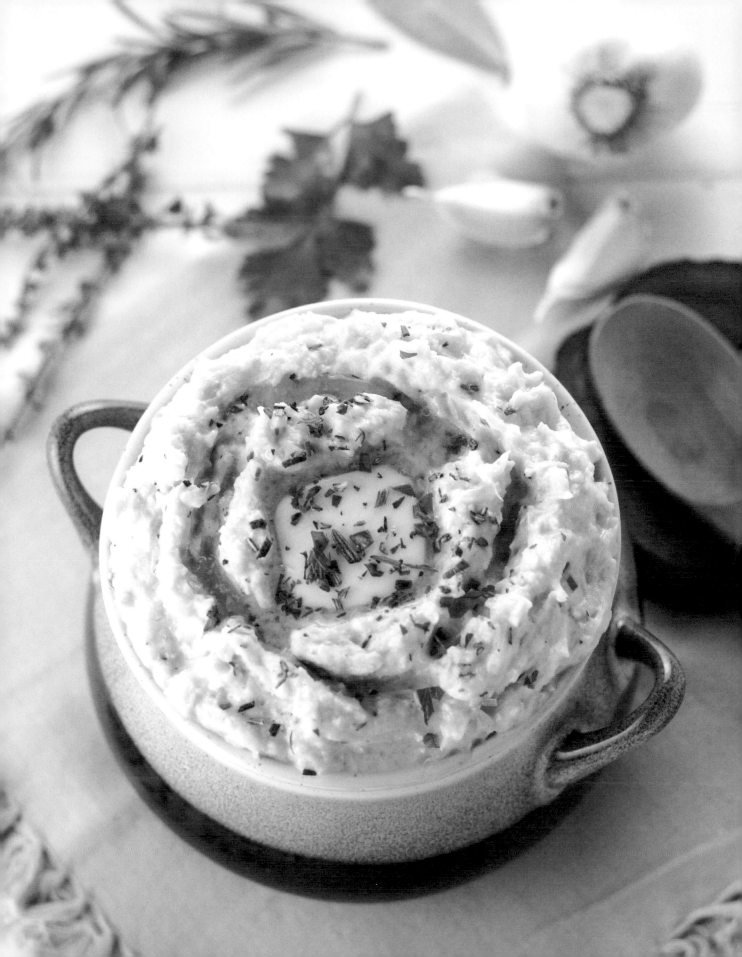

Cranberry Pecan Cauliflower Rice Stuffing

NET CARBS
3.2g

 makes 10 servings · prep time: 10 minutes · cook time: 30 minutes

I began writing this book around the holidays. We happened to be hosting Thanksgiving that year, so I took it as an opportunity to test out some of the recipes for the book on those closest to me. This was one of those recipes. My initial thought was to stuff this inside the turkey, but as it turned out, I didn't make a turkey. While the spread of food made for a nontraditional Thanksgiving dinner, everyone left with happy stomachs.

ingredients

¾ cup raw pecans

2 tablespoons butter or ghee

1 shallot, thinly sliced

1 cup chicken stock

6 cups riced cauliflower (see page 76)

2 sprigs fresh thyme

1 bay leaf

1 teaspoon sea salt

½ teaspoon ground black pepper

2 tablespoons chopped fresh flat-leaf parsley

½ cup grated Parmesan cheese

¼ cup no-sugar-added dried cranberries

directions

1. Preheat the oven to 350°F. Spread the pecans in a single layer on a rimmed baking sheet and roast them for 8 minutes.

2. Meanwhile, heat the butter in a large skillet over medium heat. Add the shallot and sauté until it is soft and translucent.

3. Add the stock to the skillet and, using a rubber spatula, scrape and mix in any bits that are stuck to the bottom of the pan.

4. Add the riced cauliflower, thyme, bay leaf, salt, and pepper to the skillet. Cook for about 15 minutes, until all of the liquid has evaporated and the cauliflower is completely cooked and tender.

5. Remove the thyme sprigs and bay leaf and discard. Mix in the roasted pecans, Parmesan cheese, and dried cranberries. Taste and add more salt and pepper, if desired.

6. Store leftovers in the refrigerator for up to 1 week.

CALORIES: 127 · FAT: 10g · PROTEIN: 4.4g · TOTAL CARBS: 5.5g · DIETARY FIBER: 2.3g · NET CARBS: 3.2g

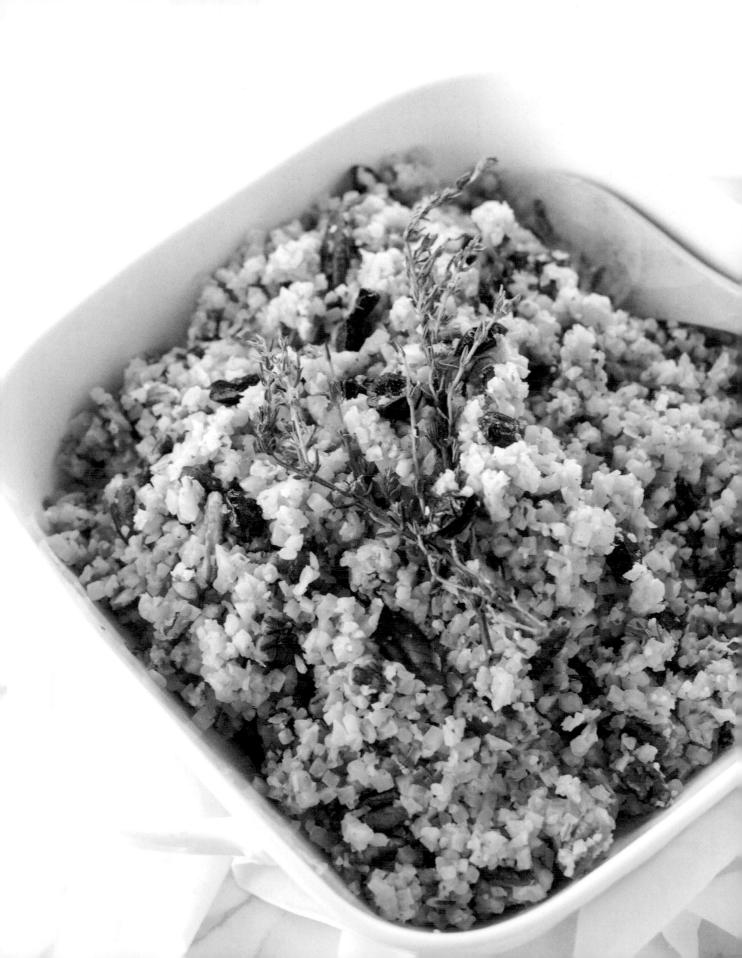

Chorizo and Garlic Brussels Sprouts

makes 6 servings · prep time: 10 minutes · cook time: 10 minutes

The spiciness of the chorizo complements the burst of freshness from the lemon juice perfectly in this dish! If you are using Mexican-style fresh (raw) chorizo, precook it in a separate pan until the sausage is nice and golden brown before adding it to the Brussels sprouts in Step 3.

ingredients

2 tablespoons olive oil

1½ pounds Brussels sprouts, ends trimmed and halved

¼ teaspoon sea salt

¼ teaspoon ground black pepper

6 ounces Spanish-style dry-cured chorizo, halved lengthwise and sliced into half-moons

2 cloves garlic, thinly sliced

2 tablespoons fresh lemon juice

¼ teaspoon smoked paprika

Lemon wedges, for serving (optional)

tip: Whether or not this recipe is Paleo compliant will depend on the brand of chorizo you use. Be sure to read the labels and look for the cleanest ingredients possible.

directions

1. Heat the olive oil in a large skillet over medium heat.

2. Place the Brussels sprouts cut side down in the skillet, sprinkle with the salt and pepper, and sear for 3 to 4 minutes, until they are golden brown and slightly crispy on the bottom.

3. Add the chorizo, garlic, lemon juice, and paprika to the pan and mix until the Brussels sprouts are evenly coated. Cook for 5 more minutes or until the Brussels sprouts are crisp-tender.

4. Store leftovers in the refrigerator for up to 1 week.

CALORIES: 143 · FAT: 10.7g · PROTEIN: 7.5g · TOTAL CARBS: 4g · DIETARY FIBER: 1.5g · NET CARBS: 2.5g

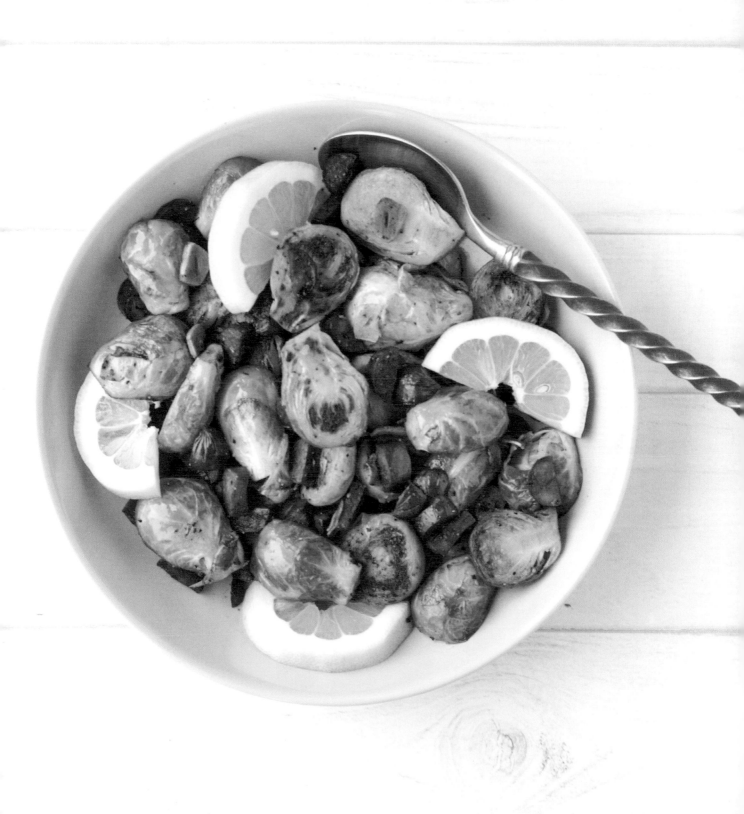

Charred Asian Asparagus and Peppers

   makes 4 servings · prep time: 15 minutes · cook time: 7 minutes

Many classic Asian dishes have sugar in them. This is meant to create a perfect harmony of sweet, salty, and sour components in the dish. The unfortunate thing is that here in the United States, we take it too far and add way too much sugar to just about everything we eat. I made the teaspoon of erythritol in this recipe optional, but it really does add to the flavor of the dish, balancing out the coconut aminos and the rice wine vinegar.

ingredients

1 large bunch asparagus, trimmed

1 small yellow bell pepper, seeded and thinly sliced

1 small red bell pepper, seeded and thinly sliced

4 tablespoons coconut aminos or gluten-free soy sauce, divided

2 tablespoons toasted sesame oil, divided

2 tablespoons unseasoned rice wine vinegar, divided

2 cloves garlic, minced

1 teaspoon grated fresh ginger

Pinch of red pepper flakes

1 teaspoon powdered erythritol (optional)

2 green onions, sliced on the bias, for garnish

1 tablespoon toasted sesame seeds, for garnish

directions

1. Place the asparagus and bell peppers in a large shallow bowl.

2. In a small bowl, combine 2 tablespoons of the coconut aminos, 1 tablespoon of the sesame oil, and 1 tablespoon of the vinegar. Pour the mixture over the asparagus and bell peppers and toss to coat; set aside to marinate.

3. Make the sauce: In a separate small mixing bowl, combine the remaining 2 tablespoons of coconut aminos, remaining tablespoon of sesame oil, and remaining tablespoon of vinegar with the garlic, ginger, red pepper flakes, and erythritol, if using. Whisk until combined, then set aside.

4. Heat a large grill pan over medium-high heat. Place the asparagus and bell peppers in the pan and pour any remaining liquid over the top. Grill, turning, until slightly charred, 5 to 7 minutes.

5. Transfer the asparagus and bell peppers to a serving dish and pour the sauce over the top. Top with the green onions and sesame seeds before serving.

CALORIES: 112 · FAT: 7.8g · PROTEIN: 1.8g · TOTAL CARBS: 8.5g · DIETARY FIBER: 2g · NET CARBS: 6.5g

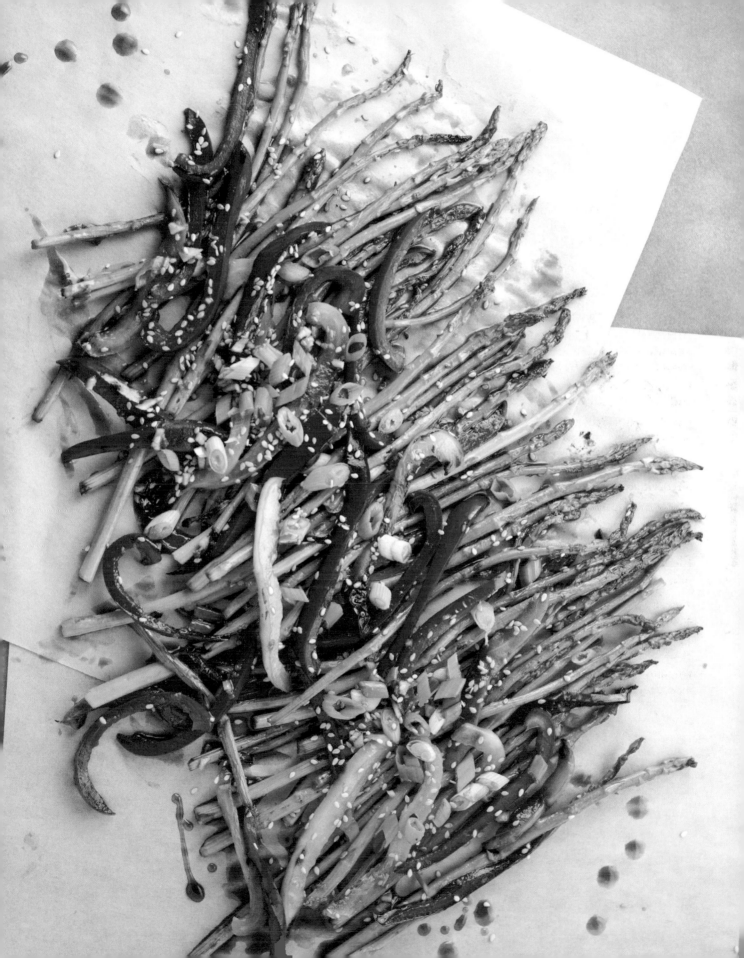

Butter Roasted Radishes

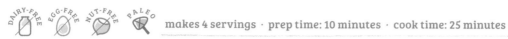

DAIRY-FREE · EGG-FREE · NUT-FREE · PALEO   makes 4 servings · prep time: 10 minutes · cook time: 25 minutes

While I was growing up, radishes were just the things I picked out of my salads at dinner. They tasted bitter and watery and I wanted nothing to do with them. Not until much later in life did I realize that roasting them replaces that bitterness with a subtle sweetness and that they make an excellent low-carb substitute for roasted potatoes. Try throwing them in a beef stew or chowder instead of potatoes. I think you will be pleasantly surprised by how much you enjoy them.

ingredients

1 pound radishes (about 2 pounds with greens)

6 tablespoons (¾ stick) butter or ghee, melted

1 teaspoon Italian seasoning

½ teaspoon garlic powder

½ teaspoon sea salt

tip: To make this recipe dairy-free and Paleo compliant, use ghee rather than butter.

directions

1. Preheat the oven to 375°F. Line a rimmed baking sheet with parchment paper.

2. Prepare the radishes: Slice the tip off each end of the radish, remove the greens (if attached), then halve.

3. In a large mixing bowl, combine the melted butter, Italian seasoning, garlic powder, and salt. Add the radishes to the bowl and toss until they are well coated.

4. Spread the radishes in a single layer on the prepared baking sheet. Bake for 20 to 25 minutes, until they are golden brown and slightly crispy. Taste and add more salt, if needed.

CALORIES: 172 · FAT: 17.5g · PROTEIN: 1g · TOTAL CARBS: 4.3g · DIETARY FIBER: 1.8g · NET CARBS: 2.5g

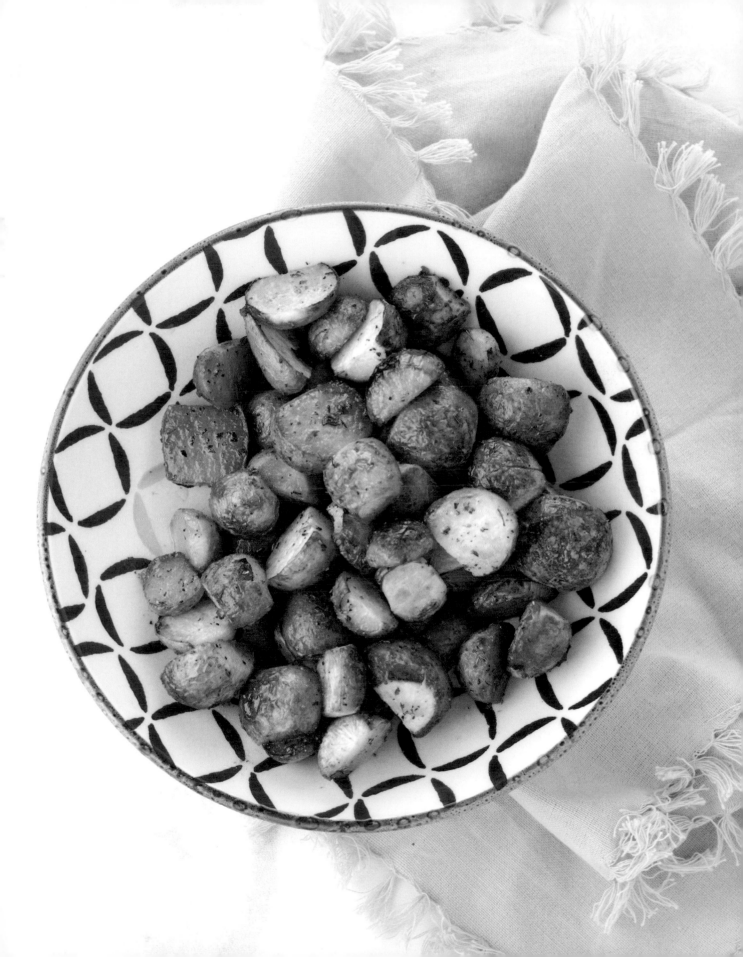

Brussels Sprouts au Gratin with Ham

 EGG-FREE NUT-FREE makes 6 servings · prep time: 20 minutes · cook time: 50 minutes

NET CARBS
4.2g

Do you have a food from your childhood that traumatized you? I sure do! When I was a kid, the quickest way to turn me off my dinner was to serve Brussels sprouts. In my under-developed brain, it was the equivalent of torture. I was not allowed to leave the table until I cleaned my plate. There were nights when I would literally spend hours staring at and roll-ing around the soggy Brussels sprouts on my plate. When I was desperate to leave the table, I would attempt to get them down without tasting them. I would puff my cheeks up with air and try to chew them without letting them touch my tongue. When that didn't work, I would take a big swig of my no-longer-cold milk and try to wash them down. I gagged every time. Here was the problem: My mother bought frozen Brussels sprouts and then boiled them until they were a soggy, flavorless mess. They were so overcooked that they weren't even green anymore. It took me years to recover from this trauma and give Brus-sels sprouts their day in court. When cooked properly, they have a wonderful crisp-tender texture with a subtle sweetness. Of course, adding cheese and garlic never hurts. Try pre-paring them like this, and you may decide they deserve a get-out-of-jail-free card.

ingredients

1½ pounds Brussels sprouts, trimmed and halved

2 tablespoons olive oil

Sea salt and ground black pepper

1 tablespoon butter or ghee

2 cloves garlic, minced

¾ cup heavy cream

1½ cups shredded sharp cheddar cheese, divided

1 cup shredded Gruyère cheese, divided

Pinch of ground nutmeg

10 ounces ham, diced (about 2 cups)

½ cup grated Parmesan cheese

Tip: This dish would also be amazing made with broccoli.

directions

1. Preheat the oven to 400°F. Line a rimmed baking sheet with a silicone baking mat or parchment paper.

2. Place the Brussels sprouts in a single layer on the prepared baking sheet. Drizzle with the olive oil and sprinkle with a little salt and pepper. Roast for 30 minutes, until they are crisp-tender.

3. While the Brussels sprouts are roasting, heat the butter and garlic in a saucepan over medium heat. Cook until the garlic is soft and fragrant.

4. To the saucepan, add the cream, 1 cup of the cheddar cheese, ½ cup of the Gruyère cheese, and nutmeg. Bring to a boil over medium heat, then reduce the heat to low and allow to simmer, stirring occasionally, until the sauce begins to thicken.

5. Transfer the roasted Brussels sprouts to a 13 by 9-inch baking dish and top with the ham. Pour the cheese sauce over the top.

6. Top the casserole with the remaining ½ cup of cheddar cheese, remaining ½ cup of Gruyère cheese, and Parmesan cheese. Bake for an additional 15 minutes, until the cheese is melted.

7. Finish by broiling the casserole for 3 to 5 minutes, until the cheese on top is bubbling and golden brown and the Brussels sprouts are just starting to char.

8. Store leftovers in the refrigerator for up to 1 week.

CALORIES: 288 · FAT: 22g · PROTEIN: 18g · TOTAL CARBS: 5.7g · DIETARY FIBER: 1.5g · NET CARBS: 4.2g

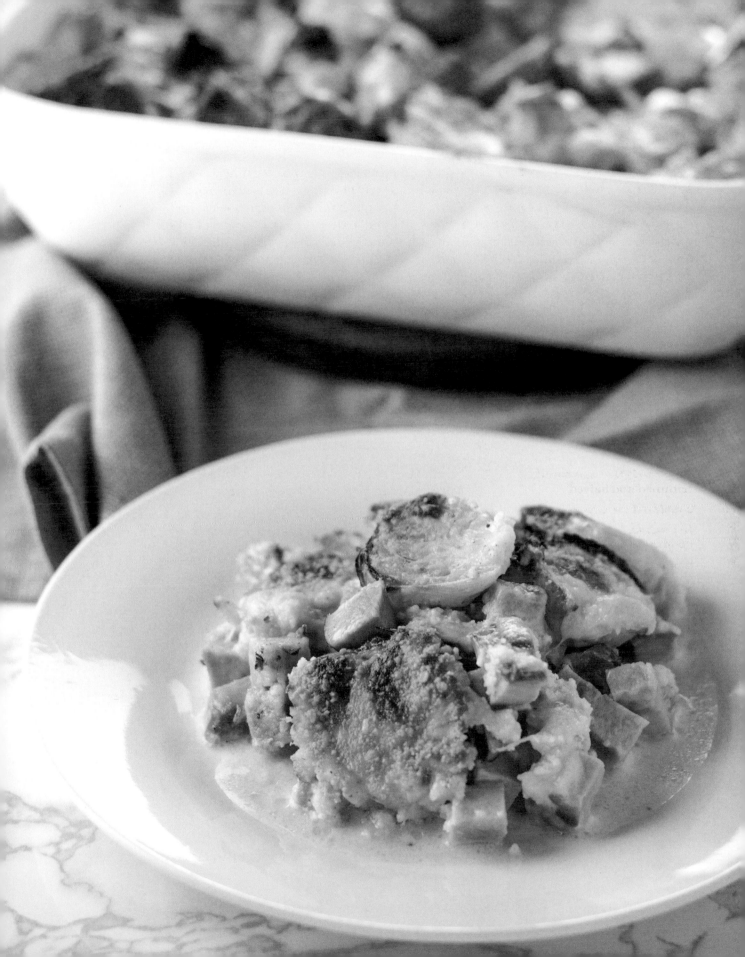

Lemon Caper
Whole Roasted Cauliflower

   makes 6 servings · prep time: 15 minutes · cook time: 40 minutes

While in Tampa for a couple of days before departing on a cruise, my husband and I ate at an amazing steakhouse. One of the things on the side dish menu was a whole roasted cauliflower. It came with a giant steak knife sticking out of it. I knew at that moment that I wanted to do something with a whole roasted cauliflower for this book. The steakhouse version was perfectly seasoned and then dry-roasted. I wanted to change things up a bit and make a mouthwatering sauce from one of my favorite combinations—the fresh flavors of lemon, butter, and capers. Yum!

ingredients

1 large head cauliflower, trimmed but left whole

1 large lemon, sliced

¼ cup (½ stick) butter or ghee, melted

¼ cup capers

2 tablespoons olive oil

1 tablespoon Dijon mustard

1 tablespoon fresh lemon juice

1 teaspoon chopped fresh chives

½ teaspoon garlic powder

½ teaspoon onion powder

½ teaspoon sea salt

¼ teaspoon ground black pepper

directions

1. Preheat the oven to 400°F. Line a large ovenproof skillet with parchment paper.

2. Place the whole head of cauliflower in the lined skillet. Surround the head of cauliflower with the lemon slices.

3. In a small mixing bowl, combine the remaining ingredients. Pour the mixture over the top of the cauliflower and make sure it is evenly covered.

4. Roast the cauliflower for 20 minutes.

5. Remove the skillet from the oven and spoon the sauce over the top until the entire head of cauliflower is coated again. Roast for an additional 20 minutes, until the cauliflower is fork-tender and lightly browned.

6. Slice the cauliflower into wedges and drizzle some of the pan sauce over each slice before serving.

tip: To make this dish dairy-free and Paleo compliant, use ghee rather than butter.

CALORIES: 143 · FAT: 12.5g · PROTEIN: 2g · TOTAL CARBS: 6.8g · DIETARY FIBER: 2.3g · NET CARBS: 4.5g

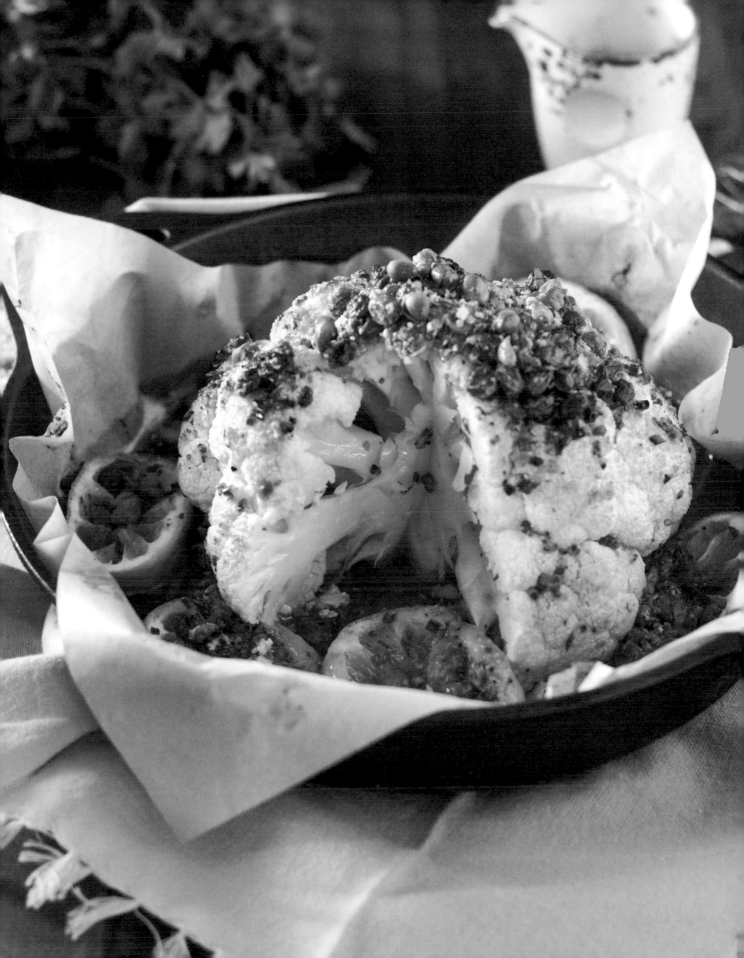

Sautéed Mushrooms with Garlic Mascarpone Cream Sauce

makes 6 servings · prep time: 15 minutes · cook time: 15 minutes

This is the perfect side dish for when you are short on time and ingredients. It comes together quickly and complements just about any main dish. Want to jazz it up? Try adding a tablespoon or two of Walnut Avocado Pesto (page 340).

ingredients

2 tablespoons butter or ghee

1 pound cremini mushrooms, quartered

3 cloves garlic, minced

½ teaspoon sea salt

¼ teaspoon ground black pepper

8 ounces mascarpone cheese

¼ cup chopped fresh flat-leaf parsley

tip: Don't have mascarpone? You can substitute full-fat cream cheese.

directions

1. Melt the butter in a large skillet over medium heat. Add the mushrooms, garlic, salt, and pepper and sauté until the mushrooms are tender and have released their liquid, about 10 minutes.

2. Mix in the mascarpone cheese, stirring to coat each mushroom.

3. Stir in the parsley. Cook for an additional 2 to 3 minutes. Taste and add more salt and pepper, if desired.

CALORIES: 138 · FAT: 11.8g · PROTEIN: 4.2g · TOTAL CARBS: 3.3g · DIETARY FIBER: 0 · NET CARBS: 3.3g

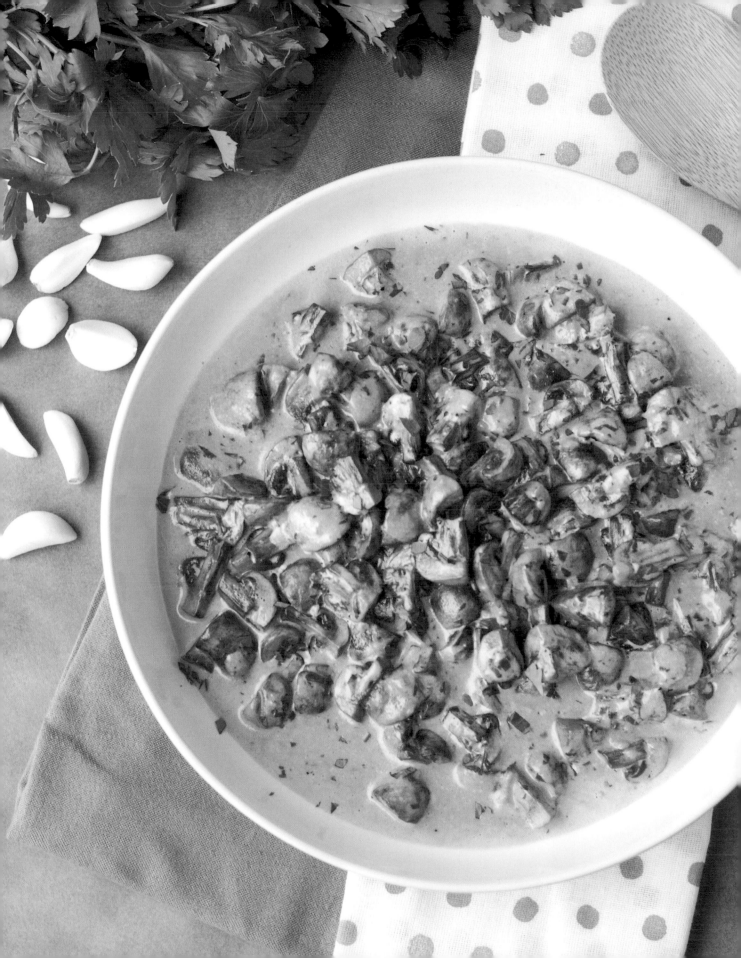

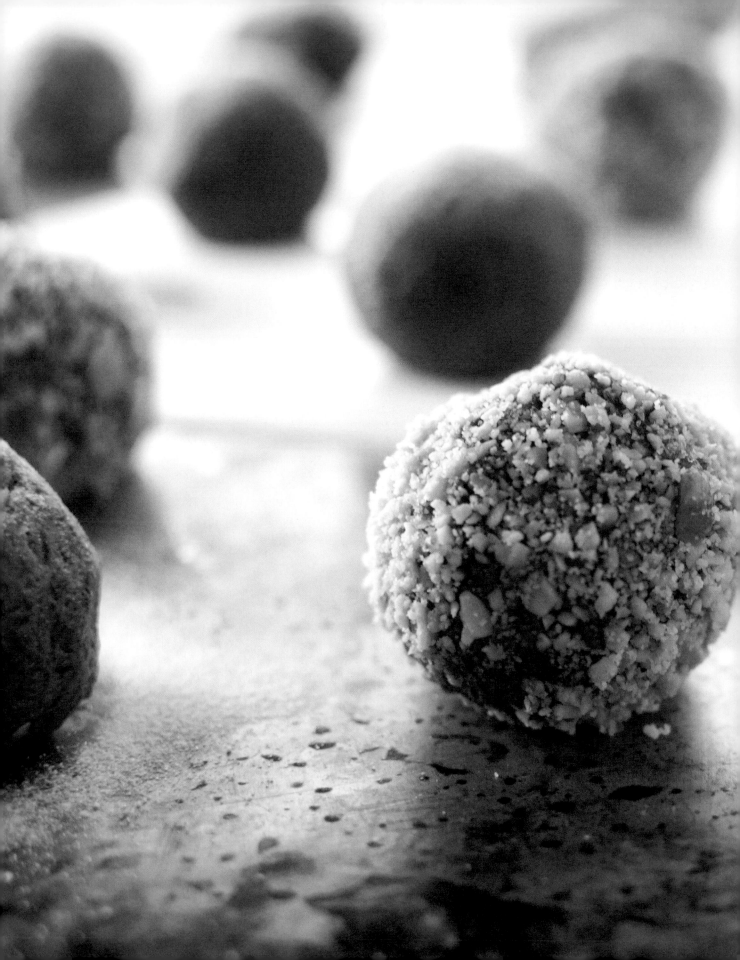

Sweet Treats

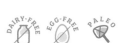

Salted Caramel Nut Brittle

DAIRY-FREE · EGG-FREE · PALEO

makes 10 servings (3 to 4 pieces per serving)
prep time: 10 minutes · cook time: 20 minutes

If I had to choose one recipe from this book that my family unanimously loves and actually fights over, this would be it! In fact, I ended up making a second batch within twenty-four hours because we devoured the first one. This brittle makes a great holiday gift. Make several tins of it and hand them out to family and friends…although I feel I must warn you, you might have trouble parting with it!

ingredients

2 cups roasted, salted mixed nuts

¾ cup granular erythritol

2 tablespoons water

1 teaspoon pure vanilla extract

1½ teaspoons Maldon sea salt flakes

tip: To make this brittle Paleo compliant, use coconut sugar in place of the erythritol, but please note that doing so will greatly increase the overall carb count of the recipe.

directions

1. Preheat the oven to 350°F. Line a rimmed baking sheet with a silicone baking mat or parchment paper.

2. Spread the nuts in a single layer on the prepared baking sheet and roast for 8 minutes. Remove the nuts from the oven and set aside to cool.

3. In a medium saucepan, combine the erythritol and water. Mix with a fork until all of the erythritol is moistened.

4. Cook over medium-high heat until the sugar melts. Continue cooking for 5 to 10 minutes, swirling (not stirring) the sugar constantly until the mixture turns golden brown in color.

5. Remove the pan from the heat and carefully add the vanilla extract; the caramel will be very hot, and the vanilla will bubble up. Swirl the pan to combine the vanilla with the sugar. Add the nuts to the caramel and, working quickly, use two spoons to coat all of the nuts in the caramel.

6. Pour the brittle mixture onto the prepared baking sheet and spread in an even layer. Sprinkle the sea salt flakes over the top and let cool.

7. Once the brittle is completely cool and the caramel has hardened, break the brittle into 1-inch pieces. Store in an airtight container in the pantry for up to 2 weeks.

CALORIES: 136 · FAT: 13.6g · PROTEIN: 4g · TOTAL CARBS: 5.6g · DIETARY FIBER: 1.6g · NET CARBS: 4g · ERYTHRITOL: 14g

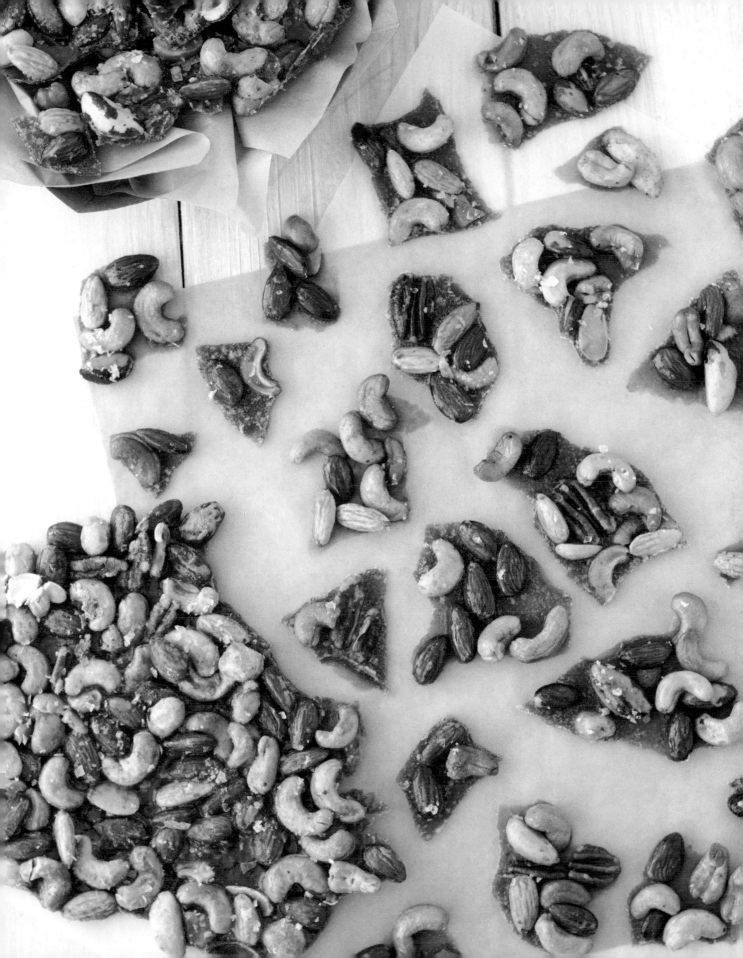

Dark Chocolate Mousse

makes 2 cups (½ cup per serving) · prep time: 10 minutes, plus 3 to 4 hours to set
cook time: 15 minutes

This recipe is a little more labor-intensive than most of the recipes in the book, but I assure you that it is worth it and that this is a dish you will make over and over again. The mousse is rich and decadent, and even your non-keto friends and family will enjoy it.

ingredients

⅔ cup sugar-free dark chocolate chips

1 tablespoon unsalted butter

4 tablespoons water, divided

⅛ teaspoon sea salt

2 large egg yolks

2 tablespoons granular erythritol

½ cup heavy cream

½ cup Fresh Whipped Cream (page 327) (optional)

1 ounce unsweetened baking chocolate, grated or shaved, for garnish (optional)

tip: Try mixing a drop or two of sugar-free mint extract into the finished mousse to make a chocolate mint version.

directions

1. Set up a double boiler by placing a heatproof bowl on top of a saucepan filled with about 1 inch of water. Make sure that the bowl is not touching the water and is suspended above the water line by the rim of the pan. Bring the water to a simmer.

2. To the bowl, add the chocolate chips, butter, 2 tablespoons of the water, and salt. Whisk until the mixture is melted and smooth. Remove the bowl from the pan and set aside.

3. In a separate double boiler setup, combine the egg yolks, remaining 2 tablespoons of water, and erythritol in the heatproof bowl placed over a saucepan of simmering water. Whisk until the mixture is foamy and hot to the touch, about 3 minutes.

4. Pour the warm egg mixture into the warm chocolate mixture and whisk until it is smooth and the ingredients are well incorporated. Fill a larger bowl half full with ice water and place the smaller bowl with the mousse in the ice water. Whisk occasionally until the mixture has cooled to room temperature or cooler, about 5 minutes.

5. Pour the heavy cream into a separate mixing bowl. Using a hand mixer, whip the cream until it holds soft peaks. Using a rubber spatula, fold the whipped cream into the chocolate mixture little by little until it is well combined and there are no visible streaks.

6. Transfer the mixture to 4 small single-serving dishes. Cover and refrigerate for 3 to 4 hours, until set.

7. Serve topped with whipped cream and chocolate shavings, if using.

CALORIES: 142 · FAT: 14g · PROTEIN: 2.5g · TOTAL CARBS: 7.5g · DIETARY FIBER: 3g · NET CARBS: 4.5g · ERYTHRITOL: 6g

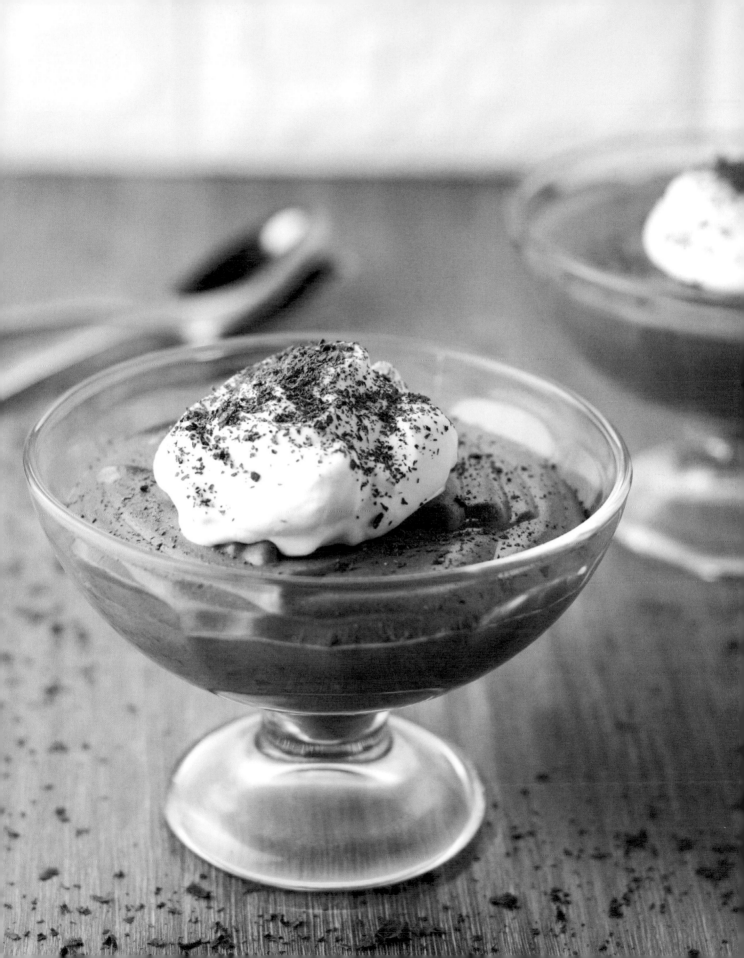

Maple Butter Pecan Truffles

 EGG-FREE

makes 20 truffles (2 per serving) · prep time: 20 minutes, plus up to 3 hours to freeze

These truffles are sinfully delicious! I like to make an afternoon of it and make a batch of these, the Lemon Coconut Cheesecake Bites on page 312, and the Chocolate Peanut Butter Cheesecake Balls on page 316 at the same time. Then I keep them all in the freezer and pop one in my mouth whenever I have a taste for a sweet treat. They do the trick every time.

ingredients

2 tablespoons butter, softened

1½ ounces cream cheese, softened (3 tablespoons)

1 cup powdered erythritol

1 teaspoon pure vanilla extract

1 teaspoon sugar-free maple extract

1 cup finely chopped toasted pecans, divided

1 tablespoon coconut oil

½ cup sugar-free dark chocolate chips

tip: If you do not have a microwave or do not wish to use one, you can set up a double boiler to melt the chocolate chips and coconut oil. See page 304 for instructions for setting up a double boiler.

directions

1. In a large mixing bowl, use a hand mixer to mix together the butter, cream cheese, erythritol, vanilla extract, maple extract, and half of the pecans until the ingredients are well combined. Freeze the mixture for 1 hour.

2. Line a large plate with parchment paper. Remove the mixture from the freezer and, using a tablespoon, scoop the mixture and roll into twenty 1-inch balls. Place the balls on the prepared plate and put them back in the freezer for another hour.

3. In a microwave-safe bowl, combine the coconut oil and chocolate chips and microwave until the chocolate is melted. Use a rubber spatula to mix the ingredients until smooth. Let cool just slightly before using.

4. Pierce each frozen ball with a toothpick, then dip it into the melted chocolate mixture and swirl to coat. Place the chocolate-dipped ball back on the plate and sprinkle with the remaining pecans. Repeat this process with the rest of the balls.

5. Freeze for an additional 30 minutes to an hour before serving. Store leftovers in an airtight container in the freezer for up to 2 months. Enjoy frozen or let thaw for a few minutes before eating.

CALORIES: 128 · FAT: 13.2g · PROTEIN: 1.6g · TOTAL CARBS: 4.4g · DIETARY FIBER: 2.2g · NET CARBS: 2.2g · ERYTHRITOL: 19.2g

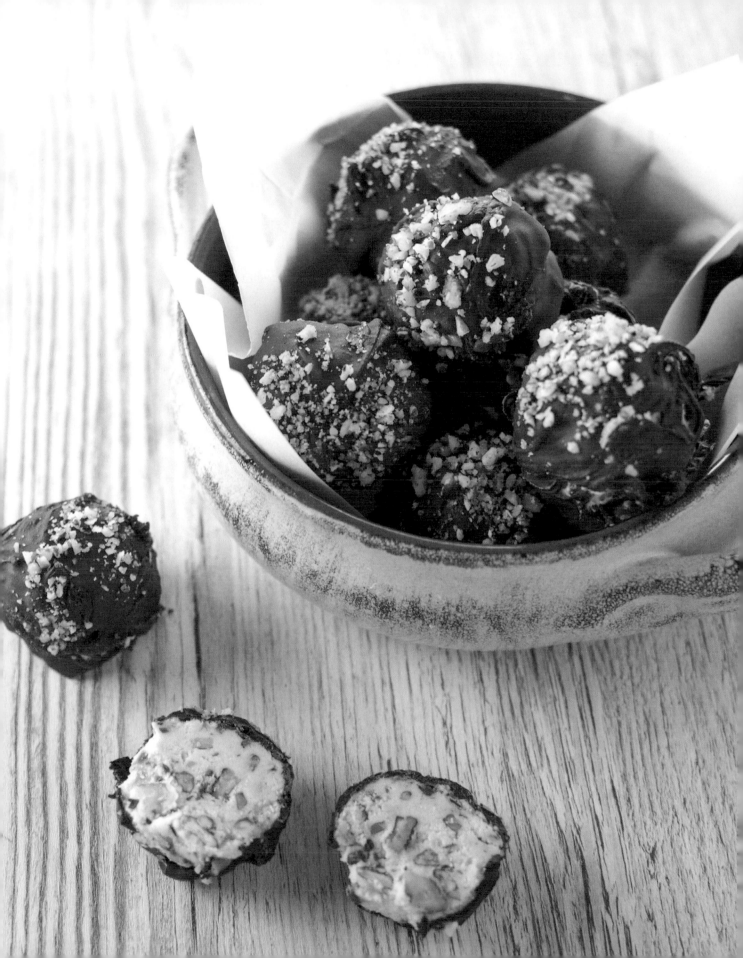

Mason Jar Chocolate Ice Cream

NET CARBS
2g

   makes 1 pint (½ cup per serving) · prep time: 5 minutes, plus 3 hours to freeze

Aside from the simplicity of this recipe, my favorite thing about this ice cream is how adaptable it is. Want plain vanilla? Skip the cocoa powder and add a little more vanilla extract. Want salted caramel? Add a little sea salt and caramel extract and omit the cocoa powder. Use this recipe as a base and then get creative with it. The flavor combinations are endless.

ingredients

1 cup heavy cream

2 tablespoons powdered erythritol

1 tablespoon unsweetened cocoa powder, or more to taste

1 teaspoon pure vanilla extract

2 tablespoons sugar-free dark chocolate chips (optional)

tip: If your arms get tired from all the shaking, you can always whip the ice cream mixture with an immersion blender and then fold in the chocolate chips, if using.

directions

1. Place all of the ingredients in a wide-mouth pint-sized mason jar. Screw the lid on and shake vigorously until the liquid has doubled in volume and fills the jar; this should take about 5 minutes.

2. Freeze until set but still creamy, at least 3 hours.

3. Scoop and enjoy!

CALORIES: 210 · FAT: 22.5g · PROTEIN: 1.5g · TOTAL CARBS: 2.5g · DIETARY FIBER: 0.5g · NET CARBS: 2g · ERYTHRITOL: 6g

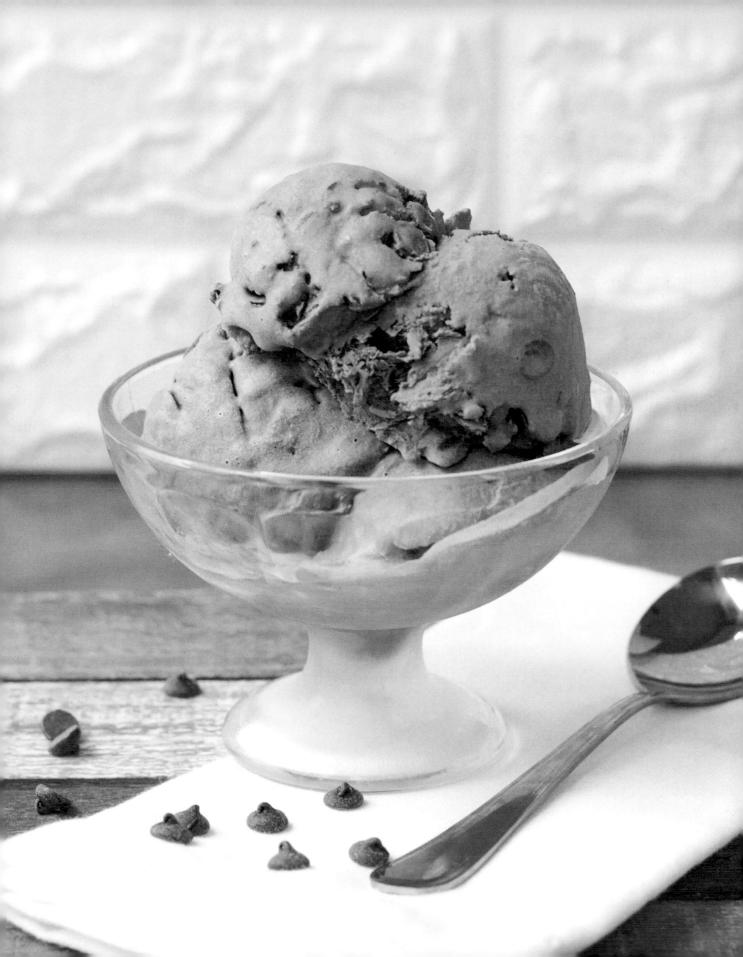

Lemon Curl

makes 2¾ cups (¼ cup per serving) · prep time: 5 minutes, plus 3 to 4 hours to chill
cook time: 15 minutes

I love lemon curd. Its fresh, bright flavor and pudding-like texture enhance countless desserts or even breakfasts. (It is a fantastic topping for the Lemon Ricotta Pancakes on page 124.) But it's also great eaten straight up, with a spoon!

ingredients

½ cup (1 stick) butter, softened

1½ cups granular erythritol

4 large whole eggs

2 large egg yolks

1 cup fresh lemon juice (about 4 large lemons)

1 tablespoon grated lemon zest

tip: If the leftover lemon curd starts to take on a gritty texture from the granular erythritol, slowly warm it in a saucepan over low heat. This will take it back to a smooth texture, after which it's ready to be enjoyed warm or cold. Alternatively, you can try making this recipe with powdered erythritol.

directions

1. Place the butter and erythritol in a mixing bowl and mix with a hand mixer on medium speed until well blended, about 45 seconds.

2. Add the whole eggs and egg yolks, one at a time, mixing just until blended in after each addition.

3. Gradually add the lemon juice to the butter mixture, mixing on low speed until well blended. Stir in the lemon zest. The mixture may look curdled at this stage; this is normal.

4. Transfer the mixture to a large saucepan and cook over medium-low heat, whisking constantly, until it thickens, about 15 minutes.

5. Transfer the lemon curd to a bowl and place plastic wrap directly on the warm curd to prevent a film from forming. Chill until firm, 3 to 4 hours. Store in an airtight container in the refrigerator for up to 2 weeks.

CALORIES: 117 · FAT: 11g · PROTEIN: 2.9g · TOTAL CARBS: 2.5g · DIETARY FIBER: 0 · NET CARBS: 2.5g · ERYTHRITOL: 26g

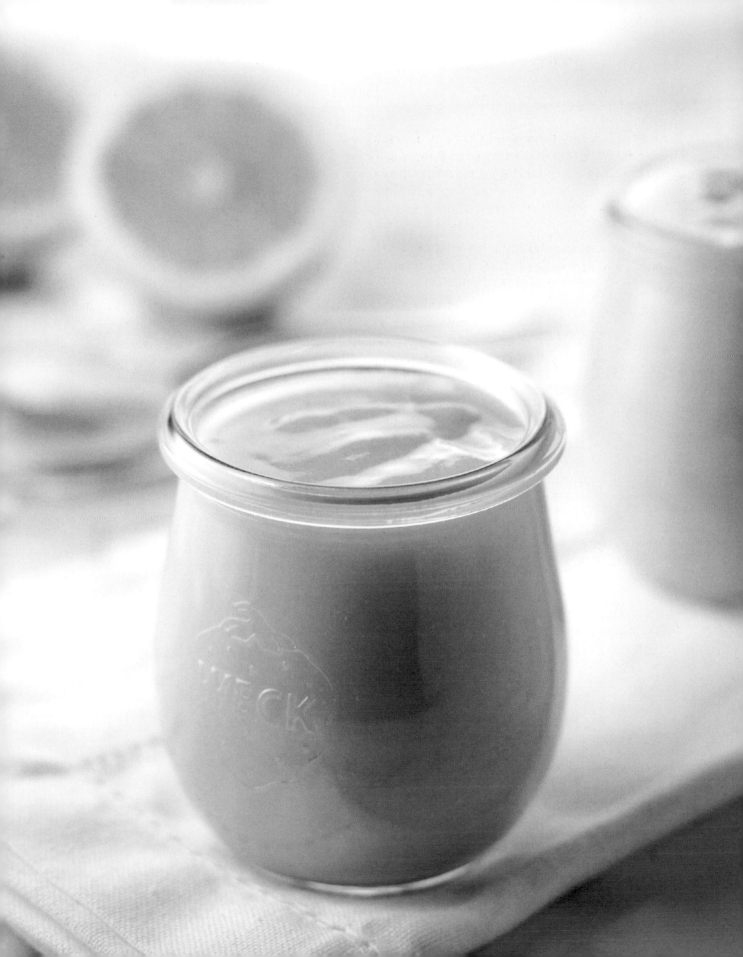

Lemon Coconut Cheesecake Bites

 EGG-FREE · NUT-FREE · makes 20 bites (2 per serving) · prep time: 20 minutes, plus 2 hours to set

Have you ever heard the phrase "That will stick to your ribs"? No, it doesn't refer to things actually sticking to your rib cage; it means eating something that will leave you feeling satiated for a long time. When I am feeling hungry between meals or have a craving for something sweet, eating something small but with a high fat content usually does the trick. This recipe fits the bill—it is sweet *and* has a high fat content. These cheesecake bites stick to my ribs, and I'm sure they will stick to yours, too.

ingredients

2 cups unsweetened coconut flakes, divided

1 (8-ounce) package full-fat cream cheese, softened

Juice of 1 lemon

¾ cup powdered erythritol

1 teaspoon pure vanilla extract

Grated zest of 1 lemon

directions

1. Put the coconut in a food processor and pulse until it is finely shredded.

2. In a large mixing bowl, combine 1 cup of the shredded coconut, cream cheese, lemon juice, erythritol, and vanilla extract. Using a hand mixer, mix until the ingredients are well combined. Refrigerate the mixture for 2 hours.

3. Combine the remaining 1 cup of shredded coconut and the lemon zest and spread it in a thin layer on a plate.

4. Line a rimmed baking sheet or large plate with parchment paper. Remove the cheesecake mixture from the refrigerator and, using a tablespoon, form it into 1- to 1½-inch balls. Roll each ball in the coconut and lemon zest mixture and place on the parchment paper.

5. Freeze the cheesecake bites for 15 minutes before eating. Store in the freezer for up to 2 months. Let thaw just slightly before eating.

CALORIES: 161 · FAT: 16g · PROTEIN: 2.2g · TOTAL CARBS: 4.5g · DIETARY FIBER: 1.6g · NET CARBS: 2.9g · ERYTHRITOL: 14.4g

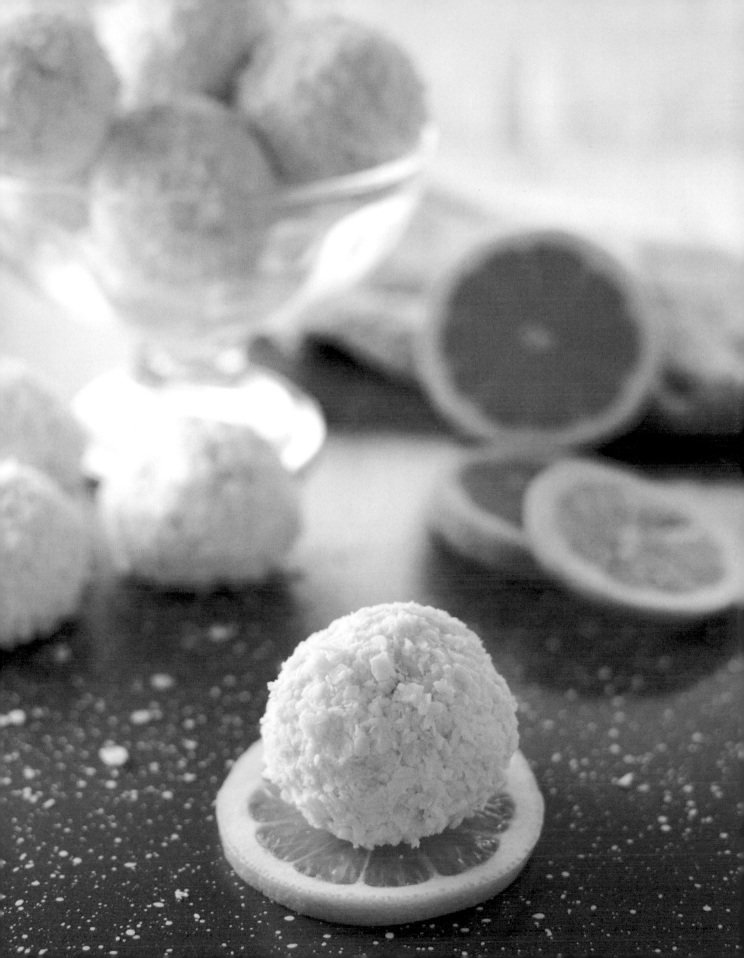

Flourless Chewy Chocolate Chip Cookies

 makes 14 cookies (1 per serving) · prep time: 10 minutes · cook time: 9 minutes

Ooey gooey chewy chocolate chip cookies. That's a mouthful...a mouthful of delicious cookies. Because these cookies are flourless, there is no grainy nut flour texture, only smooth and creamy goodness. I love to make a double batch and take them with me to gatherings where I know there will be sweet indulgences that I won't be able to partake in. With this recipe, you can have your cookie and eat it, too.

ingredients

1 cup creamy salted almond butter

⅔ cup powdered erythritol

1 large egg

1 teaspoon pure vanilla extract

1 teaspoon baking soda

⅓ cup sugar-free dark chocolate baking chips

directions

1. Preheat the oven to 350°F. Line a cookie sheet with a silicone baking mat or parchment paper.

2. In a large mixing bowl, combine the almond butter, erythritol, egg, vanilla extract, and baking soda. Using a rubber spatula, mix until the ingredients are well combined. Fold in the chocolate chips.

3. Shape the dough into 1½- to 2-inch balls. This will produce 14 good-sized cookies. You can make them smaller to yield more cookies.

4. Place the balls of dough on the prepared cookie sheet about 2 inches apart and press to flatten slightly. Bake for 9 minutes, until the edges are firm but the centers are still soft.

5. Remove the cookie sheet from the oven and place it on a cooling rack. Allow the cookies to cool on the pan before eating. Store in an airtight container in the pantry for up to 2 weeks.

CALORIES: 132 · FAT: 11g · PROTEIN: 4.5g · TOTAL CARBS: 4.7g · DIETARY FIBER: 2.9g · NET CARBS: 1.8g · ERYTHRITOL: 9g

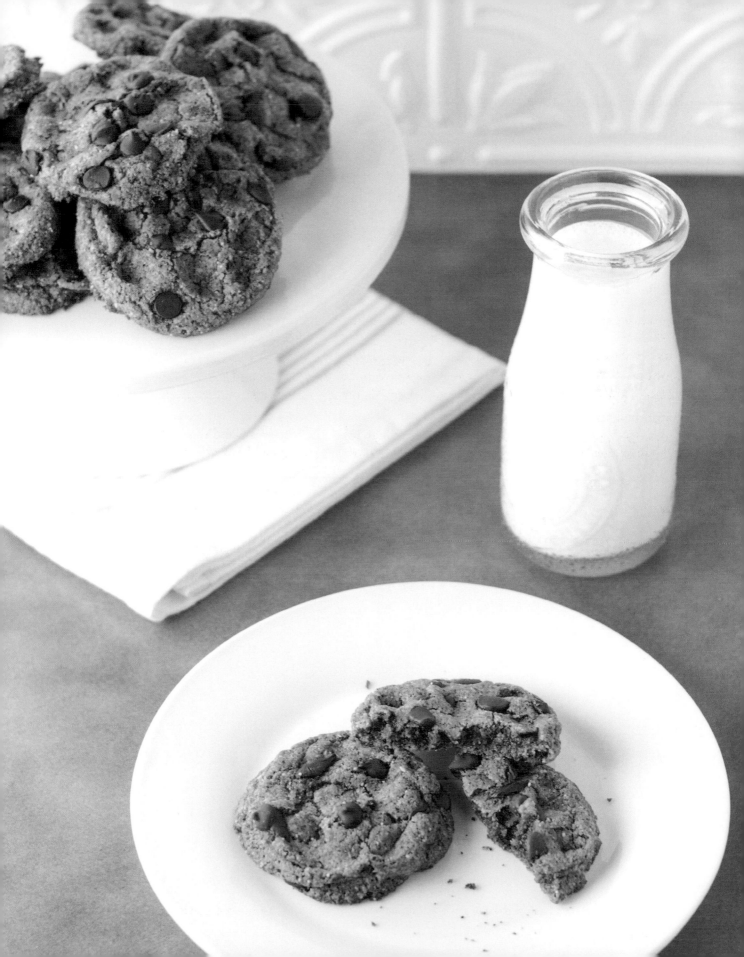

Chocolate Peanut Butter Cheesecake Balls

NET CARBS
3.6g

 makes 20 cheesecake balls (2 per serving) · prep time: 15 minutes, plus 3 hours to set

If you were to come to our house for dinner, there is a good chance that you would hear Jon or the kids ask if we have any chocolate meatballs. These are the meatballs they would be referring to. We pretty much always have a batch of these in the freezer. They are the perfect quick fix for a sweet tooth.

ingredients

1 (8-ounce) package full-fat cream cheese, softened

¾ cup reduced-sugar creamy peanut butter

¼ cup powdered erythritol, plus extra for dusting

2 tablespoons unsweetened cocoa powder, plus extra for dusting

1 teaspoon pure vanilla extract

1 cup sugar-free dark chocolate chips (optional)

¼ cup crushed roasted mixed nuts (optional)

directions

1. Put the cream cheese, peanut butter, erythritol, cocoa powder, and vanilla extract in a large mixing bowl. Using a hand mixer, mix until the ingredients are well combined.

2. Using a rubber spatula, fold in the chocolate chips, if using. Refrigerate the mixture for 2 hours.

3. Line a rimmed baking sheet or large plate with parchment paper. Using a tablespoon, scoop up some of the mixture and form it into a 1- to 1½-inch ball. Place the ball on the parchment paper. Repeat the process until the mixture is gone, making a total of 20 balls.

4. Dust each ball with either powdered erythritol or cocoa powder or roll the balls in crushed nuts, if using.

5. Freeze for 1 hour to set before eating. Store in the freezer for up to 2 months. Let thaw just slightly before eating.

CALORIES: 208 · FAT: 18.3g · PROTEIN: 6.4g · TOTAL CARBS: 5.2g · DIETARY FIBER: 1.6g · NET CARBS: 3.6g · ERYTHRITOL: 4.8g

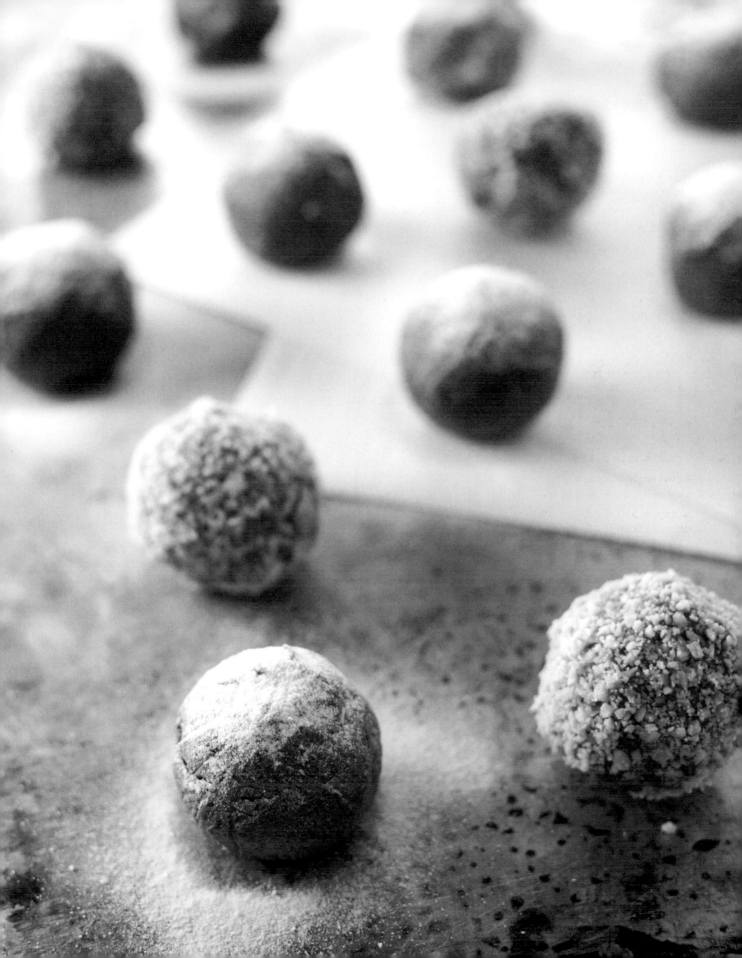

Chocolate-Covered Maple Bacon

  EGG-FREE   NUT-FREE   makes 10 pieces (1 per serving) · prep time: 10 minutes, plus 30 minutes to set
cook time: 10 minutes

Say it with me…chocolate-covered maple bacon. Need I say more? I make several batches of this recipe for our annual holiday party, and it is always the first thing gone from the food table. Honestly, how can you go wrong when combining bacon and chocolate? I've even been known to dip these in peanut butter. Yes, I went there.

ingredients

½ cup sugar-free dark chocolate chips

1 tablespoon coconut oil

1 teaspoon sugar-free maple extract

10 slices thick-cut bacon, cooked crisp

directions

1. Line a large plate with wax paper or parchment paper.

2. Pour 1 inch of water into a medium saucepan and bring to a gentle boil over medium-high heat. Place a heatproof glass bowl on top of the pan. Make sure that the bowl is not touching the water and that it is the right size to rest on the rim of the pan, allowing no steam to escape.

3. Put the chocolate chips, coconut oil, and maple extract in the glass bowl. Using a rubber spatula, stir until the chocolate is melted and smooth.

4. Dip half of each slice of bacon into the chocolate, coating it generously. Place the dipped bacon on the lined plate. Repeat this process with the remaining slices of bacon.

5. Transfer the plate to the refrigerator for 30 minutes to allow the chocolate to harden. Store in an airtight container in the refrigerator for up to 2 weeks.

CALORIES: 67 · FAT: 5.7g · PROTEIN: 3.3g · TOTAL CARBS: 2.7g · DIETARY FIBER: 1.2g · NET CARBS: 1.5g

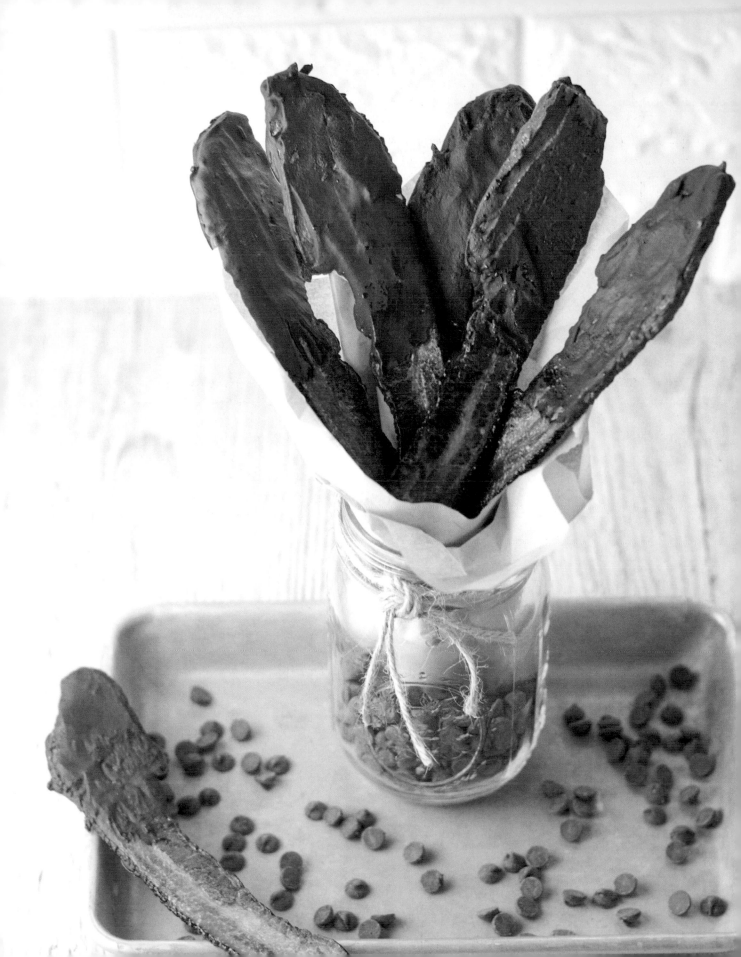

Chocolate Chip Cookie Dough Bites

makes 8 cookie dough bites (1 per serving) · prep time: 10 minutes

One taste of these cookie dough bites and you will be transported back to childhood memories of trying to reach your little hand into the mixing bowl to steal even one small bit of cookie dough. These bites have all of those same amazing flavors, without all the sugar and carbs. That's a win-win! You can lower the carbs even further by omitting the chocolate chips. That leaves you with more of a sugar cookie–type base. From there, try using different extracts to add different flavors—almond, caramel, and lemon, to name a few.

ingredients

¼ cup (½ stick) butter, softened

2 tablespoons plus 1 teaspoon granular erythritol, or more to taste

¼ cup blanched almond flour

¼ cup coconut flour

Pinch of sea salt

3 tablespoons heavy cream

1½ teaspoons pure vanilla extract

3 tablespoons sugar-free dark chocolate chips

directions

1. In a large mixing bowl, using a hand mixer, cream the butter and erythritol until the butter is creamy and the sweetener is completely mixed in.

2. To the creamed mixture, add the almond flour, coconut flour, salt, cream, vanilla extract, and chocolate chips. Mix until the ingredients are well combined. If the mixture is crumbly, form it into a ball. If the mixture is too dry, add water, little by little, until you get the right texture. But note that it should be very thick, just like raw cookie dough.

3. Use an ice cream scoop or a tablespoon to scoop the mixture into 8 equal-size cookie dough bites. Store in the refrigerator for up to 4 days.

CALORIES: 111 · FAT: 10.6g · PROTEIN: 1.5g · TOTAL CARBS: 4g · DIETARY FIBER: 2.2g · NET CARBS: 1.8g · ERYTHRITOL: 3.5g

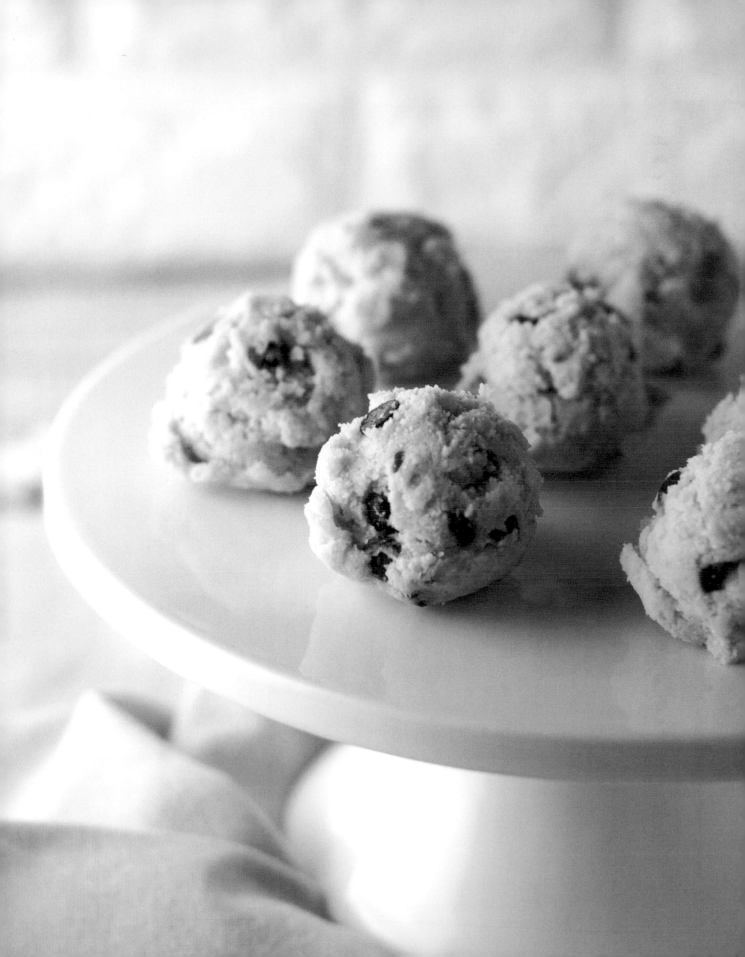

Chewy Peanut Butter Cookies

 makes 18 cookies (1 per serving) · prep time: 10 minutes · cook time: 10 minutes

Historically, I have always gravitated towards savory foods, but if there is a peanut butter cookie in my presence, my inner cookie monster is unleashed. There is nothing quite like a warm peanut butter cookie straight out of the oven. And there is something so satisfying about making the crisscross marks on top. It's like childhood and adulthood all wrapped into one. If you like a crunchier cookie, try adding chunky peanut butter. These are easy to make and ready in under 20 minutes.

ingredients

1 large egg

1 cup reduced-sugar creamy peanut butter

½ cup granular erythritol

2 teaspoons pure vanilla extract

½ teaspoon baking powder

½ teaspoon sea salt

directions

1. Preheat the oven to 350°F. Line a cookie sheet with a silicone baking mat or parchment paper.

2. Place all of the ingredients in a large mixing bowl. Using a hand mixer, mix until the ingredients are well combined and form a thick dough.

3. Shape the dough into 1- to 1½-inch balls (18 total). Place the dough balls on the cookie sheet, about 2 inches apart. Use a fork to flatten the cookies and make crisscross marks on top.

4. Bake for 10 minutes, until the edges are firm but the centers are still soft.

5. Remove the cookie sheet from the oven and place it on a cooling rack. Allow the cookies to cool on the pan before eating. Store in an airtight container in the pantry for up to 2 weeks.

CALORIES: 97 · FAT: 8g · PROTEIN: 3.8g · TOTAL CARBS: 2.7g · DIETARY FIBER: 0.9g · NET CARBS: 1.8g · ERYTHRITOL: 5g

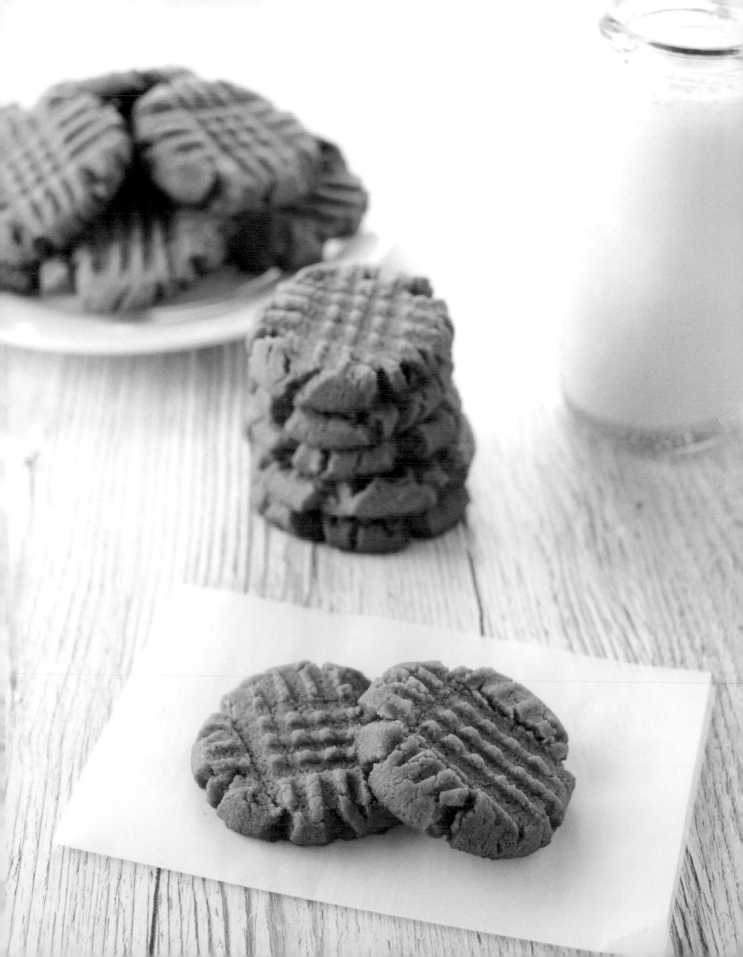

Blueberry Mojito Ice Pops

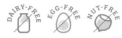

makes 10 ice pops (1 per serving) · prep time: 10 minutes, plus 3 to 4 hours to freeze cook · time: 10 minutes

Nothing takes you back to childhood quite like an ice pop on a hot summer day. But instead of chasing after a truck playing "The Entertainer," you'll be running to your own freezer! These pops are the perfect blend of sweet and tart. For an adults-only version, try adding a little bit of rum to the mixture.

ingredients

¾ cup water

½ cup fresh lime juice

⅓ cup granular erythritol

25 fresh mint leaves

2 limes

½ cup frozen blueberries

¼ cup soda water

Special equipment:

10 (3-ounce) ice pop molds

directions

1. In a small saucepan over high heat, combine the water, lime juice, erythritol, and mint leaves. Bring to a boil, then quickly remove the pan from the heat. Whisk vigorously for 1 to 2 minutes, until the sugar has completely dissolved.

2. Using a slotted spoon, remove the mint leaves and discard. Let the mixture cool.

3. Slice each lime into 5 wheels, for a total of 10 wheels.

4. Divide the blueberries evenly among 10 ice pop molds. Place a lime slice in each mold.

5. Divide the cooled ice pop mixture evenly among the molds, pouring the liquid over the fruit, filling each mold three-quarters of the way full. Top off each mold with a splash of soda water.

6. Place a Popsicle stick in each mold and freeze for 3 to 4 hours, until frozen solid. Store in the freezer for up to 2 weeks.

CALORIES: 12 · FAT: 0.2g · PROTEIN: 0.2g · TOTAL CARBS: 3.6g · DIETARY FIBER: 0.7g · NET CARBS: 2.9g · ERYTHRITOL: 6g

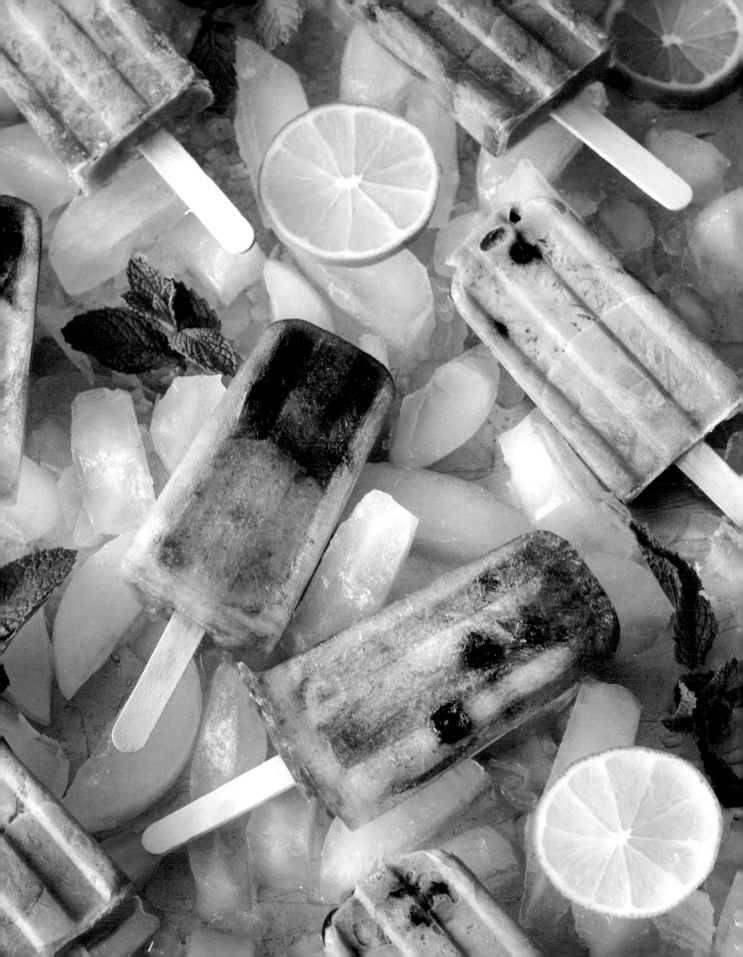

Almond Joy Chia Seed Pudding

 DAIRY-FREE · EGG-FREE · **makes 4 servings · prep time: 10 minutes, plus 1 to 2 hours to refrigerate**

How can you go wrong when combining the flavors of chocolate, almond, and coconut? Answer: you can't! Chia seeds help you feel full and satisfied while also reducing cravings between meals. They also help balance insulin levels in the body. There is definitely a reason people call them a superfood. While chia seeds may look like a high-carb food, they are also very high in fiber, making their effective carb count zero grams.

ingredients

2 cups unsweetened almond milk or coconut milk

½ cup unsweetened coconut flakes, divided

¼ cup unsweetened cocoa powder

¼ cup powdered erythritol

1 teaspoon pure vanilla extract

⅓ cup chia seeds

2 tablespoons crushed roasted almonds

¼ cup sugar-free dark chocolate chips (optional)

tip: If you are not a fan of the texture of chia seeds, you can add them to the blender in Step 1 for a smoother consistency.

directions

1. Combine the milk, ¼ cup of the coconut flakes, cocoa powder, erythritol, and vanilla extract in a blender. Mix until the ingredients are well combined.

2. Pour the mixture into a large mixing bowl. Add the chia seeds and whisk vigorously for 1 to 2 minutes.

3. Transfer the pudding to 4 individual serving bowls or cups and refrigerate for 1 to 2 hours.

4. Top with the almonds, remaining ¼ cup of coconut flakes, and chocolate chips, if desired, before serving.

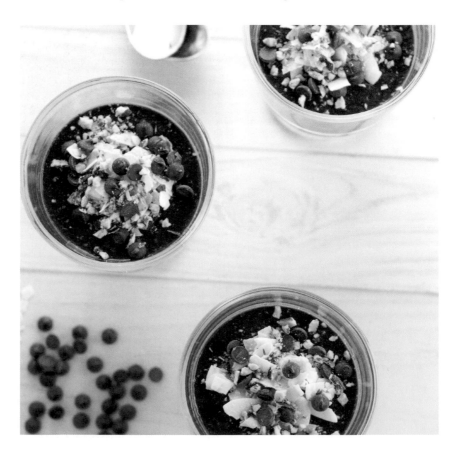

CALORIES: 172 · FAT: 12.3g · PROTEIN: 6.5g · TOTAL CARBS: 12.8g · DIETARY FIBER: 10.3g · NET CARBS: 2.5g · ERYTHRITOL: 12g

Fresh Whipped Cream

  makes 2½ cups (¼ cup per serving) · prep time: 5 minutes

Not only is this whipped cream perfect for dishes like Lemon Ricotta Pancakes (page 124) and Dark Chocolate Mousse (page 304), but I also love to put a big spoonful of it in my coffee. It just feels like an extra special treat.

ingredients

1 cup heavy cream

1 tablespoon plus 1 teaspoon powdered erythritol

1 teaspoon pure vanilla extract

directions

Place all of the ingredients in a large mixing bowl. Using a hand mixer, whip until stiff peaks form, 3 to 4 minutes. Store in an airtight container in the refrigerator for up to 1 week.

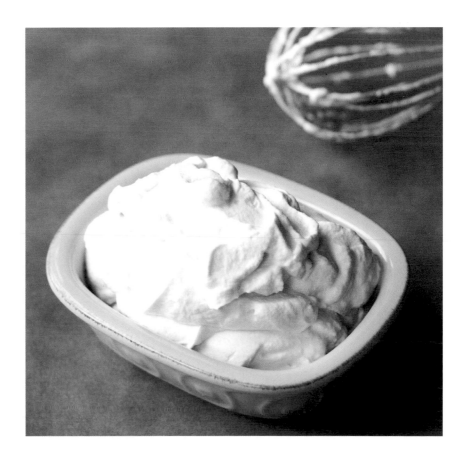

CALORIES: 83 · FAT: 9g · PROTEIN: .5g · TOTAL CARBS: 0.7g · DIETARY FIBER: 0 · NET CARBS: 0.7g · ERYTHRITOL: 1.3g

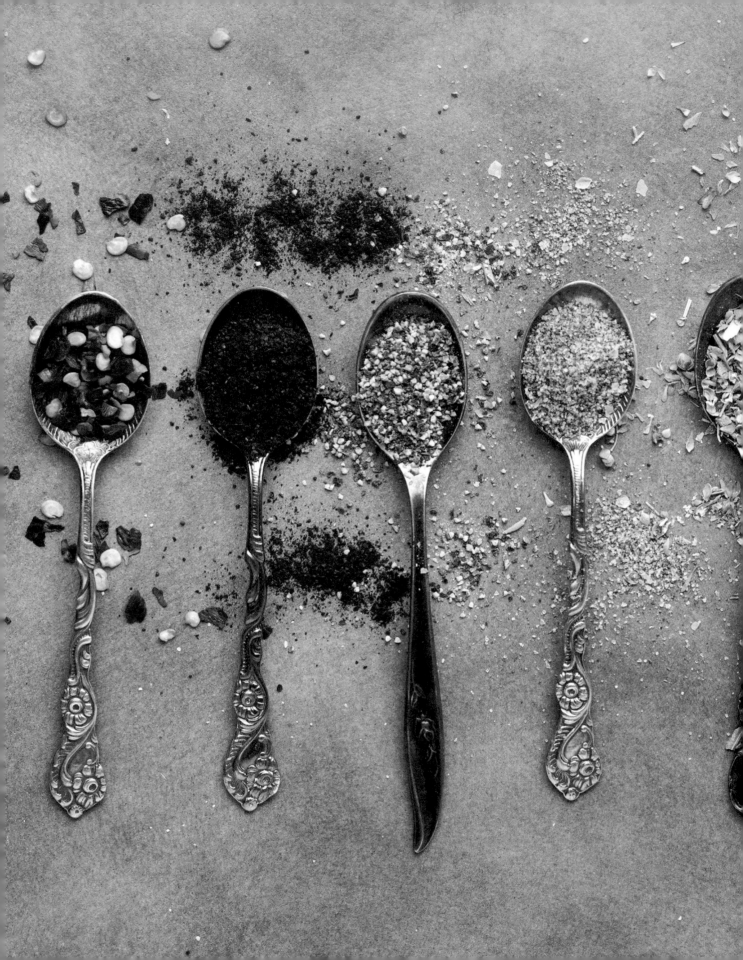

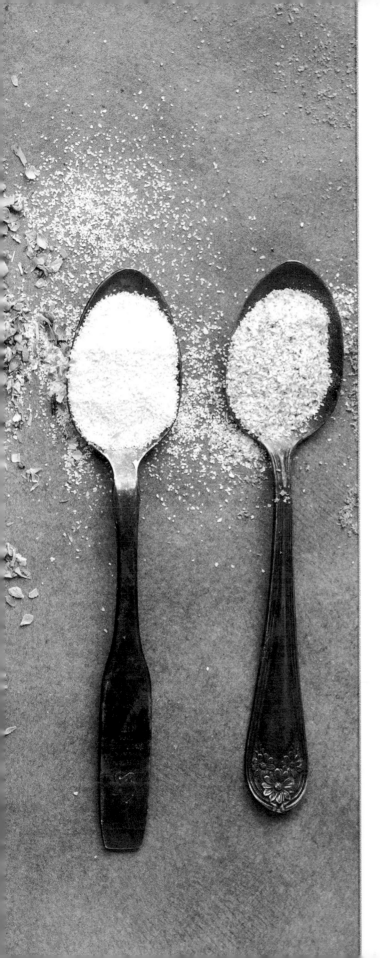

Dressings, Sauces, Seasonings & More

Thousand Island Dressing

NET CARBS
0.7g

 makes 2 cups (2 tablespoons per serving) · prep time: 10 minutes

Thousand Island dressing is a staple in many homes and restaurants. It often goes by other names, like fry sauce or secret sauce, and even gets used in place of Russian dressing in a lot of recipes. It is simple to make and contains only ingredients that you probably already have in your home. Once you make your own, you will never want to use store-bought versions again.

ingredients

1 cup mayonnaise, store-bought or homemade (page 336)

½ cup reduced-sugar ketchup

2 tablespoons Dijon mustard

2 tablespoons Worcestershire sauce

1 tablespoon chopped fresh chives

1 tablespoon chopped fresh flat-leaf parsley

½ teaspoon chopped fresh dill weed

¼ cup dill pickle relish

directions

Place all of the ingredients in a food processor and pulse just until the ingredients are well incorporated. Store in the refrigerator for up to 2 weeks.

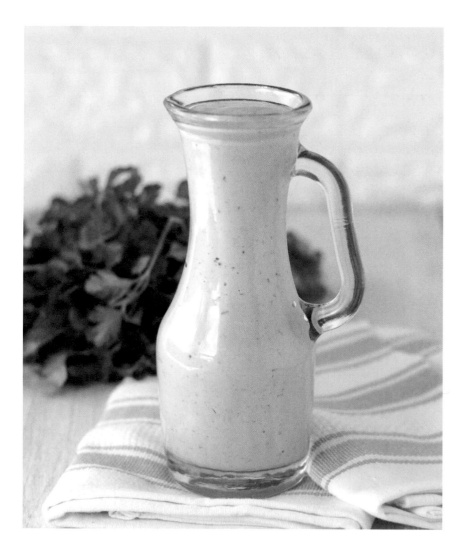

CALORIES: 95 · FAT: 10g · PROTEIN: 0 · TOTAL CARBS: 0.7g · DIETARY FIBER: 0 · NET CARBS: 0.7g

Garlic Parmesan Caesar Dressing

NUT-FREE makes 1½ cups (2 tablespoons per serving) · prep time: 10 minutes

Okay, so I realize that not everyone is a vampire slayer like my husband Jon and I are when it comes to garlic. Sometimes, I swear, it's like we are in some sort of weird garlic-eating contest, competing to see who can smell the worst. I joked with the crew at Victory Belt that this book could have just as easily been titled *The Big Book of Garlic: Kitchen Adventures of a Low-Carb Vampire Slayer*. Perhaps I found a title for my next book? At any rate, if you are not a fan of strong garlic flavors, I would recommend cutting the amount in half in this recipe.

ingredients

1 cup mayonnaise, store-bought or homemade (page 336)

½ cup grated Parmesan cheese

2 tablespoons fresh lemon juice

4 cloves garlic, minced

3 anchovy fillets, minced

1 tablespoon Worcestershire sauce

1 teaspoon Dijon mustard

½ teaspoon ground black pepper

directions

In a mixing bowl, combine all of the ingredients and whisk until well incorporated. Store in the refrigerator for up to 2 weeks.

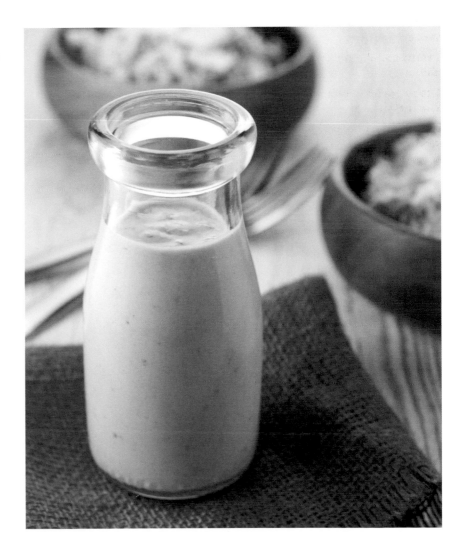

CALORIES: 172 · FAT: 17.5g · PROTEIN: 2.2g · TOTAL CARBS: 1.2g · DIETARY FIBER: 0 · NET CARBS: 1.2g

Ranch Dressing

NUT-FREE · makes 2½ cups (2 tablespoons per serving) · prep time: 10 minutes

I'm pretty sure I could sit down and easily write a love letter to ranch dressing. It is my go-to condiment for just about everything. For years I ate store-bought ranch. I'm sure you know the brand. I'll give you a hint: it's a lot like a hard-to-see, low area of land between hills or mountains. But have you ever actually read the label on a bottle of store-bought ranch? If not, do it! You will be appalled by the long list of ingredients, not to mention the number of ingredients you can't even pronounce or begin to identify. Homemade is the way to go. Once you make this ranch dressing, you won't go back.

ingredients

1 cup mayonnaise, store-bought or homemade (page 336)

1 cup full-fat sour cream

3 cloves garlic, minced

2 tablespoons chopped fresh flat-leaf parsley

2 tablespoons chopped fresh chives

1 tablespoon chopped fresh dill weed

1 tablespoon apple cider vinegar

1 teaspoon dried minced onions

½ teaspoon sea salt

¼ teaspoon ground black pepper

tip: I like to keep all of my homemade salad dressings and condiments in mason jars with screw-on pour spouts.

directions

Combine all of the ingredients in a large mixing bowl and whisk until the ingredients are well incorporated. Refrigerate, covered, for at least 1 hour before serving. This will allow time for the flavors to really come together. Store in the refrigerator for up to 2 weeks.

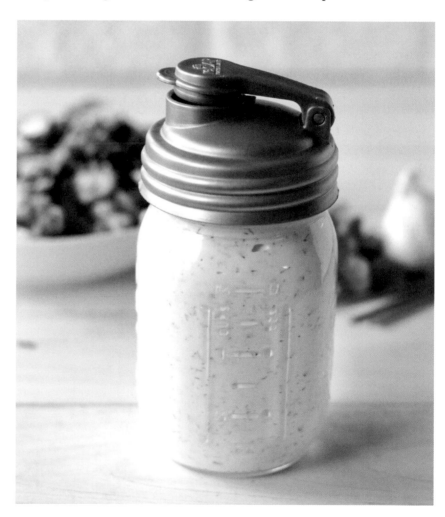

CALORIES: 110 · FAT: 12g · PROTEIN: 0.6g · TOTAL CARBS: 1g · DIETARY FIBER: 0.1g · NET CARBS: 0.9g

NET CARBS
0.8g

Avocado Green Goddess Dressing

NUT-FREE

makes 3 cups (2 tablespoons per serving) · prep time: 10 minutes

The addition of avocado gives this green goddess dressing a silkier, creamier texture. It is fresh, bright, and herbaceous—everything I love about a homemade dressing. When you make it, be sure to make the Green Goddess Chicken Dip on page 154, too.

ingredients

1 cup mayonnaise, store-bought or homemade (page 336)

1 cup full-fat sour cream

2 cloves garlic, minced

3 large green onions, chopped

3 large basil leaves, chopped

3 tablespoons chopped fresh chives

3 tablespoons chopped fresh flat-leaf parsley

1 medium avocado, peeled and pitted

3 anchovy fillets

2 tablespoons fresh lemon juice

1 tablespoon unseasoned rice wine vinegar

2 teaspoons dried tarragon

½ teaspoon mustard powder

Sea salt and ground black pepper (optional)

directions

Place all of the ingredients, except the salt and pepper, in a food processor and pulse until the ingredients are well incorporated and the dressing is smooth and creamy. Taste and add salt and pepper, if desired. Store in the refrigerator for up to 2 weeks.

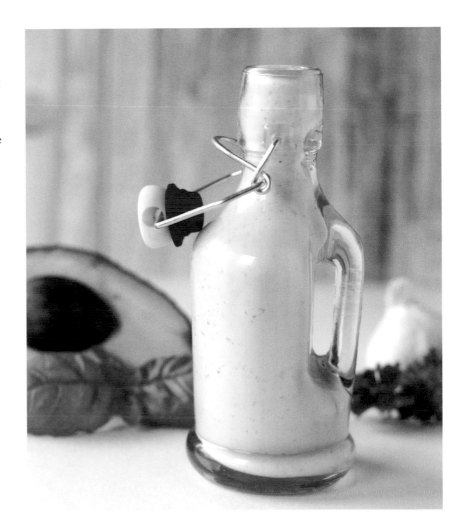

CALORIES: 94 · FAT: 10g · PROTEIN: 0.6g · TOTAL CARBS: 1.3g · DIETARY FIBER: 0.5g · NET CARBS: 0.8g

Asian Vinaigrette

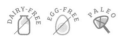 makes ¾ cup (1 tablespoon per serving) · prep time: 10 minutes

I love to serve this dressing with the Asian Chicken Salad on page 196, but it is also an amazing marinade for chicken or shrimp. I like to marinate shrimp in this dressing overnight, then skewer the shrimp and cook them on the grill.

ingredients

¼ cup coconut aminos or gluten-free soy sauce

¼ cup unseasoned rice wine vinegar

2 tablespoons avocado oil

1 tablespoon toasted sesame oil

1 clove garlic, minced

1 teaspoon grated fresh ginger

2 tablespoons unsalted almond butter

directions

Place all of the ingredients in a food processor and pulse to emulsify. Use immediately or store in the refrigerator for up to 2 weeks.

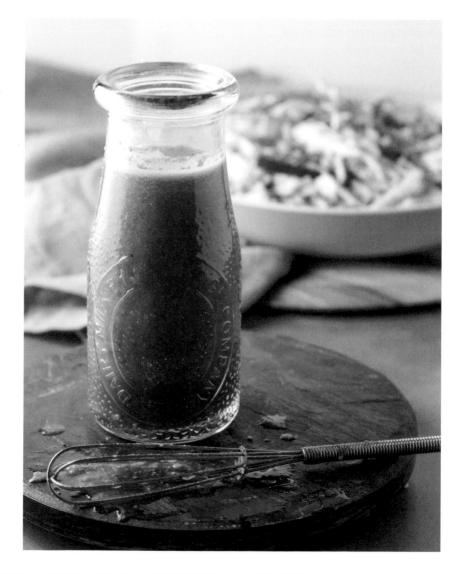

CALORIES: 55 · FAT: 5g · PROTEIN: 0.6g · TOTAL CARBS: 2.3g · DIETARY FIBER: 0.3g · NET CARBS: 2g

Dill Pickle Vinaigrette

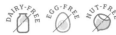 DAIRY-FREE · EGG-FREE · NUT-FREE · PALEO · makes 3 cups (2 tablespoons per serving) · prep time: 10 minutes

This is one of my favorite dressings for light summer salads. It is fresh and bright without being too heavy. It also makes a great marinade for chicken.

ingredients

1½ cups avocado oil

1 cup dill pickle juice

⅓ cup finely chopped dill pickles

2 tablespoons spicy brown or Dijon mustard

4 cloves garlic, minced

1 tablespoon dried minced onions

½ teaspoon sea salt, or more to taste

¼ teaspoon ground black pepper

directions

In a mixing bowl, combine all of the ingredients and whisk until well incorporated. Alternatively, you can combine the ingredients in a large mason jar with a lid and shake to combine (and then store it in the same jar). Store in the refrigerator for up to 3 weeks. Shake well before using.

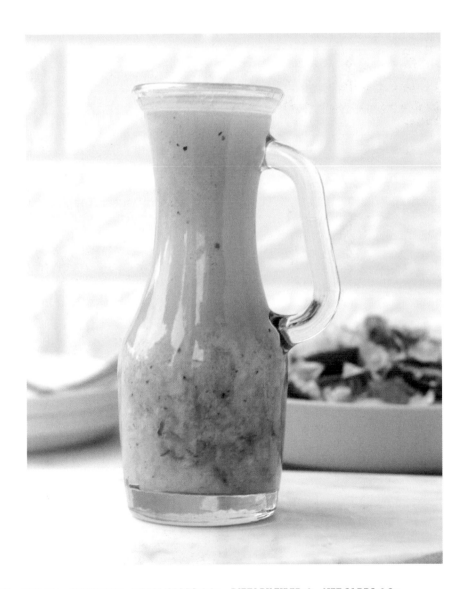

CALORIES: 129 · FAT: 14g · PROTEIN: 0 · TOTAL CARBS: 0.3g · DIETARY FIBER: 0 · NET CARBS: 0.3g

2-Minute Mayo

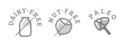

makes 1½ cups (2 tablespoons per serving) · prep time: 2 minutes

I have an almost embarrassing love affair with mayonnaise. I have loved it ever since I was a kid. If left to my own devices, I would eat a heaping mound of mayonnaise smeared on a piece of white bread. While my dietary choices have drastically changed since childhood, my love of mayo remains unwavering. One of my favorite things about mayonnaise is that you can use it to add creaminess to dishes without adding dairy.

ingredients

2 teaspoons fresh lemon juice

1 large egg

½ teaspoon mustard powder

½ teaspoon sea salt

Pinch of black pepper

1 cup avocado oil

Special equipment:

Immersion blender (see tip)

tip: For me, the success of getting this mayonnaise to set up as it should is highly dependent upon using an immersion blender. I have not been able to achieve the same thick consistency when using a blender or food processor.

directions

1. Starting with the lemon juice and ending with the oil, put the ingredients, one at a time and in the order listed, in a wide-mouth pint-sized mason jar. Let the ingredients rest for 20 seconds or so.

2. Insert an immersion blender into the jar, placing it all the way at the bottom. Turn it on high speed and leave it at the bottom of the jar for about 20 seconds. The mayonnaise will immediately begin to set up and fill the jar.

3. When the mayonnaise is almost all the way set, slowly lift the immersion blender towards the top of the jar without taking the blades out of the mayonnaise. Then slowly push it back towards the bottom of the jar. Repeat this up-and-down motion a couple of times until the ingredients are well incorporated. Store in the refrigerator for up to 2 weeks.

CALORIES: 172 · FAT: 19g · PROTEIN: 0.5g · TOTAL CARBS: 0 · DIETARY FIBER: 0 · NET CARBS: 0

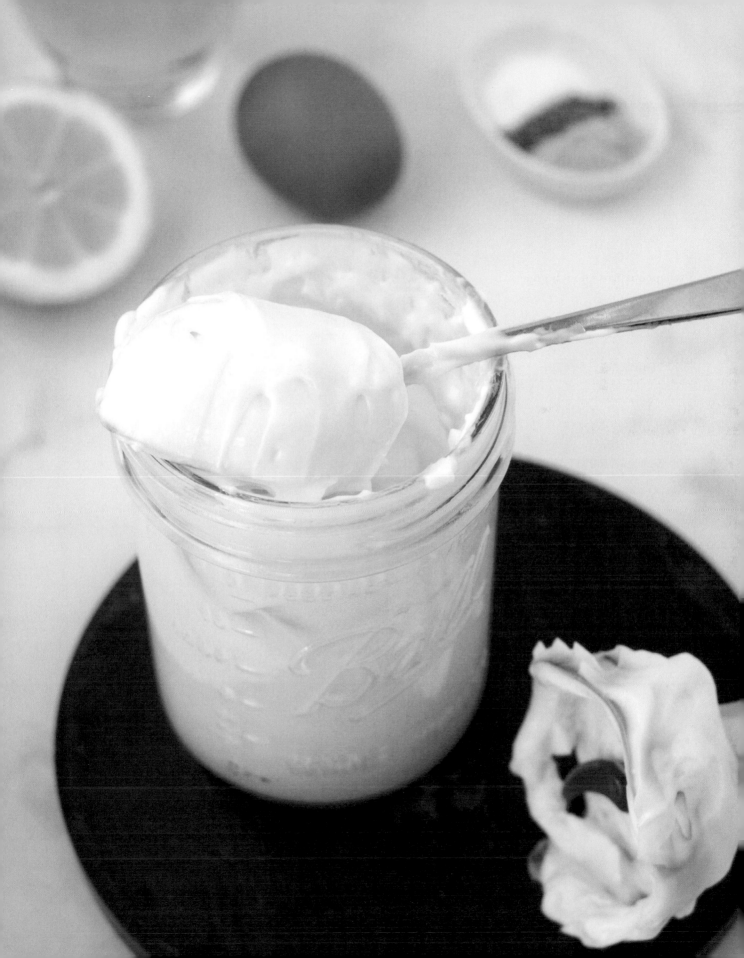

Cajun Mayo

makes 1 cup plus 2 tablespoons (2 tablespoons per serving)
prep time: 5 minutes

Not only is this mayo amazing as a spread, but it is also a great dip for pork rinds or fresh veggies. I also like to spread it over chicken or fish and then bake. It gives the chicken or fish a wonderfully creamy texture without any added dairy and makes for a super simple yet flavorful meal.

ingredients

1 cup mayonnaise, store-bought or homemade (page 336)

3 tablespoons Cajun Seasoning (page 351)

directions

Combine the mayonnaise and Cajun seasoning and mix until the ingredients are well incorporated. Store in the refrigerator for up to 2 weeks.

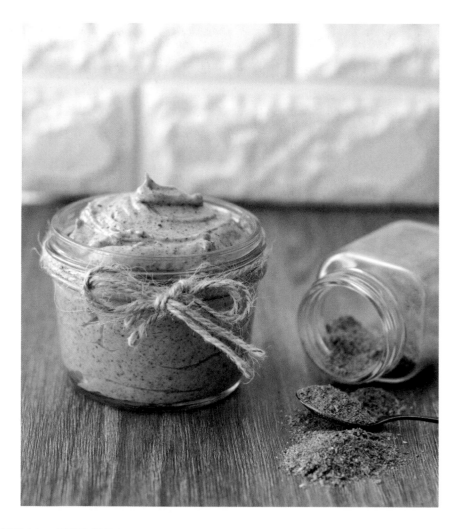

CALORIES: 167 · FAT: 18g · PROTEIN: 0.2g · TOTAL CARBS: 0.8g · DIETARY FIBER: 0.2g · NET CARBS: 0.6g

Garlic Dill Tartar Sauce

NET CARBS
0.6g

makes 2½ cups (2 tablespoons per serving) · prep time: 10 minutes

I think the tartar sauce world is divided into two distinct camps: those who like a little sweetness and those who prefer to keep it savory. I fall into the latter camp. If there were a third camp, it would be the "I'll put that on anything and everything" camp. And I definitely fall into that category as well. Not only is this sauce great on any type of seafood, but you also can use it as a salad dressing or as a base for deviled eggs. The first time I made this sauce, I may or may not have used almost the entire jar just for deviled eggs. Okay, I did! I definitely did.

ingredients

2 cups mayonnaise, store-bought or homemade (page 336)

3 cloves garlic, minced

Juice of ½ lemon

1 tablespoon spicy brown mustard

¼ cup fresh flat-leaf parsley leaves

1 tablespoon chopped fresh dill weed

1 medium dill pickle, chopped

½ teaspoon sea salt

¼ teaspoon ground black pepper

directions

Combine all of the ingredients in a food processor and pulse just until the ingredients are well incorporated. Store in the refrigerator for up to 2 weeks.

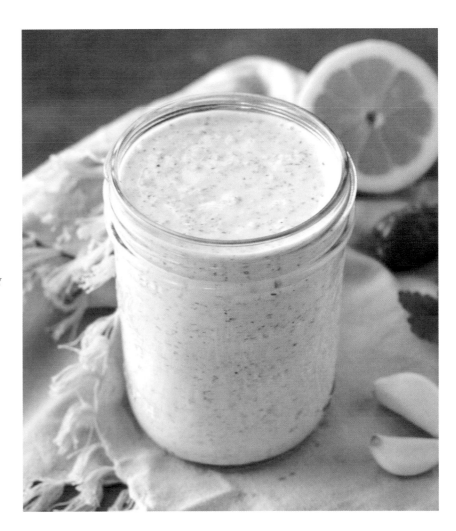

tip: If you like a little sweetness to your tartar sauce, try replacing half of the dill pickle with a little sweet relish. It will up the carbs just a bit, but it will give you the flavor you are after.

CALORIES: 164 · FAT: 18g · PROTEIN: 0.2g · TOTAL CARBS: 0.7g · DIETARY FIBER: 0.1g · NET CARBS: 0.6g

Walnut Avocado Pesto

makes 4½ cups (¼ cup per serving) · prep time: 10 minutes

Pesto is so versatile and works in a multitude of dishes. Besides using it in Creamy Avocado Pesto Deviled Eggs (page 162) and Creamy Pesto Chicken Zucchini Pasta (page 250), I like to eat it with eggs for breakfast, along with some goat cheese. It is also fantastic on salmon or in meatballs. The sky is the limit with this herbaceous beauty.

ingredients

1 medium avocado, halved, pitted, and cubed

2 cloves garlic

1 cup fresh basil leaves

1 cup fresh flat-leaf parsley leaves

⅓ cup grated Parmesan cheese

½ cup raw walnuts

Juice of ½ lemon

¼ cup chopped green onions

¼ cup water, or more if desired (see tip)

½ teaspoon sea salt

¼ teaspoon ground black pepper

Pinch of red pepper flakes

¼ cup avocado oil or olive oil

tip: If the pesto is thicker than you like, add water little by little until it reaches your desired consistency. Be careful not to water it down too much or you will diminish its amazing flavor.

directions

1. Put all of the ingredients, except the oil, in a food processor. Pulse until everything is finely chopped and begins to form a paste.

2. With the food processor running, slowly pour in the oil. Continue to pulse until smooth. Store in the refrigerator for up to 2 weeks.

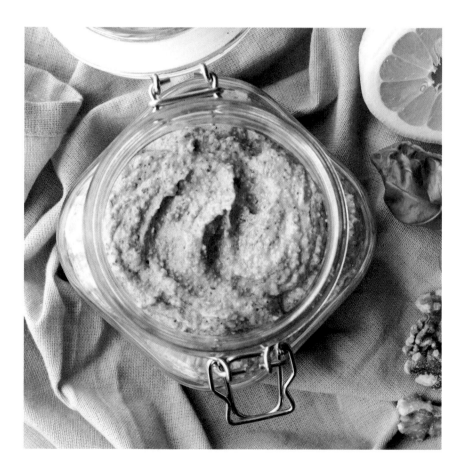

CALORIES: 75 · FAT: 7.2g · PROTEIN: 1.6g · TOTAL CARBS: 1.8g · DIETARY FIBER: 1g · NET CARBS: 0.8g

Bacon Jam

 makes 2 cups (¼ cup per serving) · prep time: 15 minutes · cook time: 35 minutes

The first time I made this jam, I went through the whole batch in just a couple of days because I put it on everything I ate. From my morning eggs to my lunchtime salad to my steak for dinner, it was all covered in bacon jam. I also really like this jam on Chicken Cordon Bleu Pizza (page 256) and in Baked Egg Jars (page 108).

ingredients

10 slices bacon, diced

1 tablespoon butter or ghee

1 large onion, thinly sliced (about 1½ cups)

Leaves from 2 sprigs fresh thyme

½ teaspoon ground black pepper

Pinch of cayenne pepper

1 tablespoon cooking sherry

1 tablespoon brown sugar erythritol (optional)

tip: This jam freezes well for later use. Allow it to thaw fully before reheating it on the stovetop.

directions

1. Heat a large skillet over medium heat. Put the bacon in the skillet and cook until it is crisp. Using a slotted spoon, remove the bacon from the pan and set aside; retain half of the drippings in the pan.

2. Reduce the heat to medium-low. To the bacon drippings, add the butter, onion, thyme, black pepper, and cayenne. Cook until the onions are caramelized, 25 to 30 minutes.

3. Mix in the reserved bacon, sherry, and brown sugar erythritol, if using, and cook for an additional 5 to 10 minutes, until the sherry has evaporated and the erythritol has had time to caramelize. Store the jam in the refrigerator for up to 1 week.

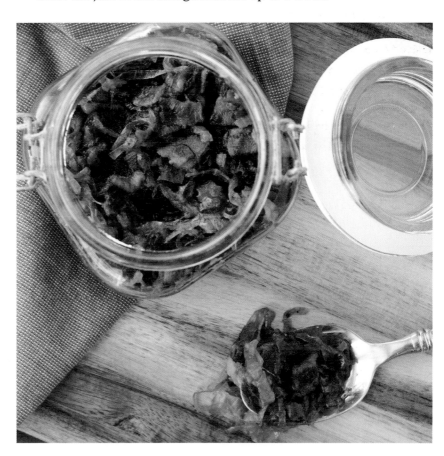

CALORIES: 72 · FAT: 5.3g · PROTEIN: 4g · TOTAL CARBS: 1.8g · DIETARY FIBER: 0.4g · NET CARBS: 1.4g

Garlic Parmesan Cream Sauce

  makes 2 cups (¼ cup per serving) · prep time: 5 minutes · cook time: 10 minutes

Given how fast this sauce comes together, it is amazing how much flavor it has. It is terrific on chicken or fish and even over zucchini noodles or spaghetti squash. When reheating it, I recommend using the stovetop and adding a little heavy cream to help bring it back to life.

ingredients

1 cup heavy cream

1 cup grated Parmesan cheese

6 cloves garlic, minced

Sea salt and cracked black pepper (optional)

directions

1. In a small saucepan over medium-high heat, whisk together the cream, Parmesan cheese, and garlic until well combined.

2. Bring the sauce to a boil, then reduce the heat to low and simmer, stirring occasionally, until thickened, about 5 minutes. Taste and add salt and pepper, if needed. Store in the refrigerator for up to 1 week.

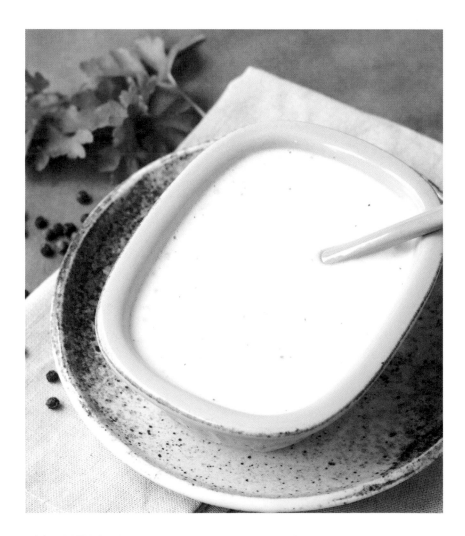

CALORIES: 160 · FAT: 15g · PROTEIN: 5.5g · TOTAL CARBS: 2g · DIETARY FIBER: 0 · NET CARBS: 2g

Pizza Sauce

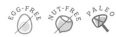

makes 1¼ cups (2 tablespoons per serving)
prep time: 5 minutes · cook time: 15 minutes

It's amazing to me how many store-bought versions of things we use as a society when they are so easy to make at home. Making your own pizza sauce will save you money, and not only does it taste better, but it is better for you, too. Next time you are at the grocery store, look at the ingredient list on the back of a jar of pizza sauce. It might just be enough to make you never want to buy it again.

ingredients

1 (8-ounce) can tomato sauce

1 (6-ounce) can tomato paste

2 tablespoons grated Parmesan cheese

1 clove garlic, minced

1 teaspoon dried basil

1 teaspoon dried minced onions

¼ teaspoon smoked paprika

⅛ teaspoon red pepper flakes

1 bay leaf

tip: To make this sauce dairy-free and Paleo compliant, simply omit the Parmesan cheese.

directions

In a medium saucepan over low heat, combine all of the ingredients. Simmer, stirring frequently, for 15 minutes to allow the flavors to come together. Remove the bay leaf before using. Store in the refrigerator for up to 2 weeks.

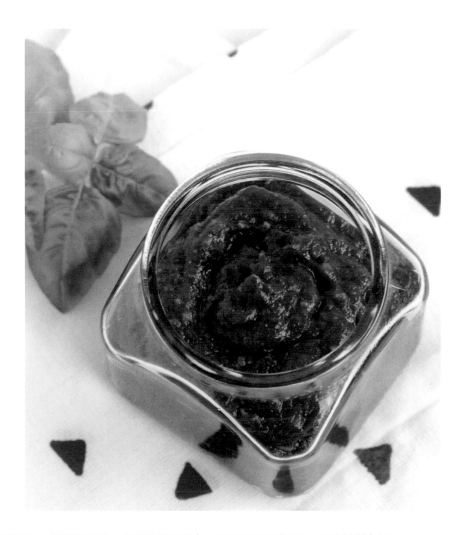

CALORIES: 28 · FAT: 0.4g · PROTEIN: 1.4g · TOTAL CARBS: 5g · DIETARY FIBER: 1.4g · NET CARBS: 3.6g

Garlic and Herb Marinara Sauce

   makes 4½ cups (¼ cup per serving)
prep time: 15 minutes · cook time: 40 minutes

Rich, vibrant flavors and textures come together to make this a perfectly versatile sauce that is sure to become a family favorite. A couple of preparation notes: If you don't want to be a total vampire slayer, reduce the garlic. Or, better yet, just force everyone around you to eat it, too. Families who smell like garlic together stay together! If using dried herbs in place of fresh, a good general rule is 1 teaspoon of dried herbs for every tablespoon of fresh herbs.

ingredients

2 tablespoons olive oil

6 cloves garlic, minced

1 (28-ounce) can fire-roasted whole San Marzano tomatoes

1 (8-ounce) can tomato sauce

1 (6-ounce) can tomato paste

1 tablespoon plus 1 teaspoon chopped fresh basil, or more to taste

1 tablespoon plus 1 teaspoon chopped fresh flat-leaf parsley, or more to taste

1 tablespoon dried minced onions

1 teaspoon dried oregano leaves

1 teaspoon sea salt

½ teaspoon ground black pepper

Pinch of red pepper flakes

1 tablespoon balsamic vinegar

directions

1. Heat the olive oil in a large saucepan over medium heat. Add the garlic and sauté until it is soft and fragrant. Watch closely so that the garlic does not get scorched, which will make it bitter.

2. Combine the fire-roasted tomatoes, tomato sauce, and tomato paste in a blender or food processor and puree until smooth. Pour the mixture into the saucepan with the sautéed garlic.

3. To the saucepan, add the basil, parsley, dried minced onions, oregano, salt, pepper, red pepper flakes, and vinegar. Stir to combine.

4. Bring to a low boil over medium heat, then reduce the heat to low and simmer, stirring occasionally, for 30 minutes to allow the flavors time to come together. Taste and add more salt, if desired. Store in the refrigerator for up to 2 weeks.

tips: You can also use an immersion blender or a potato masher to puree the tomatoes directly in the saucepan.

This sauce freezes well for later use. I recommend allowing it to thaw fully before reheating it on the stovetop.

CALORIES: 38 · FAT: 1.5g · PROTEIN: 1g · TOTAL CARBS: 5.2g · DIETARY FIBER: 1.2g · NET CARBS: 4g

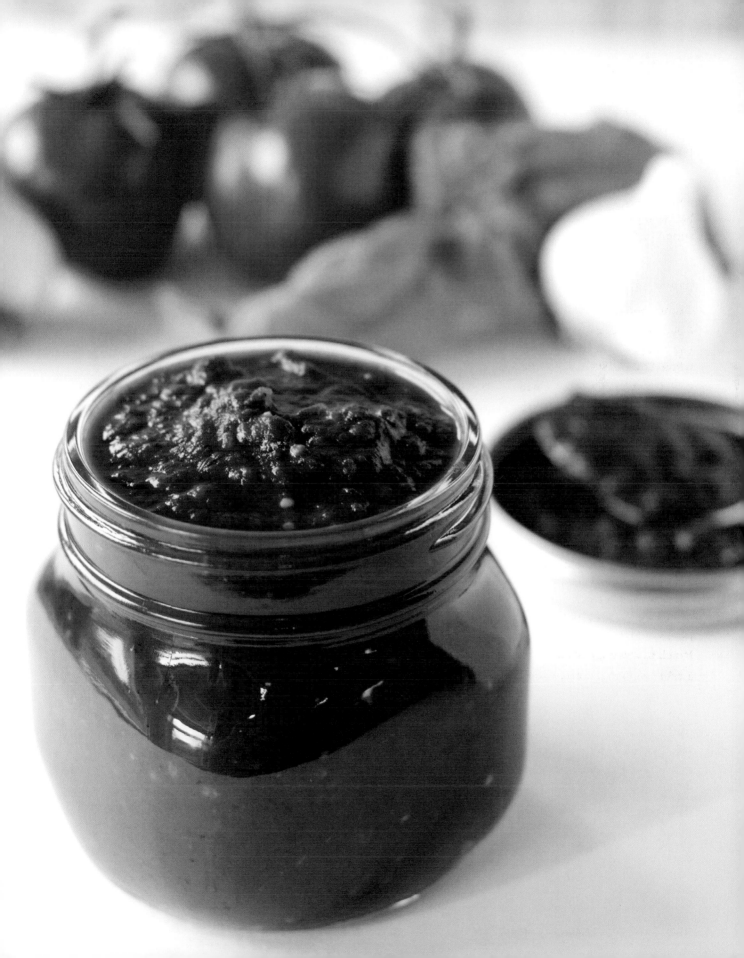

Enchilada Sauce

   DAIRY-FREE · EGG-FREE · NUT-FREE · PALEO

makes 2¼ cups (2 tablespoons per serving)
prep time: 5 minutes · cook time: 30 minutes

This sauce is truly at its best when made ahead of time. I like to make it a full day or two before I plan to use it to let the flavors come together in rich, delicious harmony.

ingredients

3 tablespoons olive oil

3 cloves garlic, minced

3 tablespoons coconut flour

2 tablespoons chili powder

1 teaspoon dried minced onions

1 teaspoon dried oregano leaves

1 teaspoon ground cumin

1 teaspoon onion powder

½ teaspoon dried basil

½ teaspoon ground black pepper

1 teaspoon sea salt

1 (8-ounce) can tomato sauce

2 tablespoons tomato paste

1 teaspoon apple cider vinegar

2 cups chicken stock

tip: I like to make a batch of this sauce and freeze it in ice-cube trays for the perfect preportioned sauce bomb. Add a cube or two to chicken, beef, or pork for a quick-and-easy weeknight meal.

directions

1. Heat the olive oil in a large saucepan over medium heat. Add the garlic and sauté until it is soft and fragrant. Stir in the coconut flour until completely combined.

2. Mix in the spices, salt, tomato sauce, tomato paste, vinegar, and stock.

3. Bring to a boil over medium heat, then reduce the heat to low and simmer for 30 minutes, stirring occasionally, to allow the flavors time to come together. Store in an airtight container in the refrigerator for up to 2 weeks.

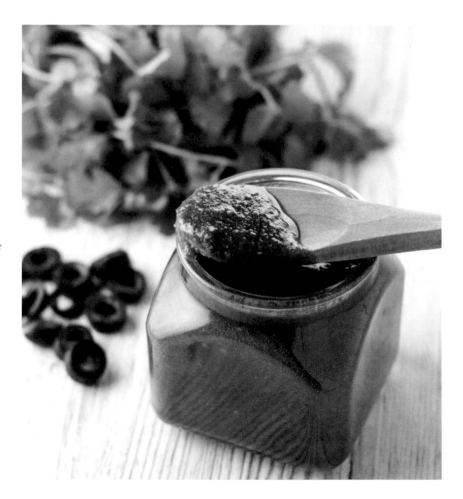

CALORIES: 39 · FAT: 2.6g · PROTEIN: 1.2g · TOTAL CARBS: 2.5g · DIETARY FIBER: 1g · NET CARBS: 1.5g

Not-So-Secret Burger Sauce

makes ¾ cup (1 tablespoon per serving) · prep time: 10 minutes

Once you taste this sauce, you won't want to eat anything else on your burgers ever again. The hint of spiciness in this recipe perfectly complements the sweetness of the Bacon Jam (page 341) on the Best-Ever Fork and Knife Pub Burger on page 260. This just might become your go-to condiment for everything.

ingredients

½ cup mayonnaise, store-bought or homemade (page 336)

2 tablespoons reduced-sugar ketchup

2 teaspoons Sriracha sauce

1 teaspoon Dijon mustard

1 teaspoon Worcestershire sauce

1 clove garlic, minced

¼ teaspoon ground black pepper

tip: Try mixing a little of this sauce into your scrambled eggs. Delish!

directions

In a mixing bowl, whisk all of the ingredients together until well combined. Store in the refrigerator for up to 2 weeks.

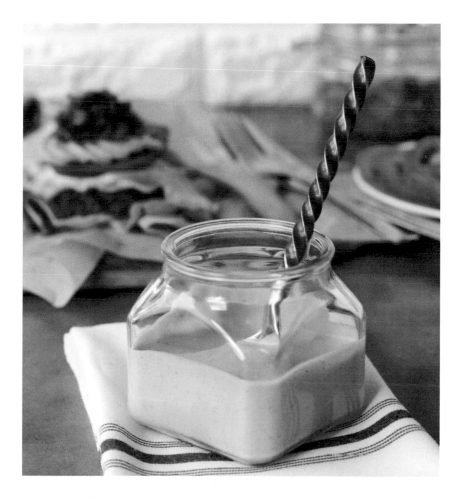

CALORIES: 63 · FAT: 7g · PROTEIN: 0 · TOTAL CARBS: 0.7g · DIETARY FIBER: 0 · NET CARBS: 0.7g

Cranberry Ginger Quick Jam

NET CARBS
0.9g

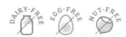 DAIRY-FREE · EGG-FREE · NUT-FREE

makes 2 cups (1 tablespoon per serving)
prep time: 10 minutes · **cook time:** 20 minutes

Not only is this quick jam delicious on dishes like Easy Peasy Maple Blender Pancakes (page 134), but it is amazing for savory dishes, too. It is the perfect addition to your holiday table as a cranberry sauce. Between this and the recipes for Cranberry Pecan Cauliflower Rice Stuffing (page 286), Creamy Herbed Slow Cooker Cauliflower Mash (page 284), and Green Beans with Shallots and Pancetta (page 276), your holiday sides are set. All you need is the turkey, and you are in low-carb holiday business.

ingredients

1 (12-ounce) bag fresh cranberries

¾ cup granular erythritol, or more to taste

2 tablespoons water

1 tablespoon grated lemon zest

1 tablespoon fresh lemon juice

1 tablespoon balsamic vinegar

1 teaspoon grated fresh ginger

directions

1. Put all of the ingredients in a saucepan and cook over medium heat until the cranberries begin to pop, about 10 minutes. Use a fork to smash the berries as they pop.

2. Reduce the heat to low and simmer until thickened, about 10 minutes. Store in a jar in the refrigerator for up to 2 weeks.

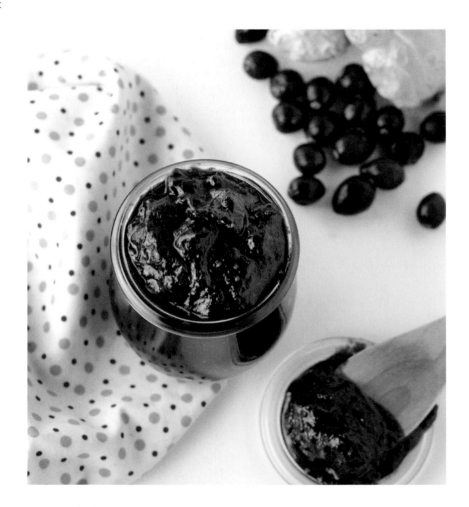

CALORIES: 6 · FAT: 0 · PROTEIN: 0 · TOTAL CARBS: 1.3g · DIETARY FIBER: 0.4g · NET CARBS: 0.9g · ERYTHRITOL: 4g

Seasoning Salt

    makes 6 tablespoons (½ teaspoon per serving) · prep time: 5 minutes

I always have a batch of this seasoning salt prepared. I keep it in a pinch bowl next to the stove, and when I am whipping up a random meal without a recipe, I use it for everything savory that I make.

ingredients

2 tablespoons garlic powder

2 tablespoons onion powder

1 tablespoon sea salt

2 teaspoons ground black pepper

1 teaspoon Italian seasoning

directions

Mix all of the ingredients together and store in an airtight container or spice jar. Shake well before using.

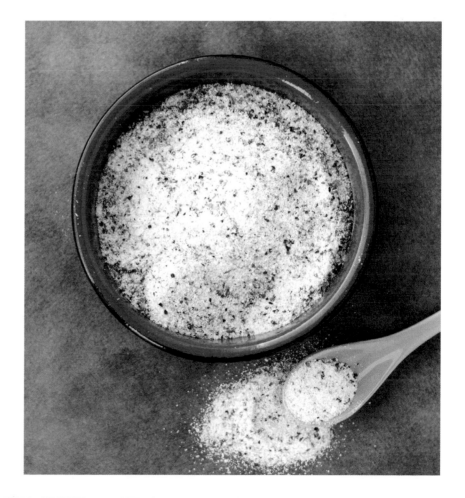

CALORIES: 3 · FAT: 0 · PROTEIN: 0.1g · TOTAL CARBS: 0.7g · DIETARY FIBER: 0.1g · NET CARBS: 0.6g

Mexican Seasoning Blend

NET CARBS
0.6g

   makes ⅓ cup (1 teaspoon per serving) · prep time: 5 minutes

This is a great multipurpose seasoning blend for anything Mexican inspired. From Steak Fajita Bowls (page 210) to Fiesta Cauliflower Rice (page 282), this blend has you covered! Jazz up your Taco Tuesday, or even throw it in Mexican Chicken Soup (page 180). But don't eat too much, or after your fiesta, you might need a siesta.

ingredients

2 tablespoons chili powder

1 tablespoon ground cumin

2 teaspoons celery salt

1 teaspoon garlic powder

1 teaspoon onion powder

1 teaspoon smoked paprika

½ teaspoon dried oregano leaves

½ teaspoon ground black pepper

¼ teaspoon red pepper flakes

directions

Mix all of the ingredients together and store in an airtight container or spice jar. Shake well before using.

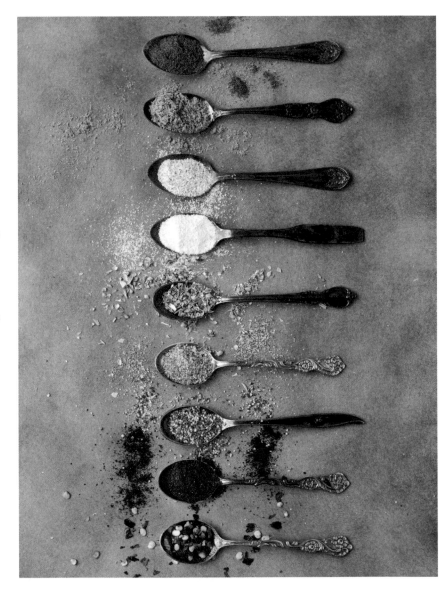

tip: To make taco meat, use ¼ cup of the seasoning blend for each pound of meat. Simply brown 1 pound of ground beef, ground turkey, or the meat of your choice and drain the excess grease. Add ⅔ cup water and ¼ cup seasoning blend to the pan, then reduce the heat to low and simmer for 3 to 4 minutes, until thickened.

CALORIES: 7 · FAT: 0.3g · PROTEIN: 0.3g · TOTAL CARBS: 1g · DIETARY FIBER: 0.4g · NET CARBS: 0.6g

Cajun Seasoning

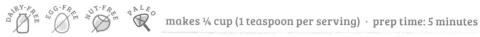

DAIRY-FREE · EGG-FREE · NUT-FREE · PALEO · makes ¼ cup (1 teaspoon per serving) · prep time: 5 minutes

This seasoning is great for so much more than just Cajun Mayo (page 338) and Sausage, Shrimp, and Chicken Jambalaya (page 224). I love to season chicken breasts with it and then grill them for a fresh and light blackened chicken salad. I also like to add it to my breakfast scrambles to spice things up a bit.

ingredients

2 teaspoons smoked paprika

2 teaspoons garlic powder

1½ teaspoons onion powder

1 teaspoon celery salt

1 teaspoon ground black pepper

1 teaspoon cayenne pepper

1 teaspoon dried oregano leaves

½ teaspoon dried rubbed sage

½ teaspoon red pepper flakes

Pinch of sea salt

tip: To tone down the heat just a bit, reduce the cayenne and red pepper flakes by half, or omit them altogether.

directions

Mix all of the ingredients together and store in an airtight container or spice jar. Shake well before using.

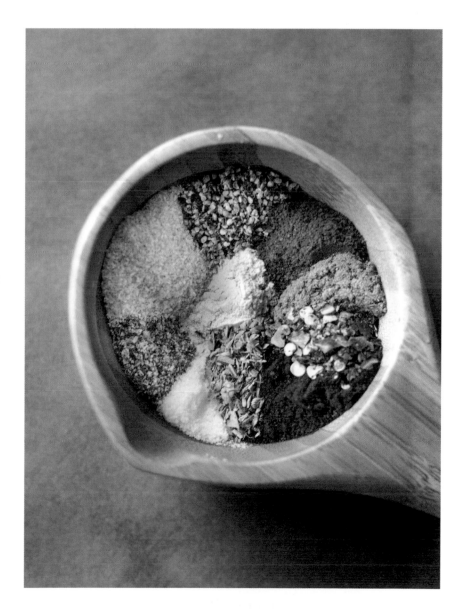

CALORIES: 7 · FAT: 0 · PROTEIN: 0.2g · TOTAL CARBS: 0.8g · DIETARY FIBER: 0.2g · NET CARBS: 0.6g

Everything Bagel Seasoning

   makes 1 cup (2 tablespoons per serving) · prep time: 5 minutes

Am I going too far if I say that this Everything Bagel Seasoning is everything? I have been putting it on just about everything, so I'd say it's a fair assessment. One of my favorite ways to use this seasoning is on my morning eggs. Try it! You won't be disappointed.

ingredients

¼ cup toasted sesame seeds

3 tablespoons plus 1 teaspoon poppy seeds

3 tablespoons plus 1 teaspoon dried minced onions

3 tablespoons plus 1 teaspoon dried garlic flakes

2 tablespoons coarse sea salt

directions

Mix all of the ingredients together and store in an airtight container or spice jar. Shake well before using.

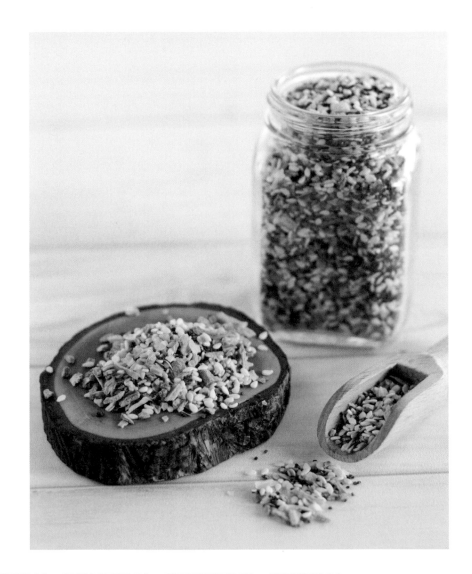

CALORIES: 61 · FAT: 1.5g · PROTEIN: 0.8g · TOTAL CARBS: 3.5g · DIETARY FIBER: 0.9g · NET CARBS: 2.6g

Barbecue Dry Rub

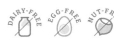 makes about ⅓ cup · prep time: 5 minutes

This rub is amazing on the Barbecue Dry Rub Ribs on page 244. For a spicier rub, add a little cayenne pepper.

ingredients

1 tablespoon plus 1 teaspoon smoked paprika

1 tablespoon garlic powder

1 tablespoon onion powder

1 tablespoon brown sugar erythritol

2 teaspoons chili powder

2 teaspoons sea salt

tip: Combine this rub with some reduced-sugar ketchup to make barbecue sauce.

directions

Mix all of the ingredients together and store in an airtight container or spice jar. Shake well before using.

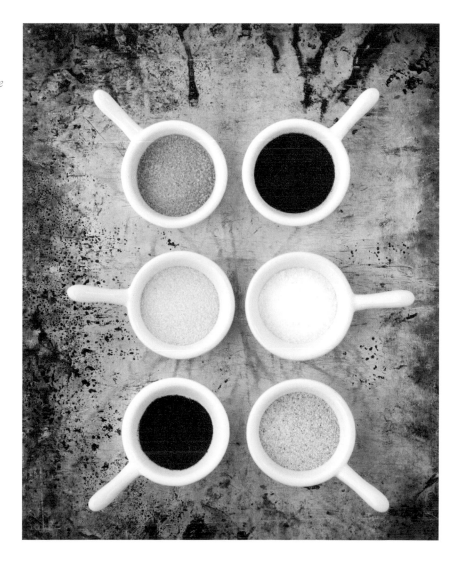

Per Batch

CALORIES: 163 · FAT: 1g · PROTEIN: 3g · TOTAL CARBS: 15g · DIETARY FIBER: 4g · NET CARBS: 11g · ERYTHRITOL: 9g

Savory Breading Mix

EGG-FREE

makes just over 1 cup (2 tablespoons per serving) · prep time: 5 minutes

ingredients

½ cup grated Parmesan cheese

½ cup blanched almond flour

2 teaspoons Italian seasoning

1 teaspoon garlic powder

1 teaspoon onion powder

½ teaspoon sea salt

directions

Mix all of the ingredients together for same-day use.

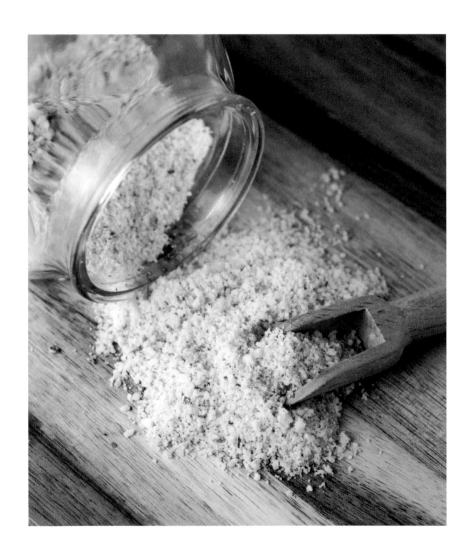

Per Serving (2 Tablespoons)
CALORIES: 69 · FAT: 5.3g · PROTEIN: 4g · TOTAL CARBS: 2.3g · DIETARY FIBER: 0.9g · NET CARBS: 1.4g

Per Batch
CALORIES: 554 · FAT: 42g · PROTEIN: 32g · TOTAL CARBS: 18g · DIETARY FIBER: 7g · NET CARBS: 11g

Nut-Free Keto Breading Mix

  makes 1½ cups (2 tablespoons per serving) · prep time: 5 minutes

This breading is incredibly versatile. It is amazing for breading chicken tenders, the Dill Pickle Juice Brined Fish and Chips on page 246, or anything else you would want to bread and deep-fry or bake. It is also terrific as a binding agent for things like meatloaf or any other savory recipe that calls for breadcrumbs.

ingredients

1 cup crushed pork rinds

½ cup grated Parmesan cheese

1 teaspoon Italian seasoning

½ teaspoon garlic powder

½ teaspoon onion powder

¼ teaspoon sea salt, or more to taste

tip: For a dairy-free version, simply swap out the Parmesan cheese for blanched almond flour.

directions

Mix all of the ingredients together for same-day use.

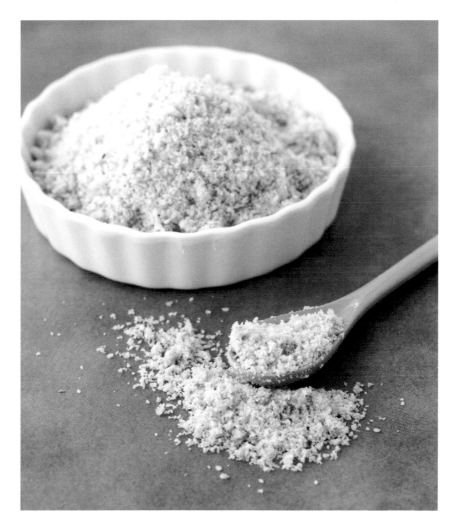

Per Serving (2 Tablespoons)
CALORIES: 52 · FAT: 3.3g · PROTEIN: 5g · TOTAL CARBS: 0.3g · DIETARY FIBER: 0 · NET CARBS: 0.3g

Per Batch
CALORIES: 625 · FAT: 39g · PROTEIN: 60g · TOTAL CARBS: 4g · DIETARY FIBER: 0 · NET CARBS: 4g

Pizza Crust

NET CARBS
16g

makes one 12-inch crust · prep time: 10 minutes · cook time: 12 minutes

This pizza crust recipe is so versatile. You can use the dough to make a calzone, the Everything Bagel Dogs on page 212, or even the Beef and Chorizo Empanadas on my website, peaceloveandlowcarb.com. If you omit the seasonings and add a little sweetener and cinnamon, you can even make sweet dishes like cinnamon rolls and Danish pastries. It truly is a magical recipe in the low-carb world.

ingredients

1½ cups shredded low-moisture, part-skim mozzarella cheese

1½ ounces full-fat cream cheese (3 tablespoons)

1 large egg

¾ cup blanched almond flour

½ teaspoon garlic powder

½ teaspoon onion powder

½ teaspoon Italian seasoning

¼ teaspoon sea salt

¼ teaspoon ground black pepper

tip: If you are not using the pizza crust right away, store it in the refrigerator for up to 1 week. Alternatively, you can freeze it for later use.

directions

1. Preheat the oven to 425°F. Line a 12-inch pizza pan with parchment paper.

2. In a large microwave-safe mixing bowl, combine the mozzarella and cream cheese. Microwave for 1 minute, then stir to combine. Return to the microwave and heat for 1 additional minute.

3. Add the egg, almond flour, garlic powder, onion powder, Italian seasoning, salt, and pepper to the mixing bowl. Using your hands, mix until the ingredients are well incorporated. If you are having a hard time mixing the ingredients together, put the bowl back in the microwave for another 20 to 30 seconds to soften. If the dough starts sticking to your hands, wet your hands slightly and continue working the dough.

4. Place the dough on the prepared pizza pan and, using your hands, spread it into a thin, even layer, covering the pan. If the dough gets too stringy and unworkable, simply put it back in the microwave for 1 minute to soften.

5. Bake on the middle rack of the oven for 10 to 12 minutes, until golden brown. Watch the crust to make sure that it doesn't bubble up. Use a toothpick to pop any bubbles, if necessary.

Per Crust

CALORIES: 1219 · FAT: 95g · PROTEIN: 75g · TOTAL CARBS: 25g · DIETARY FIBER: 9g · NET CARBS: 16g

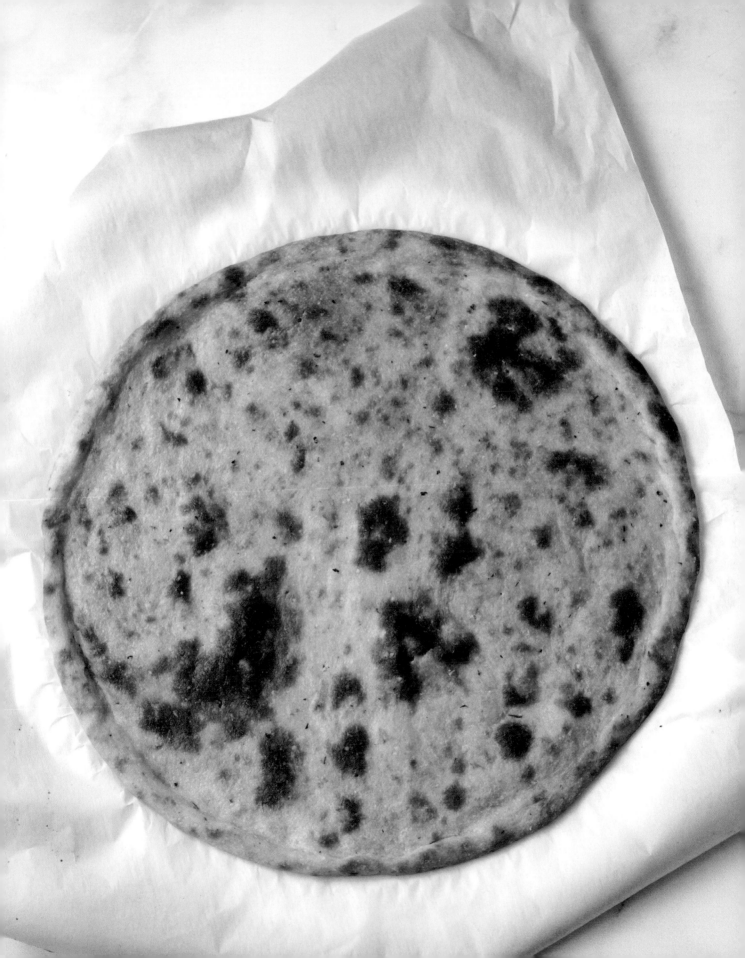

Nut-Free Pizza Crust

 makes one 12-inch crust · prep time: 10 minutes · cook time: 22 minutes

This was one of the very first recipes I made for my blog back in 2012. We have been using it ever since. It is a great option for those with a nut allergy or those who find that eating too much almond flour stalls weight loss. Not only is this crust nut-free, but it comes in at just over 1 gram of carbs per slice (if sliced into eighths). Would you believe me if I told you that this pizza crust also makes an excellent noodle replacement? No? Check out the "Just Like the Real Thing" Lasagna recipe on page 240.

ingredients

4 ounces full-fat cream cheese (½ cup), softened

2 large eggs

½ teaspoon garlic powder

½ teaspoon onion powder

½ teaspoon Italian seasoning

¼ cup grated Parmesan cheese

1¼ cups shredded low-moisture, part-skim mozzarella cheese

tip: If you are not using the pizza crust right away, store it in the refrigerator for up to 1 week. Alternatively, you can freeze it for later use.

directions

1. Preheat the oven to 375°F. Line a 12-inch pizza pan with parchment paper. Alternatively, you can make the crust in a baking dish lined with parchment paper or a silicone baking mat, or even in a lined casserole dish. Work with what you have.

2. In a mixing bowl, using a hand mixer, combine the cream cheese, eggs, garlic powder, onion powder, and Italian seasoning. There will be some small clumps, but it should be mostly smooth.

3. Using a rubber spatula, fold in the Parmesan and mozzarella cheeses.

4. Transfer the dough to the lined pizza pan. Spread out the dough in a thin, even circle, covering the pan. For a thicker crust, make a smaller circle.

5. Bake for 22 minutes, flipping the crust after 12 to 14 minutes. To flip the crust without breaking it, I place a second piece of parchment paper over top of the crust and slide my hands under the bottom piece of parchment, picking it up from the bottom, flipping it over with the new sheet of parchment paper now under the crust, on top of the pizza pan.

Per Crust
CALORIES: 1057 · **FAT:** 81g · **PROTEIN:** 69g · **TOTAL CARBS:** 11g · **DIETARY FIBER:** 0 · **NET CARBS:** 11g

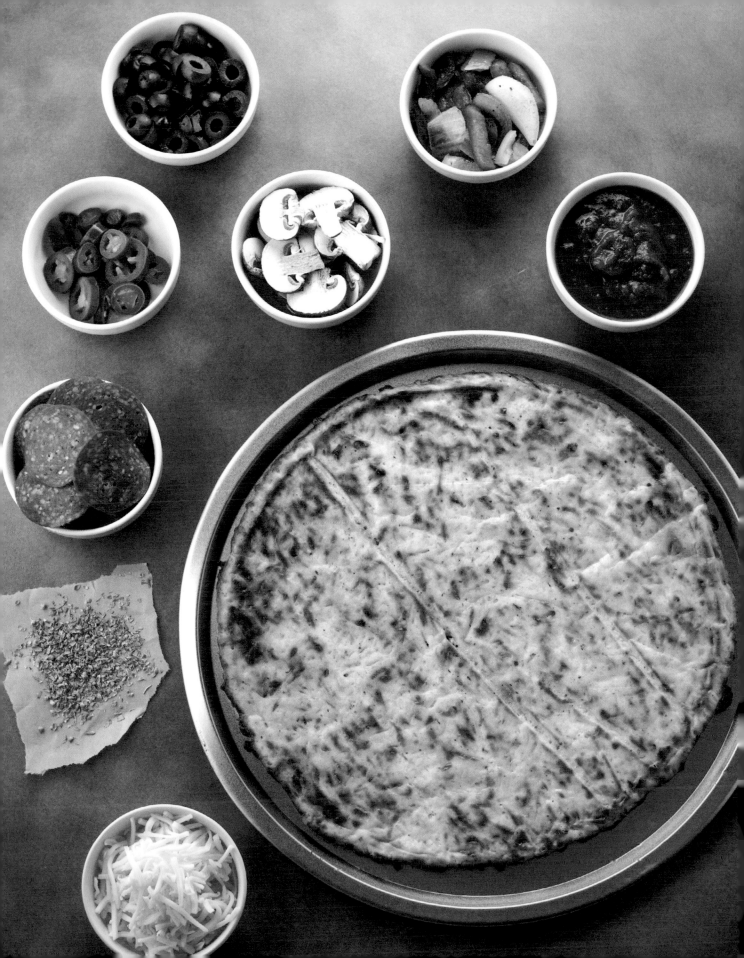

Acknowledgments

To the entire crew at Victory Belt: I can't thank you enough for being so accessible, accommodating, positive, and just generally awesome to work with. You make this process easy and fun—just as it should be!

To my husband, Jon: I could fill every page of this book with reasons that I love you. I did something seriously right in this life to deserve you. Every day I feel blessed to be able to do life with you.

To my five crazy pups: Thank you for being the best kitchen floor cleaners a girl could ask for. When I look at all of you, all I can think is, "Who rescued who?" I'm so lucky I get to be your human. I promise you that if this book does well, I will buy you all the new toys and treats your hearts' desire. (Let's be honest, I'll do that anyway.)

To Erin Finney: Thanks for being my person. You are my favorite person to make silly faces with and to talk about everything and nothing with. My world is a far greater place because you are in it.

To my sister, Pamela: Thanks for always being my biggest cheerleader and reminding me that I can do anything I set my mind to. You are the kindest, most compassionate human I have ever met and I am infinitely lucky to call you my sister and friend. You are also one hell of a coffee mug picker-outer.

To the Pritchows and Cantellays: I lied when I said that I named recipes after each of you. Sorry about that. Thanks for being the best travel partners ever and for making me laugh until I cry every single time we hang out.

To my dear friend and work PIC, Hayley Bubs: Thank you for all the years of loyal friendship, fun, and laughter. But mostly, thank you for having enough faith in me to take a huge leap of faith in your life and career. I promise not to let you down! P.S. Please leave a dollar on the toilet.

To Crystal Fazio: There is no one in the world I would rather drink wine and sing country music at the top of my lungs with. Thank you for always being an amazing friend and loving me even when I didn't feel lovable.

Convenient Conversions

CONVERTING FAHRENHEIT TEMPERATURES TO CELSIUS

Fahrenheit	Celsius
275°	140°
300°	150°
325°	165°
350°	180°
375°	190°
400°	200°
425°	220°
450°	230°
475°	240°
500°	260°

LIQUID OR VOLUME EQUIVALENTS

This	Is Equal to This	Is Equal to This	Is Equal to This
1 pinch	⅛ teaspoon		
1 tablespoon	3 teaspoons	¹⁄₁₆ cup	½ fluid ounce
2 tablespoons		⅛ cup	1 fluid ounce
4 tablespoons		¼ cup	2 fluid ounces
5 tablespoons + 1 teaspoon		⅓ cup	
6 tablespoons		⅜ cup	3 fluid ounces
8 tablespoons		½ cup	4 fluid ounces
10 tablespoons + 2 teaspoons		⅔ cup	
12 tablespoons		¾ cup	6 fluid ounces
16 tablespoons		1 cup	8 fluid ounces
2 cups	1 pint	½ quart	16 fluid ounces
4 cups	2 pints	1 quart	32 fluid ounces
16 cups	8 pints	4 quarts	1 gallon

DRY OR WEIGHT EQUIVALENTS

This	Is Equal to This	Is Equal to This
½ ounce	About 15 grams	
1 ounce	About 30 grams	
2 ounces	55 grams	
3 ounces	85 grams	
4 ounces	125 grams	¼ pound
8 ounces	240 grams	½ pound
12 ounces	375 grams	¾ pound
16 ounces	455 grams	1 pound
32 ounces	910 grams	2 pounds

Allergen Index

RECIPES	PAGE	DAIRY-FREE	EGG-FREE	NUT-FREE	PALEO
Oven-Roasted Cabbage Wedges with Dijon Bacon Vinaigrette	272	✓	✓	✓	✓
Mascarpone Creamed Greens	274		✓	✓	
Green Beans with Shallots and Pancetta	276	✓	✓	✓	✓
Ginger Lime Slaw	278	✓	✓	✓	✓
Dill Pickle Coleslaw	280	✓		✓	✓
Parmesan Roasted Broccoli	281		✓	✓	
Fiesta Cauliflower Rice	282	✓	✓	✓	✓
Creamy Herbed Slow Cooker Cauliflower Mash	284		✓	✓	
Cranberry Pecan Cauliflower Rice Stuffing	286		✓		
Chorizo and Garlic Brussels Sprouts	288	✓	✓	✓	✓
Charred Asian Asparagus and Peppers	290	✓	✓	✓	✓
Butter Roasted Radishes	292	✓	✓	✓	✓
Brussels Sprouts au Gratin with Ham	294		✓	✓	
Lemon Caper Whole Roasted Cauliflower	296	✓	✓	✓	✓
Sautéed Mushrooms with Garlic Mascarpone Cream Sauce	298		✓	✓	
Salted Caramel Nut Brittle	302	✓	✓		✓
Dark Chocolate Mousse	304			✓	
Maple Butter Pecan Truffles	306		✓		
Mason Jar Chocolate Ice Cream	308		✓	✓	
Lemon Curd	310			✓	
Lemon Coconut Cheesecake Bites	312		✓	✓	
Flourless Chewy Chocolate Chip Cookies	314	✓			
Chocolate Peanut Butter Cheesecake Balls	316		✓		
Chocolate-Covered Maple Bacon	318		✓	✓	
Chocolate Chip Cookie Dough Bites	320				
Chewy Peanut Butter Cookies	322	✓			
Blueberry Mojito Ice Pops	324	✓	✓	✓	
Almond Joy Chia Seed Pudding	326	✓	✓		
Fresh Whipped Cream	327		✓	✓	
Thousand Island Dressing	330	✓		✓	
Garlic Parmesan Caesar Dressing	331			✓	
Ranch Dressing	332			✓	
Avocado Green Goddess Dressing	333			✓	
Asian Vinaigrette	334	✓	✓	✓	✓
Dill Pickle Vinaigrette	335	✓	✓	✓	✓
2-Minute Mayo	336	✓		✓	✓
Cajun Mayo	338	✓		✓	✓
Garlic Dill Tartar Sauce	339	✓		✓	✓
Walnut Avocado Pesto	340		✓		
Bacon Jam	341	✓	✓		
Garlic Parmesan Cream Sauce	342		✓	✓	
Pizza Sauce	343		✓	✓	
Garlic and Herb Marinara Sauce	344	✓	✓	✓	✓
Enchilada Sauce	346	✓	✓	✓	✓
Not-So-Secret Burger Sauce	347	✓		✓	
Cranberry Ginger Quick Jam	348	✓	✓	✓	
Seasoning Salt	349	✓	✓	✓	✓
Mexican Seasoning Blend	350	✓	✓	✓	✓
Cajun Seasoning	351	✓	✓	✓	✓
Everything Bagel Seasoning	352	✓	✓	✓	✓
Barbecue Dry Rub	353	✓	✓	✓	
Savory Breading Mix	354		✓		
Nut-Free Keto Breading Mix	355		✓	✓	
Pizza Crust	356				
Nut-Free Pizza Crust	358			✓	

Recipe Thumbnail Index

BREAKFAST

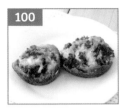 100
Sausage, Egg, and Cheese Pinwheels

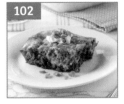 102
Cheesy Chorizo Breakfast Bake

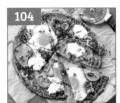 104
Breakfast Pizza

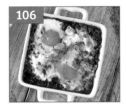 106
Baked Eggs with Chorizo and Ricotta

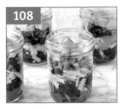 108
Baked Egg Jars

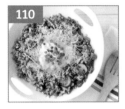 110
13 Jon's Special

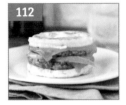 112
Sausage and Egg Breakfast Sandwich

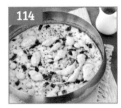 114
Reuben Frittata

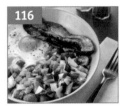 116
Radishes O'Brien

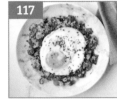 117
Pastrami Breakfast Hash

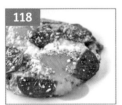 118
Pizza Eggs

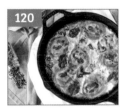 120
Pancetta, White Cheddar, and Spinach Frittata

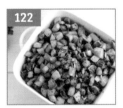 122
Oven-Roasted Garlic and Herb Home Fries

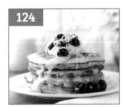 124
Lemon Ricotta Pancakes

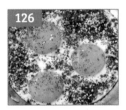 126
Kyndra's Favorite Buttery Herbed Eggs

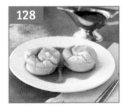 128
French Toast Egg Puffs

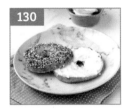 130
Keto Everything Bagels

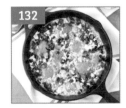 132
Creamy Herbed Bacon and Egg Skillet

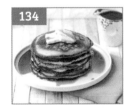 134
Easy Peasy Maple Blender Pancakes

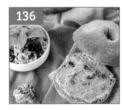 136
Cranberry Cream Cheese Spread

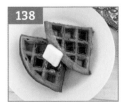 138
Chocolate Peanut Butter Waffles

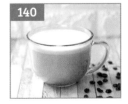 140
Boosted Coffee

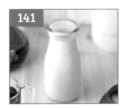 141
Vanilla Coffee Creamer

SNACKS AND STARTERS

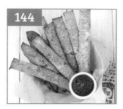
144
Parmesan Italian Breadsticks

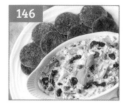
146
Warm Mediterranean Goat Cheese Dip

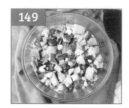
148
Tuna Salad Pickle Boats

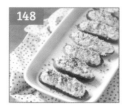
149
Avocado Feta Salsa

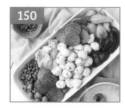
150
Marinated Mozzarella Balls

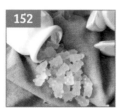
152
Sour Lemon Gummy Snacks

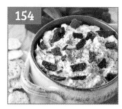
154
Green Goddess Chicken Dip

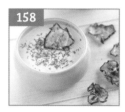
156
Garlic Dill Quick Pickled Brussels Sprouts

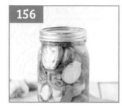
158
Garlic Dill Baked Cucumber Chips

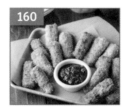
160
Fried Mozzarella Sticks

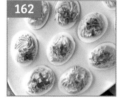
162
Creamy Avocado Pesto Deviled Eggs

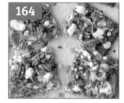
164
Buffalo Chicken Flatbread

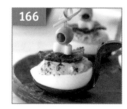
166
Bloody Mary Deviled Eggs

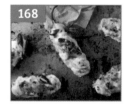
168
Bacon Chicken Ranch Jalapeño Poppers

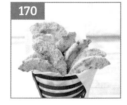
170
Baked Avocado Fries

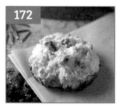
172
Asiago Rosemary Bacon Biscuits

SOUPS AND SALADS

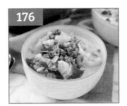
Zuppa Toscana

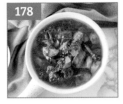
Smoked Sausage and Kale Soup

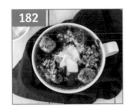
Mexican Chicken Soup

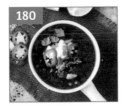
Italian Wedding Soup

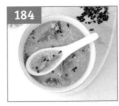
Egg Drop Soup

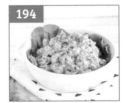
Cheesy Ham and Cauliflower Soup

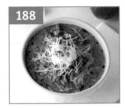
Creamy Lasagna Soup

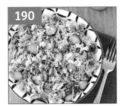
Mac Daddy Salad

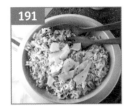
Shaved Brussels Sprouts Caesar Salad

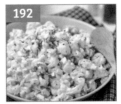
Roasted Cauliflower Mock Potato Salad

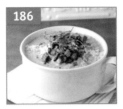
Dill Chicken Salad

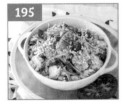
Creamy Cucumber Salad

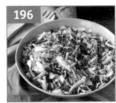
Asian Chicken Salad

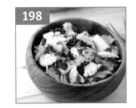
Creamy Caesar Salad with Garlic Parmesan Cheese Crisps

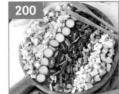
Cobb Salad

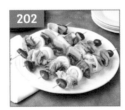
Chef Salad Skewers

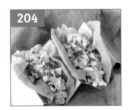
Deviled Ham and Egg Salad Wraps

MAIN DISHES

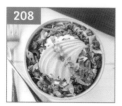 **208** Warm Taco Slaw

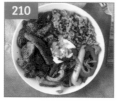 **210** Steak Fajita Bowls

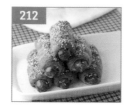 **212** Everything Bagel Dogs

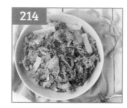 **214** Spaghetti Squash Pork Lo Mein

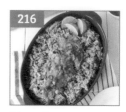 **216** Slow Cooker Spiced Pork Tenderloin

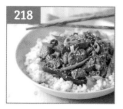 **218** Slow Cooker Chinese Five-Spice Beef

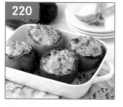 **220** Shrimp and Cheesy Cauliflower Rice Stuffed Peppers

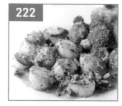 **222** Seared Scallops with Sherry Beurre Blanc

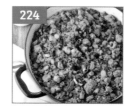 **224** Sausage, Shrimp, and Chicken Jambalaya

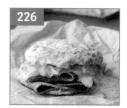 **226** Reuben Biscuit Sandwiches

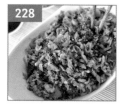 **228** Pork Egg Roll in a Bowl

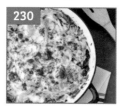 **230** Philly Cheesesteak Casserole

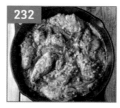 **232** Peanut Chicken Skillet

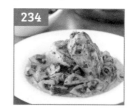 **234** Pan-Seared Chicken with Balsamic Cream Sauce, Mushrooms, and Onions

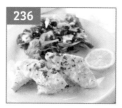 **236** Lemon Sherry Chicken

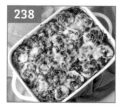 **238** Lasagna Zucchini Roll-Ups

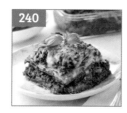 **240** "Just Like the Real Thing" Lasagna

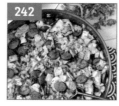 **242** Fried Cabbage with Kielbasa

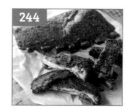 **244** Barbecue Dry Rub Ribs

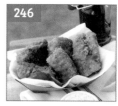 **246** Dill Pickle Juice Brined Fish and Chips

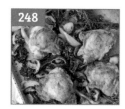 **248** Crispy Chicken Thigh and Vegetable Sheet Pan Dinner

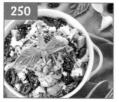 **250** Creamy Pesto Chicken Zucchini Pasta

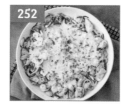 **252** Chicken Zoodle Alfredo

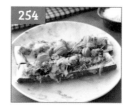 **254** Chicken Parmesan Zucchini Boats

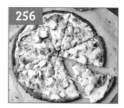 **256** Chicken Cordon Bleu Pizza

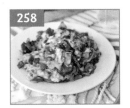

258

Cheesy Smoked
Sausage and
Cabbage Casserole

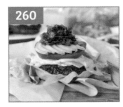

260

Best-Ever Fork and
Knife Pub Burger

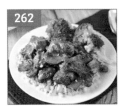

262

Beef Tips in
Mushroom Brown
Gravy

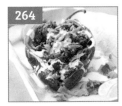

264

Beef Stuffed
Poblanos with
Lime Crema

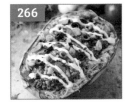

266

Beef Enchilada
Stuffed Spaghetti
Squash

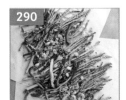

268

Asian Beef Skewers

SIDES

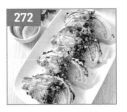

272

Oven-Roasted Cabbage
Wedges with Dijon
Bacon Vinaigrette

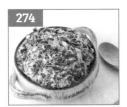

274

Mascarpone
Creamed Greens

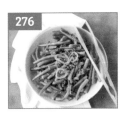

276

Green Beans
with Shallots and
Pancetta

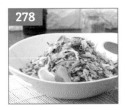

278

Ginger Lime Slaw

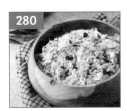

280

Dill Pickle
Coleslaw

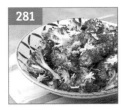

281

Parmesan Roasted
Broccoli

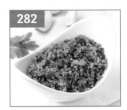

282

Fiesta Cauliflower
Rice

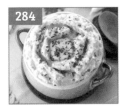

284

Creamy Herbed
Slow Cooker
Cauliflower Mash

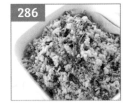

286

Cranberry Pecan
Cauliflower Rice
Stuffing

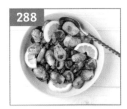

288

Chorizo and Garlic
Brussels Sprouts

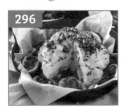

290

Charred Asian
Asparagus and
Peppers

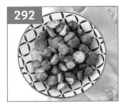

292

Butter Roasted
Radishes

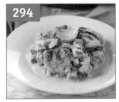

294

Brussels Sprouts
au Gratin
with Ham

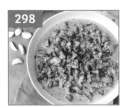

296

Lemon Caper
Whole Roasted
Cauliflower

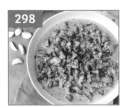

298

Sautéed Mushrooms
with Garlic Mascarpone
Cream Sauce

SWEET TREATS

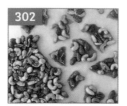
302
Salted Caramel Nut Brittle

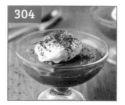
304
Dark Chocolate Mousse

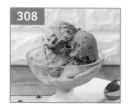
306
Maple Butter Pecan Truffles

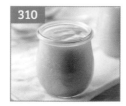
308
Mason Jar Chocolate Ice Cream

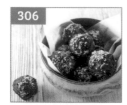
310
Lemon Curd

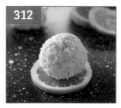
312
Lemon Coconut Cheesecake Bites

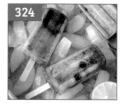
314
Flourless Chewy Chocolate Chip Cookies

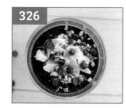
316
Chocolate Peanut Butter Cheesecake Balls

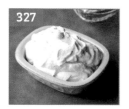
318
Chocolate-Covered Maple Bacon

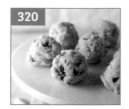
320
Chocolate Chip Cookie Dough Bites

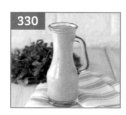
322
Chewy Peanut Butter Cookies

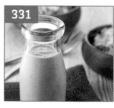
324
Blueberry Mojito Ice Pops

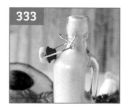
326
Almond Joy Chia Seed Pudding

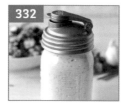
327
Fresh Whipped Cream

DRESSINGS, SAUCES, SEASONINGS, AND MORE

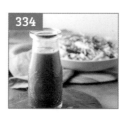
330
Thousand Island Dressing

331
Garlic Parmesan Caesar Dressing

332
Ranch Dressing

333
Avocado Green Goddess Dressing

334
Asian Vinaigrette

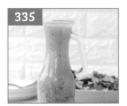

Dill Pickle
Vinaigrette

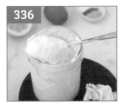

2-Minute Mayo

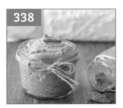

Cajun Mayo

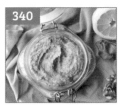

Garlic Dill
Tartar Sauce

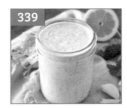

Walnut Avocado
Pesto

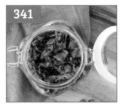

Bacon Jam

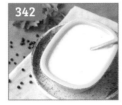

Garlic Parmesan
Cream Sauce

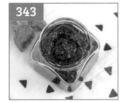

Pizza Sauce

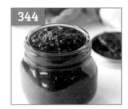

Garlic and Herb
Marinara Sauce

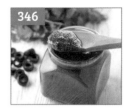

Enchilada Sauce

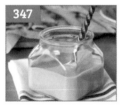

Not-So-Secret
Burger Sauce

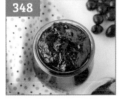

Cranberry Ginger
Quick Jam

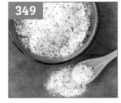

Seasoning Salt

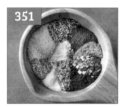

Mexican Seasoning
Blend

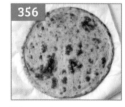

Cajun Seasoning

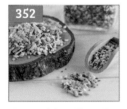

Everything Bagel
Seasoning

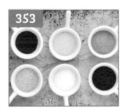

Barbecue Dry Rub

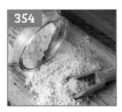

Savory
Breading Mix

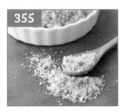

Nut-Free Keto
Breading Mix

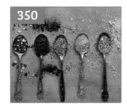

Pizza Crust

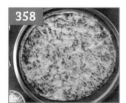

Nut-Free
Pizza Crust

General Index

Reader Testimonial

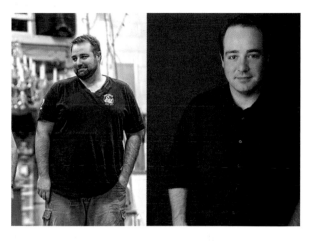

Around the age of 16 or 17, I started to gain weight. I was growing quickly and was constantly hungry. I can remember coming home from school and raiding the cupboards, then hiding the evidence so that I could still eat dinner when my family got home. My parents actually resorted to putting a lock on the downstairs pantry to keep me out. When I got my first job at a fast-food restaurant, it wasn't long before the weight gain started to accelerate. I knew how to cook, but it was so much easier to just eat at work or bring food home. My weight steadily rose, eventually reaching 350 pounds. Last year I decided enough was enough. On April 1, 2016, I went keto. Suddenly I was cooking real food for myself again, and I'll admit it was tough. I basically only ate salad for the first couple weeks because I doubted my culinary skills and just plain didn't know what to make. So I took to the internet to find new low-carb/keto recipes to help me make it through.

It wasn't long before I came across Kyndra Holley's *Peace, Love and Low Carb*. Every time I re-created one of her recipes, it turned out perfectly, and I became one of those people who started posting pictures of their food. I connected with her on social media and immediately was drawn to her electric personality, her positive energy, and her sense of humor. Listening to her talk about her own journey, watching her develop recipes, and of course making them for myself became an addiction for me. Before I knew it, the weight was starting to fly off. I was super happy and filled with energy. I was visiting *Peace, Love and Low Carb* daily and making delicious meals like Egg Roll in a Bowl, Peanut Chicken Skillet, and even Chewy Chocolate Peanut Butter and Bacon Cookies. Following Kyndra on social media not only gave a face to the delicious low-carb recipes and blog posts, but really made me feel a connection to her and her brand. She promotes kindness and well-being and speaks to how everyone's journey is different; it's all about listening to your own body. Armed with all that inspiration and knowledge, I set off on a weight-loss journey that would change my life.

Flash-forward to today. It's been 15 months since I first started down this path and about 14.5 months since I discovered Kyndra Holley. She has been such a major factor in my story, and I can't thank her enough. I was just a chubby guy from the west coast of Canada, and now here I am 104 pounds lighter, an immeasurable amount happier, and hopefully a symbol that you can do it, too! It was a lot of work and not always fun...but with a whole lot of *Peace, Love and Low Carb*...I DID IT!!

THANK YOU, KYNDRA, FOR EVERYTHING THAT YOU DO!

—Darren Rathgaber

Also by Kyndra D. Holley

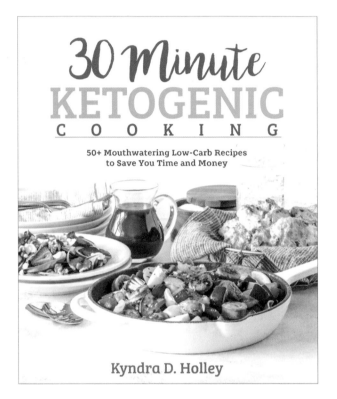

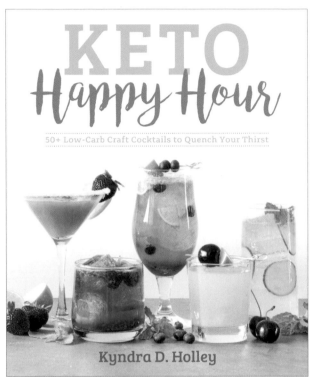